Thyroid Disease: Pathophysiology, Diagnosis and Management

Thyroid Disease: Pathophysiology, Diagnosis and Management

Editor: Dakota Marshall

AMERICAN
MEDICAL PUBLISHERS
www.americanmedicalpublishers.com

AMERICAN
MEDICAL PUBLISHERS
www.americanmedicalpublishers.com

Cataloging-in-Publication Data

Thyroid disease : pathophysiology, diagnosis and management / edited by Dakota Marshall.
p. cm.
Includes bibliographical references and index.
ISBN 978-1-63927-127-6
1. Thyroid gland--Diseases. 2. Thyroid gland--Diseases--Pathophysiology.
3. Thyroid gland--Diseases--Diagnosis. 4. Thyroid gland--Diseases--Treatment. I. Marshall, Dakota.
RC655 .T49 2022
616.44--dc23

American Medical Publishers,
41 Flatbush Avenue,
1st Floor, New York,
NY 11217, USA

ISBN 978-1-63927-127-6 (Hardback)

Contents

Preface

The medical condition that affects the function of the thyroid gland is known as thyroid disease. Generally, there are five types of thyroid diseases, namely, hypothyroidism, hyperthyroidism, structural abnormalities, tumors and subclinical hypothyroidism. Each of them has their own symptoms. Symptoms of hyperthyroidism are tiredness, weight gain, muscle cramps, slow heart rate, constipation, etc. Symptoms of hyperthyroidism include difficulty in sleeping, tremors and weight loss. Thyroid disease can be diagnosed via a blood test, ultrasound, biopsy and a radioiodine scanning and uptake study. It can be treated with the help of medications, surgery and radioiodine. This book contains some path-breaking studies in the field of thyroid disease. It includes some of the vital pieces of work being conducted across the world, on various topics related to this domain. This book aims to equip students and experts with advanced topics and upcoming concepts in this area.

The information shared in this book is based on empirical researches made by veterans in this field of study. The elaborative information provided in this book will help the readers further their scope of knowledge leading to advancements in this field.

Finally, I would like to thank my fellow researchers who gave constructive feedback and my family members who supported me at every step of my research.

Editor

1

Riedel's thyroiditis - a case report with genes' expression studies

Katarzyna Wojciechowska-Durczyńska[1], Adam Durczyński[2], Stanisław Sporny[3], Janusz Strzelczyk[2] and Andrzej Lewiński[1*]

Abstract

Background: Genetic background of Riedel's thyroiditis remains unknown. Herein, we describe our results of studies on genes expression levels in Riedel's thyroiditis.

Case report and genetic findings: We report the case of 48-year old woman with Riedel's thyroiditis who has presented unusual course of disease with non-specific cervical discomfort, though as with no pain and/or no compression symptoms. After surgery, thyroid specimens were quantitatively evaluated, regarding *PIK3CA, PIK3CD, PIK3CG, Tg, TGFB1, THRB, COL1, CDKN1C, CDH3* and *CACNA2D2* genes expression levels, by real-time PCR in the ABI PRISM® 7500 Sequence Detection System. Out of 10 above genes, in 2 cases the expression was higher than in respective Controls of unchanged thyroid tissue. In the remaining 8 cases, expression in question became comparable or lower as in Controls.

Discussion: The association between increased expression levels of *PIK3CA* and *CDH3* genes and Riedel's thyroiditis is not well-defined. However, the increased expression of *PIK3CA* and *CDH3* genes in our case report and in previous studies of other authors on various malignancies may suggest possible molecular relation between Riedel's thyroiditis and certain neoplastic processes, the relation of which requires further genetic evaluation. It is to be stressed that gene expression studies in Riedel's thyroiditis are difficult to perform, mainly due to fibrosis, resulting in scarce thyroid specimens and - in consequence - small amount of genetic material.

Keywords: Riedel?'?s thyroiditis, Genes?'? expression, Real-time PCR

Background

Riedel's thyroiditis is a rare fibrosclerotic infiltrative thyroid disorder of unclear etiology, during which normal thyroid tissues are replaced by fibrous tissue, often expanding outside the thyroid capsule. The diagnosis can be difficult to establish prior to surgical removal of the thyroid and to subsequent histopathological examination of the resected gland [1-3]. Reports on genetic findings in Riedel's thyroiditis are scarce in medical literature. Herein, we describe our results of studies on genes expression levels in Riedel's thyroiditis.

Case report

We report the case of 48-year old women, diagnosed originally as a goiter with eminently increased consistency on palpation, presented with non-specific cervical discomfort, though with no pain and/or no compression symptoms. Clinically, the thyroid was enlarged, painless, however very firm. Serum thyrotropin (TSH) and free thyroid hormones (FT3 and FT4) concentrations were in normal ranges. Prior to surgery, the result of chest X-ray examination showed no pathological changes and all biochemical laboratory tests were normal. Ultrasound examination of the thyroid gland revealed few normoechoic foci in both lobes. Based on benign cytology of the nodules (normal thyroid follicular cells and colloid - Bethesda II) and the absence of compression symptoms, a subtotal thyroidectomy was performed. During surgery, a stony hard, white thyroid was disclosed. No complications after thyroid surgery were observed. Histopathological findings led to the diagnosis of Riedel's thyroiditis, based on disappearance of thyroid follicles, which were replaced by the fibrous tissue and

* Correspondence: alewin@csk.umed.lodz.pl
[1]Department of Endocrinology and Metabolic Diseases, Polish Mother's Memorial Hospital Research Institute, Medical University of Lodz, Rzgowska St. No. 281/289, 93-338 Lodz, Poland
Full list of author information is available at the end of the article

lymphocytes infiltrations, and features of focal endoarteritis (Figures 1, 2, 3, 4). Postoperatively, the patient was treated with levothyroxine, 100 μg per day. At 4-months follow up, results TSH, FT3, FT4, PTH, calcium-phosphorus homeostasis and autoantibodies against thyroid peroxidase and TSH receptor were in normal ranges; autoantibodies against thyroglobulin (anti-Tg) were elevated. Ultrasound examination of the neck did not showed features of disease recurrence.

Genetic findings

After surgery, following conventional histopathological examination, thyroid specimen, received from patient with Riedel's thyroiditis, was quantitatively evaluated regarding *PIK3CA, PIK3CD, PIK3CG, Tg, TGFB1, THRB, COL1, CDKN1C, CDH3 and CACNA2D2* genes expression levels by real-time PCR in the ABI PRISM ®7500 Sequence Detection System. Macroscopically unchanged thyroid tissue, surgically removed from the patient with non-toxic nodular goitre (NTG), served as a control for *real-time* PCR experiment.

Total RNA from tissue was extracted by use of an RNeasy Midi Kit (Qiagen, Hilden, Germany) based on modified Chomczyński and Sacchi's according to manufacturers' recommendations. The purity of total RNA was assessed by NanoDrop® ND-100 spectrophotometr and next the RNA was used in the first strand cDNA synthesis with TaqMan® Reverse Transcripton Reagents (Applied Biosystem) according to maufacturers' instruction. Real-time PCR was performed by using *Taq*Man® Universal PCR Master Mix (Applied Biosystem) and *Taq*Man® Gene Expression Assays probe and primer mix (Applied Biosystem) according to the manufacturer' specification. Thermal cycler conditions were as follows: hold for 10 min. at 95°C, follow by two-step PCR for 50 cycles of 95°C for 15 s followed by 60°C for 1 min. Amplification reactions, in triplicate for each sample, were performed and the results were normalized to the *ACTB* gene expression level.

An analysis of relative gene expression data was performed, using the $2^{-\Delta\Delta CT}$ method on an ABI PRISM® 7500 Sequence Detection System Software. The fold change in studied gene expression, normalised to endogenous control, was calculated using: RQ = $2^{-\Delta\Delta CT}$.

Out of 10 above genes, in 2 cases [*PIK3CA* - responsible for coding alpha catalytic subunit of class I PI3K (phosphoinositide 3-kinase) and *CDH3* - responsible for coding P-cadherin] the expression was higher than in

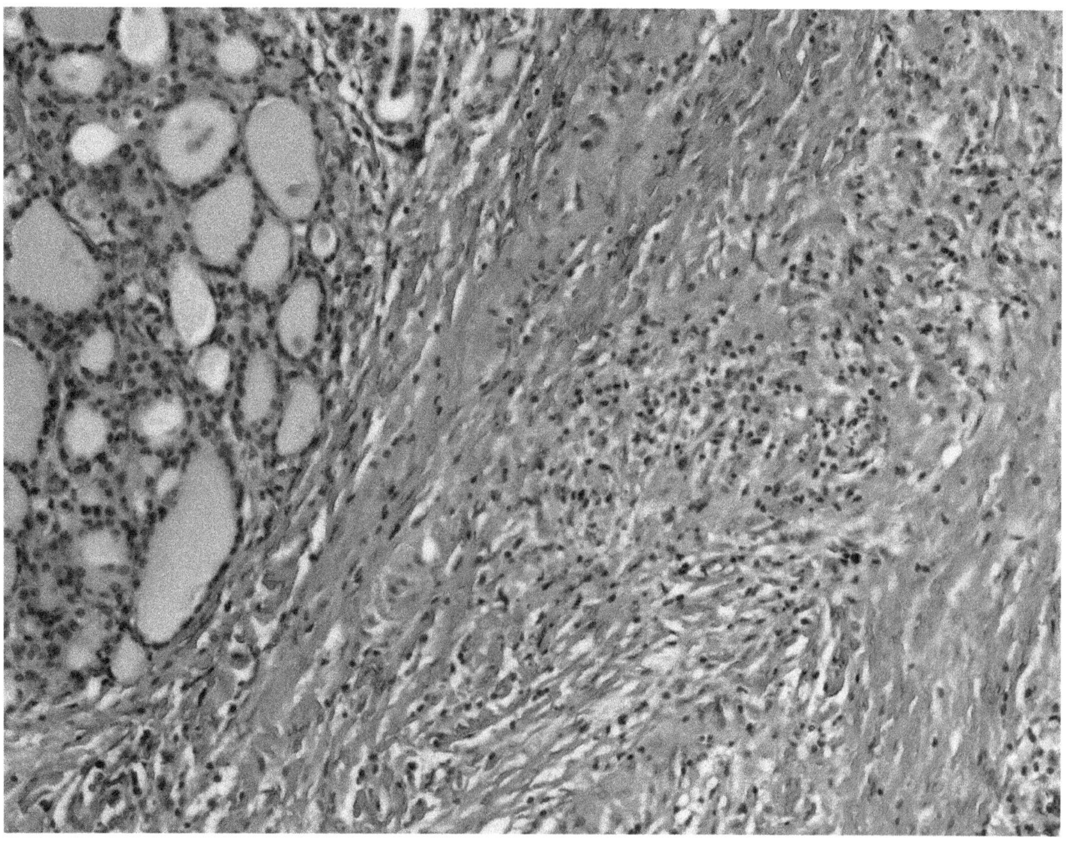

Figure 1 Thyroid parenchyma peripherally to dense connective tissue hyperplasia. HE 320 ×.

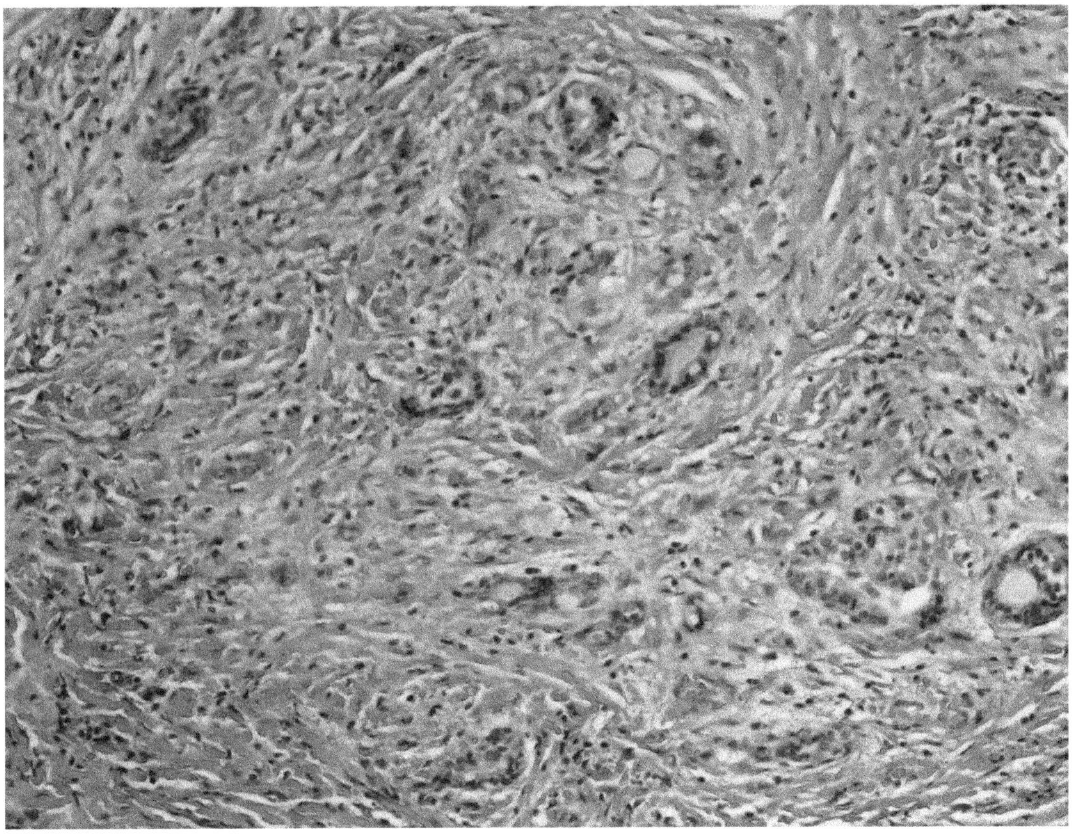

Figure 2 Thyroid parenchyma remnant among dense connective tissue. HE 320 ×.

respective Controls of unchanged thyroid tissue. In the remaining 8 cases, expression in question became comparable or lower as in Controls (Figure 5).

Discussion

Riedel's throiditis is a rare disease that most commonly occurs in females in their fifties and usually demonstrates as a goitre without clinical evidence of thyroid nodules. On palpation, thyroid demonstrates firm or stony consistency ("iron-hard thyroiditis"). Symptoms of regional compression might progressively appear. However, the clinical course of this disease is mostly variable and may include cases with no thyroid-related symptoms, as we have noted in our patient [3]. Before surgery, Riedel's thyroiditis is often difficult to differentiate from aggressive types of thyroid cancers (i.e., undifferentiated thyroid carcinoma), nevertheless, a long-term follow-up shows no disease-specific mortality [4]. Likewise in presented patient, in vast majority of cases, only histopathological, postoperative examination leads to diagnosis of Riedel's thyroiditis, due to no specific symptoms. Cytological evaluation is also of limited use in Riedel's thyroiditis, due to firm thyroid tissue consistency and scanty amount of cellular material thus often non-diagnostic thyroid specimens [5]. According to our opinion, in the case described by us, unusual course of the Riedel's thyroiditis with the absence of compressive symptoms may be related to early-stage of the disease.

A number of hypotheses have been proposed regarding etiology and pathogenesis of Riedel's thyroiditis. The disease may be associated with subacute and chronic thyroiditis, thus some authors proposed the, so called, "intrathyroidal hypothesis". According to that hypothesis, the entity may represent the late stage (i.e., the progression to fibrotic stage) of chronic inflammatory disorder [6-8]. On the contrary, the "pharmacological hypothesis" suggests that some particular medications may trigger Riedel's thyroiditis development [8]. Although not proven, inherited susceptibility and development was hypothesized, as well [8]. Nowadays, the "systemic autoimmune hypothesis" seems to have the most support and it basically views Riedel's thyroiditis as a manifestation of disordered fibroplastic proliferation because of hypersensivity reaction and consequent release of stimulating growth factors [9]. This theory considers a fibroblast not only as a final cell responsible for fibrosis, but also as a main target for well-defined systemic autoimmune attack [8]. In our case, the

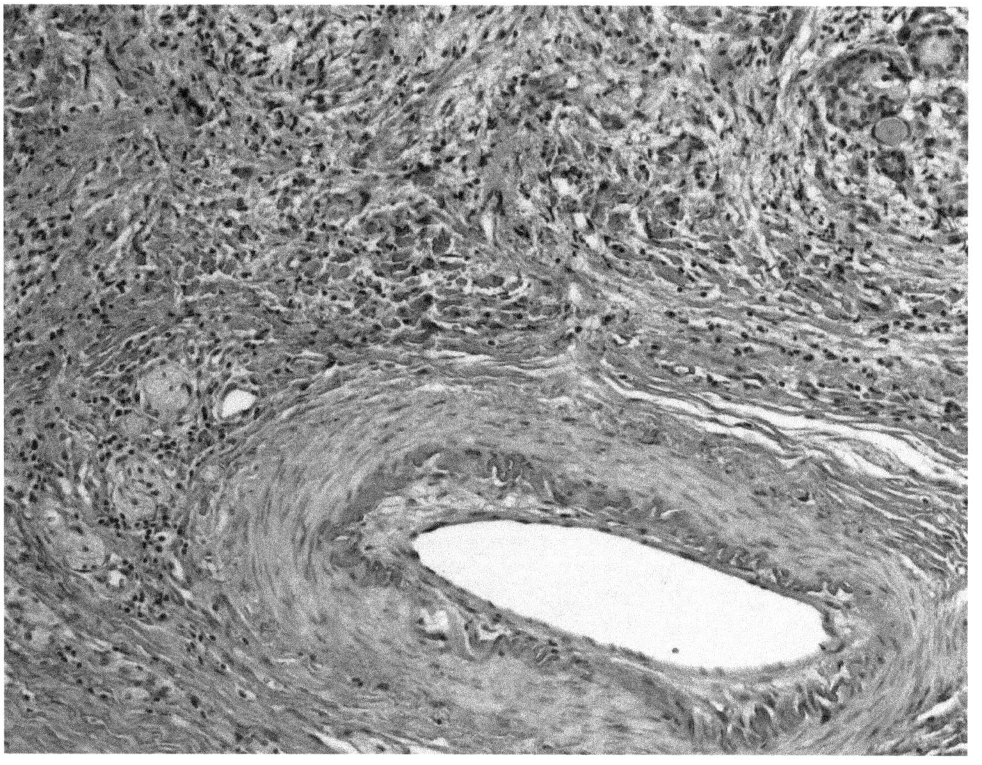

Figure 3 Arterial vessel among fibrosing thyroid parenchyma. HE 320 ×.

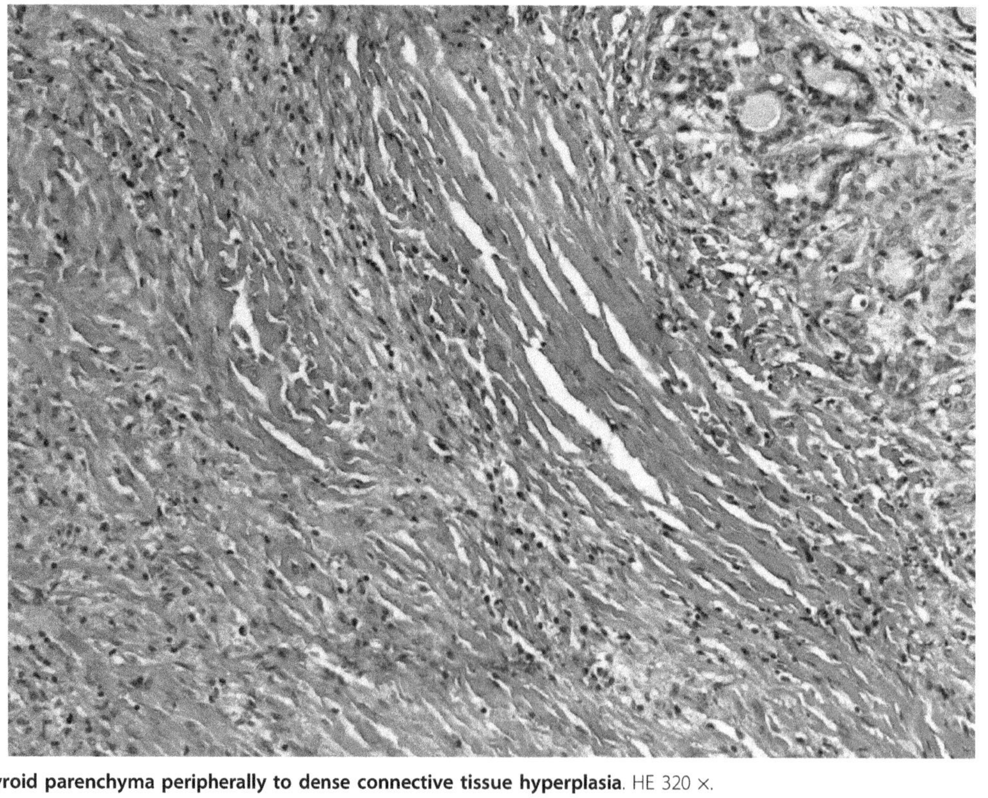

Figure 4 Thyroid parenchyma peripherally to dense connective tissue hyperplasia. HE 320 ×.

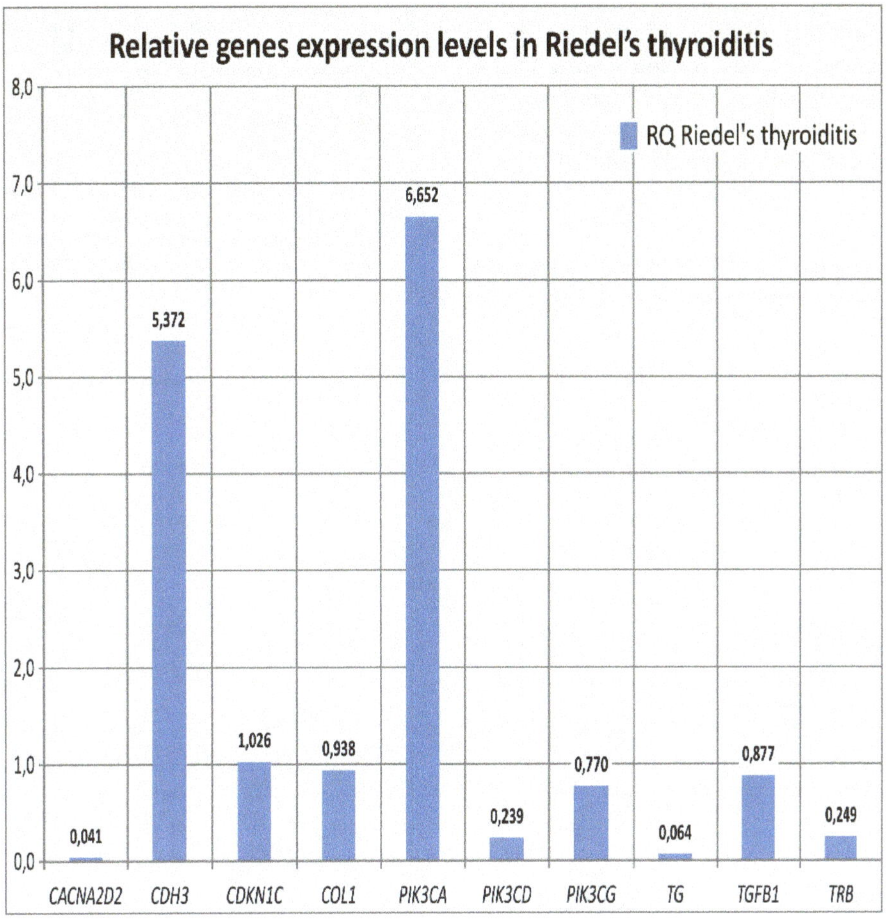

Figure 5 Real-time PCR relative quantification (RQ) of studied genes levels in Riedel's thyroiditis. Bars represents quantification values normalized to an endogenous control (β-actin) and relative to a calibrator (control sample, RQ = 1).

"systemic autoimmune hypothesis" of Riedel's thyroiditis is the most plausible, it is supported by laboratory findings of autoimmune thyroid disease (anti-Tg), which have persisted after surgery.

PI3K/Akt (phosphoinositide 3-kinase/serine-threonine protein kinase) pathway participates in cellular signaling in response to various growth factors including FGF (fibroblast growth factor). Activating mutations and amplification of *PIK3CA* gene have been associated with enhancing PIK3CA kinase activity and Akt phosphorylation. Increased PI3K/Akt expression has been observed in both Hashimoto thyroiditis and well-differentiated thyroid cancer [10,11]. Still, little is known about the precise role of *PIK3CA* in fibrosclerotic disorders, however, it has been proved that hepatic Akt expression correlated with advanced liver fibrosis in chronic hepatitis C patient [12].

Our results demonstrate that *CDH3* gene expression may increase in Riedel's thyroiditis, as well. Cadherins, such as *CDH3*, are integral membrane glycoproteins responsible for calcium-dependent cell-cell adhesion. Our contemporary knowledge about the role of P-cadherin in fibrosis and autoimmune processes is scanty and, so far, it has been only demonstrated that aberrant expression of E-cadherin/β-catenin complex is associated with a wide variety of human malignancies and fibrosis [13].

The association between increased expression levels of *PIK3CA* and *CDH3* genes and Riedel's thyroiditis is not well-defined. However, the increased expression of *PIK3CA* and *CDH3* genes in our case report and in previous studies of other authors on various malignancies may suggest possible molecular relation between Riedel's thyroiditis and certain neoplastic processes, the relation which requires further genetic evaluation.

Low expression levels of the remaining studied genes could be associated with destruction of glandular thyroid tissue. The levels of *TGFB1, COL1* and *CDKN1C* genes expression were comparable in Riedel's thyroiditis and in macroscopically unchanged tissue. It is to be emphasized that high expression levels of *TGFB1* and of *COL1A1* genes in chronic thyroiditis and its correlation with thyroid fibrosis has previously been observed [14].

These results call into question the "intrathyroidal hypothesis" of Riedel's disease pathogenesis. One should remind once again that gene expression studies in Riedel's thyroiditis are difficult to perform, mainly due to fibrosis, resulting in scarce thyroid specimens and - in consequence - small amount of genetic material.

Consent

Written informed consent was obtained from the patient for publication of this report and any accompanying images.

Author details

[1]Department of Endocrinology and Metabolic Diseases, Polish Mother's Memorial Hospital Research Institute, Medical University of Lodz, Rzgowska St. No. 281/289, 93-338 Lodz, Poland. [2]Department of General and Transplant Surgery, Medical University of Lodz, Barlicki University Hospital, Lodz, Poland. [3]Department of Dental Pathology, Medical University of Lodz, The Clinical-Didactic Centre, Lodz, Poland.

Authors' contributions

KW-D designed and coordinated the study, carried out the molecular genetic studies, writing a manuscript. AD, SS and JS participated in coordination of the study. AL senior supervision, writing a manuscript. All authors have read and approved the final manuscript.

Competing interests

The authors declare that they have no competing interests.

References

1. Schwaegerle SM, Bauer TW, Esselstyn CB Jr: **Riedel's thyroiditis.** *Am J Clin Pathol* 1988, **6**:715-722, Review.
2. Papi G, Corrado S, Cesinaro AM, Novelli L, Smerieri A, Carapezzi C: **Riedel's thyroiditis: clinical, pathological and imaging features.** *Int J Clin Pract* 2002, **1**:65-67.
3. Fontaine S, Gaches F, Lamant L, Uzan M, Bennet A, Caron P: **An unusual form of Riedel's thyroiditis: a case report and review of the literature.** *Thyroid* 2005, **1**:85-88.
4. Fatourechi MM, Hay ID, McIver B, Sebo TJ, Fatourechi V: **Invasive fibrous thyroiditis (Riedel thyroiditis): the Mayo Clinic experience, 1976-2008.** *Thyroid* 2011, **7**:765-772.
5. Junik R, Juraniec O, Pypkowski J, Krymer A, Marszałek A: **A difficult diagnosis: a case report of combined Riedel's disease and fibrosing Hashimoto's thyroiditis.** *Endokrynol Pol* 2011, **62(4)**:351-356.
6. Zelmanovitz F, Zelmanovitz T, Beck M, Cerski CT, Schmid H, Czepielewski MA: **Riedel's thyroiditis associated with high titers of antimicrosomal and antithyroglobulin antibodies and hypothyroidism.** *J Endocrinol Invest* 1994, **9**:733-737.
7. Papi G, Corrado S, Carapezzi C, De-Gaetani C, Carani C: **Riedel's thyroiditis and fibrous variant of Hashimoto's thyroiditis: a clinicopathological and immunohistochemical study.** *J Endocrinol Invest* 2003, **5**:444-449.
8. Papi G, LiVolsi VA: **Current concepts on Riedel thyroiditis.** *Am J Clin Pathol* 2004, **121**:50-63.
9. Biddinger PW: **Thyroiditis.** In *Diagnostic Pathology and molecular Genetics of the Thyroid.* Edited by: Nikiforov YE. Lippincott Williams 2009:39-59.
10. Larson SD, Jackson LN, Riall TS, Uchida T, Thomas RP, Qiu S, Evers BM: **Increased incidence of well-differentiated thyroid cancer associated with Hashimoto thyroiditis and the role of the PI3k/Akt pathway.** *J Am Coll Surg* 2007, **5**:764-773.
11. Wojciechowska-Durczyńska K, Krawczyk-Rusiecka K, Cyniak-Magierska A, Zygmunt A, Gałecka E, Lewiński A: **Relative quantification of *PIK3C* gene expression level in fine-needle aspiration biopsy thyroid specimens collected from patients with papillary thyroid carcinoma and non-toxic goitre by real-time RT-PCR.** *Thyroid Res* 2010, **3**:5.
12. Huang JF, Chuang YH, Dai CY, Yu ML, Huang CF, Hsiao PJ, Hsieh MY, Huang CI, Yeh ML, Yang JF, Lin ZY, Chen SC, Chuang WL: **Hepatic Akt expression correlates with advanced fibrosis in patients with chronic hepatitis C infection.** *Hepatol Res* 2011, **5**:430-436.
13. Tian X, Liu Z, Niu B, Zhang J, Tan TK, Lee SR, Zhao Y, Harris DC, Zheng G: **E-cadherin/β-catenin complex and the epithelial barrier.** *J Biomed Biotechnol* 2011, **2011**:567305.
14. Cyniak-Magierska A, Januszkiewicz-Caulier J, Brzeziańska E, Lewiński A: **Analysis of correlation between the process of thyroid fibrosis and TGFB1 gene expression level in fine-needle aspiration biopsy (FNAB) thyroid specimens collected from patients with Hashimoto's thyroiditis and non-toxic goitre.** *Exp Clin Endocrinol Diabetes* 2010, **7**:420-426.

2

Reference interval of thyroid stimulating hormone and free thyroxine in a reference population over 60 years old and in very old subjects (over 80 years): comparison to young subjects

Rosita Fontes[1,2*], Claudia Regina Coeli[3], Fernanda Aguiar[3] and Mario Vaisman[1]

Abstract

Background: Studies based on laboratory data about thyroid stimulating hormone (TSH) and free thyroxine (FT4) reference interval (RI) show conflicting results regarding the importance of using specific values by age groups with advancing age. Retrospective laboratory data or non-specific criteria in the selection of subjects to be studied may be factors leading to no clear conclusions. The aim of this study is to test the hypothesis that TSH and FT4 have specific RI for subjects over 60 to 80 years.

Methods: We evaluated prospectively 1200 subjects of both sexes stratified by age groups, initially submitted to a questionnaire to do the first selection to exclude those with factors that could interfere in TSH or FT4 levels. Then, we excluded those subjects with goiter or other abnormalities on physical examination, positive thyroid peroxidase antibodies (TPOAb), thyroglobulin antibodies (TGAb), and other laboratory abnormalities.

Results: TSH increased with age in the whole group. There was no statistical difference in the analysis of these independent subgroups: 20–49 *versus* 50–59 years old ($p > 0.05$), and 60–69 *versus* 70–79 years old ($p > 0.05$). Consequently, we achieved different TSH RI for the three major age groups, 20 to 59 years old: 0.4 - 4.3 mU/L, 60 to 79 years old: 0.4 - 5.8 mU/L and 80 years or more: 0.4 - 6.7 mU/L. Conversely, FT4 progressively decreases = significantly with age, but the independent comparison test between the sub-groups showed that after age 60 the same RI was obtained (0.7 - 1.7 ng/dL) although the minimum value was smaller than that defined by manufacturer. In the comparison between TSH data obtained by this study and those defined by the manufacturer (without segmentation by age) 6.5% of subjects between 60 and 79 years and 12.5% with 80 years or more would have a misdiagnosis of elevated TSH.

Conclusions: TSH normal reference range increases with age, justifying the use of different RI in subjects 60 years old and over, while FT4 decreases with age. Using specific-age RI, a significant percentage of elderly will not be misdiagnosed as having subclinical hipothyroidism.

Introduction

In recent decades there has been increased life expectancy of the population and, consequently, of the aging process. Persons older than age 60 comprise 20 per cent of the world population in the more developed regions, and from 5 to 8 per cent in the less developed regions. The oldest old, persons aged 80 years or older, is the fastest growing segment of the older population and by 2050 the number of this group is projected to be five times as large as at present [1].

Several aspects of the aging process affect the endocrine system and stimulate the use of screening programs for the detection of hormonal changes and drug interventions with hormone replacement therapies to provide better quality of life for the elderly. Evaluation of thyroid function in normal elderly is difficult, since the prevalence of non-thyroid disease and the use of medications that interfere with thyroid function is greater

* Correspondence: fontesrosita@hotmail.com
[1]Hospital Clementino Fraga Filho, Universidade Federal do Rio de Janeiro, Rua Prof. Rodolpho Paulo Rocco 255, Cidade Universitária, CEP 21941-913, Rio de Janeiro-RJ, Brazil
[2]Diagnósticos da América SA, Rio de Janeiro, Brazil
Full list of author information is available at the end of the article

than in young people. As a result, questions about the meaning of functional changes observed in the elderly are relatively common [2].

Data interpretation of thyroid function in the elderly has been changing over the past decades. In a study conducted in 1995 in a non-selected population, the authors considered that subjects of any age with some degree of TSH elevation had some grade of thyroid gland failure [3]. However, in 2002, the NHANES III study revisited this parameter data in a population excluding those with evidence of thyroid disease and, in this more uniform population, TSH still showed a progressive increase with age [4].

The International Federation of Clinical Chemistry and Laboratory Medicine (IFCC) Committee developed the theory of reference values for the "Reference Intervals and Decision Limits (CRIDL)" [5]. In 1995 the Clinical and Laboratory Standards Institute (CLSI) first published with IFCC the joint guideline "Defining, Establishing, and Verifying Reference Intervals in the Clinical Laboratory", reviewed in 2008 [6]. This document recommends application of prospective questionnaires and, if necessary, physical evaluation, of candidate subjects to be part of a control group. It also discourages the indirect approach in which database results are used to establish ranges, retroactively identifying acceptable reference populations. This has been a challenge since then, and many clinical laboratories do not have these procedures performed in accordance with the recommendations, due to the fact that they require time, additional costs, knowledge, and efforts to further clarify physicians and patients.

Recent studies have shown conflicting results regarding the decision to use reference intervals (RI) of TSH suitable for the elderly or not [7,8]. On studies with review of medical records, it is difficult to use strict inclusion and exclusion criteria in the selection of subjects representing a control group. Several bias may occur due to registration errors, and omission of information that were not actively taken from the patient. The consequent inclusion of a significant number of subjects with potential thyroid or general disease or use of interfering medications as belonging to the control group that may alter the final data obtained is a real possibility. Thus, the theme is still far from being exhausted, and this topic is relevant regarding the issue of not to hyper diagnose subclinical hypothyroidism in the elderly who actually could have higher TSH, but at appropriate levels for their age.

Likewise, as FT4 is the test of choice for the confirmation of thyroid disease, it is also relevant to assess whether there is a need for RI specific for subjects above 60 years and 80 years or older.

The aim of this study was to test the hypothesis that it is necessary to use specific RI for TSH and FT4 for subjects over 60 years old, and over 80 years old, compare the values with those of young subjects, and analyze the impact of using specific TSH RI for these age groups in the screening of thyroid dysfunction.

Materials and methods

Between March and December 2012, 1200 subjects of both sexes were evaluated prospectively distributed as follows: 120 males and 120 females in each of the following age ranges: 20–49, 50–59, 60–69, 70–79 and above 80 years, who attended a clinical laboratory to collect routine tests for which function evaluation and/or thyroid autoimmunity had not been requested. They were invited to participate in order to arrive at the laboratory on pre-determined weekdays, according to availability of the researchers. A questionnaire was applied by one of the researchers, through direct interviews with participating candidates, which consisted of: 1) Identification data, address and phone number of the participants, as well as the name and telephone number of their physician for communication in case of abnormal results; characterization of their color or race according to themselves; if they consider themselves as healthy individuals; personal or familial thyroid disease in the present or past; current medications (among these, medications containing iodine in the last six months), smoking, hospitalization due to illness or accident in the last six months (and what the disease was), and pregnancy (for females who had not had menopause). Subjects were from the metropolitan area of Rio de Janeiro, belonging to middle and upper social class, as declared income, 77% white, 18% mulatto and 5% black. Subjects with negative thyroid peroxidase antibodies (TPOAb) and thyroglobulin antibodies (TGAb), normal lipid profile, ultrasensitive C-reactive protein level (CRP), blood count, renal function, and absence of goiter on palpation were in the inclusion criteria. The measurement of urinary iodine was not done since the salt iodization in Brazil is determined by federal law [9] and the authors have shown in previous study that the intake iodine in the Rio de Janeiro population is sufficient [10]. In addition, the National Health Surveillance Agency (ANVISA), which is the regulatory agency under the Ministry of Health, conducted a review of salt iodization in the samples used in Rio de Janeiro in the year before beginning of the study confirming that it was appropriate [11].

Exclusion criteria included past or present history of thyroid disease, previous thyroid surgery, family history of thyroid disease, TSH <0.1 mU/L or >10.0 mU/L, as these results indicate a high probability of thyroid dysfunction [12], palpable goiter, smoking habit, use of medicines known as possible analytical or physiological interference on measurement of TSH or FT4 in the past three months (medicines and contrasts containing iodine in the past six months) mentioned in the list of medications and other drugs that may interfere with TSH and/or FT4 measurements [13-24], antidepressants, hospitalization in the past six months and pregnant females. As changes in thyroid morphology are significantly higher among the elderly, we assessed whether this was a factor in generating different results in the selection of subjects for the study. A thyroid ultrasonography (US) was performed on 687 subjects with exclusion of 24.1% who presented some thyroid change. More than 120 subjects still remained in each group. Comparing TSH and FT4 values between subjects who had normal US and those who did not perform US, there was no statistically significant difference (data not shown). Therefore, as this exam was not essential in the selection of subjects as controls, all of the initially selected subjects could be enrolled in the study, except those who were initially excluded and had been replaced by the same number of other subjects of the same age and sex in order of maintaining the initial number to be studied.

List of medications and other drugs that may interfere with TSH and/or FT4 measurements

2-3-dimercatopropanol, 2-4-dinitrophenol, 5-fluorouracil, 5-hydroxytryptophan
Acetazolamide, acetylsalicylic acid, alpha adrenergic blockers, aminoglutethimide, aminotriazole, amiodarone, androgens and other anabolic steroids, anphenona, anphetamines, antipyrine
Benserazide, beta adrenergic blockers, bexarotene, bromine, brompheniramine
Cadmium, carbamazepine, chromate, chromium picolinate, cimetidine, clofibrate, clomiphene, clomipramine, cobalt, complex anions, corticosteroids, cytostatics
Danazol, diphenylhydantoin, dinitrophenol, dobutamine, domperidone, dopamine and its agonists, other dopaminergic agents
Erythrosine, estrogens, ethionamide
Fenclofenac, fenoldopam, flunarizine, fluor, furosemide, fusaric acid
Growth hormone (GH), GH-Releasing hormone
Halofenate, heroin, heparin
Interleukins, iopanoic acid, other radiological contrasts, and other iodine-containing substances and drugs (potassium iodide and others), insulin-like Growth Factor-1, interferon
Ketoconazole
L-asparaginase, L-dopa inhibitors, levothyroxine, lithium, lovastatin,
Mefenamic acid, melatonin, metformin, methadone, methimazole, metoclopramide, mitotane
Nevirapine, niacin, nicotinic acid, nifedipine, NSAIDs, nitrate
O, p'-DDD, orphenadrine, opioids, oxcarbazepine
Para-aminobenzoic acid, perchlorate, perphenazine, phenidone, phenylbutazone, phenobarbital, pimozide, prazozin, primidone, propylthiouracil, pyridoxine
Quetiapine
Raloxifen, resorcinol, rifampicin, ritonavir, rubidium
Salsalate, serotonergics antagonists, somatostatin and its analogues, spironolactone, St. John's Wort, stavudine, sulfonamides, sulfonylureas, sulpiride, steroids hormones
Tamoxifen, thiocyanate, thyroid hormones and their analogs, troleandomycin, tyrosine kinase inhibitors
Valproic acid

Drugs are listed in alphabetical order and not in possible importance as interfering in TSH or thyroid hormone values.

The study was approved by the Research Ethics Committee of the Hospital Clementino Fraga Filho, Universidade Federal do Rio de Janeiro (HUCFF/UFRJ) and individuals agreed to participate by signing the informed consent form.

Collection of data and collection of samples

Serum was collected in the morning, in same species standard sampling tubes with separator gel. The measurements were done on the same day in primary tubes, after blood centrifugation at 3200 RPM for 15 min.

Biochemical data

Serum TSH, FT4, TPOAb and TGAb were measured by electrochemiluminescence immunoassays on the Roche Modular Analytics® E170 (Roche Diagnostics Australia Pty Ltd, Castle Hill, NSW, Australia).

Serum TSH concentrations were measured by an immunometric method, with an intra-assay percentage coefficient of variation (% CV) of 3.0% at concentrations of 0.040 ± 0.001 mU/L, 2.7% at 0.092 ± 0.002 mU/L and 1.1% at 9.4 ± 0.1 mU/L. The reference interval provided by the manufacturer is 0.3- 4.2 mU/L. Serum FT4, TPOAb and TGAb concentrations were measured by competitive assays. For FT4, the % CV was 1.4% at FT4 concentrations of 0.7 ± 0.01 ng/dL, 1.8% at 1.3 ± 0.02 and 2.0% at 2.7 ± 0.1 ng/dL. The reference interval provided by the manufacturer is 0.9 -1.7 ng/dL. For TPOAb the intra-assay % CV is 6.3% at TPO concentrations of 21.3 ± 1.34 IU/mL, 5.1% at 51.2 ± 2.6 IU/mL and 2.7% at 473 ± 12.7 IU/mL. According to the manufacturer, individuals without thyroid disease score lower than 34 IU/mL. For TGAb the intra-assay % CV is 4.9% at TG concentrations of 47.2 ± 2.3 IU/mL, 1.3% at 588 ± 7.4, and 1.3 at 3289 ± 42.0 IU/mL TGAb concentrations. According to the manufacturer, individuals without thyroid disease score lower than <115 IU/mL.

Statistical analysis

Data were analyzed using the program GraphPad Prism®, version 6.0 (GraphPad Software, Inc, California). In order to assess the Normal distribution of both data series (TSH and FT4) Kolmogorov–Smirnov tests were performed. Logarithmic 10 was used for analysis. TSH and FT4 were calculated for each subgroup and gender from 20 to 49 years, then, by 10-year age range until 80 years; all those aged older than 80 were grouped together. Descriptive analysis of serum TSH was reported as medians and 25% and 75% percentiles because it is not normally distributed. Two tailed Mann–Whitney test and Kruskal-Wallis test were used to compare the nonparametric TSH distributions in different subpopulations. Evaluation between two subgroups was made by independent test of Dunn multiple comparisons. Means and standard deviations were calculated for FT4, since it has showed a normal distribution. For comparing FT4 between all groups, two-way ANOVA tests were used when more than two data series were analyzed, and Student test in the case of two data series.

Outlying observations were calculated using the test proposed by Dixon. In all cases, the level of significance used was 0.05 [25]. For the RI, for both hormones 2.5% and 97.5% were taken. We used the method of Harris and Boyd [26] to decide whether it was necessary to separate the reference values for gender. According to this method, to calculate the statistical significance of the difference between the means of groups standard normal deviation (z), if the value z is less than 3 means there is no need to reference values separated by gender.

To calculate correlations between TSH and FT4 levels in all age groups, TSH data were transformed into logarithmic 10. With normal distribution the two-tailed Pearson test was used; it was considered statistically significant if a p-value was less than 0.05. Pearson test was also used to analyze, individually, correlations between TSH and age and FT4 and age.

Results

TSH data

The reference group was comprised of 50% females and 50% males. The mean age by gender in each age subgroups are in Table 1. TSH data analysis by age or gender exhibited a non-Gaussian distribution. In each age group, there was no significant difference in serum TSH median between males and females (Table 1). Therefore, considering these factors, all individuals were eligible in each group for the establishment of reference intervals. Statistical parameters of TSH measurements are listed in Figure 1 and in Table 1. Analysis of median TSH as a whole group showed that there was a significant increase of this hormone with age ($p < 0.001$), but the analysis of independent subgroups, 20–49 years old *versus* 50–59 years old ($p > 0.05$), and 60–69 years old *versus* 70–79 years old ($p > 0.05$), showed no statistically significant difference. These data confirm that different RI for three major age groups should be used: 20 to 59 years, 60–79 years and 80 years or more. RI calculated for each sub-group are shown in Table 1.

FT4 data

FT4 exhibited a Gaussian distribution. Data of FT4 measurements are shown in Figure 2, and statistical parameters are listed in Table 2. Analysis of FT4 mean ± standard deviation (SD) shows that there is a significant reduction of the hormone with age as a whole group ($p < 0.0001$). However, despite a tendency to fall in FT4 with increasing

Table 1 Statistical data of TSH measurements

	Age groups				
	20-49	**50-59**	**60-69**	**70-79**	**≥80**
Mean age females (years old)	34.3	54.1	64.2	74.4	84.4
Mean age males (years old)	35.2	53.9	64.2	74.2	86.7
Median TSH in females	1.5		1.7		2.0
Median TSH in males	1.5		1.8		2.1
z values and p values between gender	z = −1.45 p = 0.30	z = −0.60 p = 0.69	z = −0.43 p = 0.54	z = −0.78 p = 0.40	z = −0.14 p = 0.99
Minimum TSH	0.3	0.4	0.2	0.3	0.2
Maximum TSH	5.8	5.9	8.4	9.5	9.3
25% TSH percentile	1.1	1.2	1.7	1.7	2.0
75% TSH percentile	2.2	2.6	2.8	3.0	3.5
Lower 95% CI	1.6	1.8	2.0	2.1	2.5
Upper 95% CI	1.9	2.1	2.4	2.5	2.9
Median TSH assumed	1.5		1.7		2.0
Minimum and maximum TSH RI assumed	0.4 – 4.3		0.4 – 5.8		0.4 – 6.7

RI: reference interval SD: standard deviation TSH in mU/L.

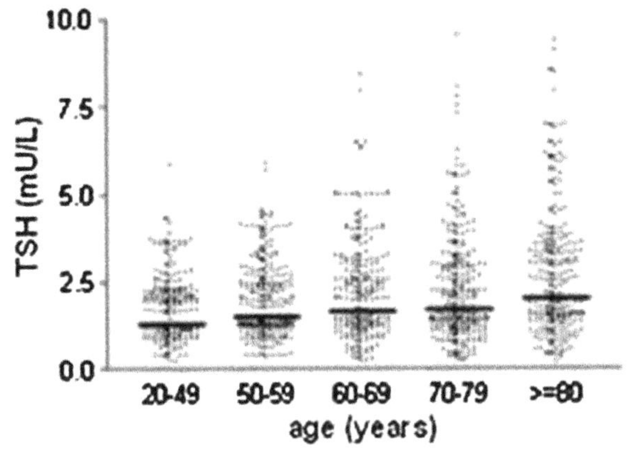

Figure 1 Graph-distribution of TSH among different age groups. The transverse line marks median values.

age, the independent comparison test between the sub-groups showed that there was no statistically significant difference between those over 60 years old. Reference intervals calculated for FT4 are shown in Table 2.

Regarding the correlation between TSH and FT4, a high level of significance was observed in all age sub-groups, independently analyzed ($p < 0.0001$), 20–49 years old: Pearson r = −0.4641, 95% confidence interval (CI) = −0.4961 to −0.2926, R squared = 0.1652; 50–59 years old: Pearson r = −0.3862, 95% CI = −0.4881 to −0.2739, R squared = 0.1492; 60–69 years old: Pearson r = −0.4653, 95% CI = −0.5583 to −0.3607, R squared = 0.2165; 70–79 years old: Pearson r = −0.4946, 95% CI = −0.5839 to −0.3934, R squared = 0.2446; 80 years old and over: Pearson r = −0.3951, 95% confidence interval = −0.4961 to −0.2835, R squared = 0.1561.

In order to assess whether the RI obtained in this study had clinical impact regarding the use of RI defined by the manufacturer in screening for thyroid disease, we compare the percentage of subjects who had TSH below or above the RI defined by age range obtained from this study with the values without segmentation by age. The results are showed in Table 3.

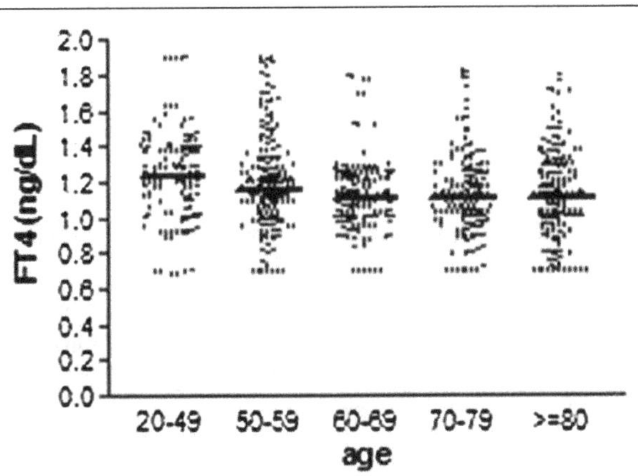

Figure 2 Graph-distribution of FT4 among different age groups. The transverse line marks median values.

Discussion

Usually, for the interpretation of a laboratory test, clinical laboratories use RI provided by the manufacturer of lab kits. The result of a patient's test is then compared to this RI in order to diagnose whether it is normal or not. TSH concentration is the most sensitive test to reliably detect thyroid function abnormalities and is used as the screening test for studying thyroid function because of the inverse log-linear relationship between circulating TSH and FT4 concentrations [27,28].

This study, conducted prospectively with a reference population, showed that TSH increases progressively and significantly with age. The value of z less than 3.0 in all age groups indicates that the same RI should be adopted for both genders. On the other hand, FT4 tends to decrease with age. In the age groups above 60 years, FT4 values are equal between males and females. In subjects younger than 60, the value of z pointed that FT4 is lower in males than in females. A study of Kratzsch et al. also reports lower FT4 in males than in females [29]. However, as in our study, z result (3.0249) is very close to the cutoff point we consider that in the clinical routine, it is appropriate to use the same RI to both genders, the same way as in older subjects.

The lower TSH limit defined in this study of 0.4 mU/L is the same for all age groups over 60 years old, and does not differ from the lower limit of younger people. This value is in accordance with previous study using third generation immunometric TSH methodology, that refers to the lower TSH reference limit as approximately 0.3 to 0.4 mU/L, irrespective of the population studied or the method used [30]. The value found in this study, very slightly higher than that reported by the manufacturer, has no impact on an eventual reclassification of how many people have low TSH, as the difference between one and other is under 2%.

Association between TSH and age is highly significant. The median is 1.5 mU/L in people under 60 years old, increases to 1.7 mU/L from 60 to 79 years old, and to 2.0 mU/L for those aged 80 or more. Upper TSH limit increases from 4.3 mU/L under 60 years old, to 5.8 mU/L in the range of 60 to 79 years old and to 6.7 mU/L in those very old subjects, over 80. So, although the manufacturer's TSH kit is suitable for subjects less than 60 years of age, the same is not true for those 60 years or more, in which the limits are significantly higher.

Within the age ranges of 60–79 years and 80 years or over, a significant percentage of subjects are reclassified as having not elevated TSH if age-specific RI is adopted. The same does not occur in young subjects. According

Table 2 Statistical data of FT4 measurements

	Age groups				
	20-49	**50-59**	**60-69**	**70-79**	**≥80**
Mean FT4 ± SD in females	1.2 ± 0.03	1.2 ± 0.24	1.1 ± 0.22	1.2 ± 0.24	1.1 ± 0.24
Mean FT4 ± SD in males	1.3 ± 0.02	1.2 ± 0.25	1.1 ± 0.23	1.1 ± 0.22	1.1 ± 0.23
z values and p values between gender	z = 3.02 p = −0.0001	z = 1.26 p = 0.28	z = 0.70 p = 0.31	z = −1.63 p = 0.08	z = 0.39 p = 0.31
Minimum level FT4	0.7	0.7	0.7	0.7	0.7
Maximum level FT4	1.9	1.9	1.8	1.8	1.8
Lower FT4 95% CI	1.2	1.2	1.1	1.1	1.1
Upper FT4 95% CI	1.3	1.2	1.2	1.2	1.2
Mean FT4 ± SD assumed for both genders	1.2 ± 0.3	1.2 ± 0.3	1.1 ± 0.2	1.1 ± 0.2	1.1 ± 0.2
Minimum and maximum FT4 RI assumed for both genders	0.7 – 1.9			0.7 – 1.7	

RI: reference interval SD: standard deviation FT4 in ng/dL.

to the RI for each age group obtained in this study, 6.5% of subjects between 60 and 70 years and 12.5% of those with 80 years or more have less misdiagnosis of elevated TSH, leading to 19% reclassification from hypothyroidism to normal, using these criteria. With regard to the effects of age on serum TSH levels, other epidemiological studies indicate that the population's mean TSH levels increase with age [4,31,32]. The NHANES III was the best designed in selecting a control population, and data obtained were similar to the current study, indicating that increase in TSH is probably a physiological event for the elderly [33,34] or that this increase may be due to the presence of TSH isoforms with low bioactivity [35]. In each scenario one can avoid excessive diagnosis of subclinical hypothyroidism in the elderly adopting specific RI. And, to clarify the second hypothesis, the answer would be the development and clinical use of technologies to quantify only isoforms with normal TSH bioactivity.

Failure to find these differences in RI between the young and the elderly reported in other studies may be due to retrospective studies based, or selection choosing populations to be reference for which strict selection criteria were not applied through specific questionnaires and appropriate physical examination to exclude factors such as thyroid dysfunction in the subject or in the family, interfering medications, other illnesses, recent hospitalizations, smoking habits and goiter.

Like TSH, FT4 has the same minimum reference value for all age groups. This value of 0.7 ng/dL however, is lower in relation to that defined by the manufacturer (0.9 ng/dL) in all groups. In relation to the maximum reference value, the level of 1.7 ng/dL is suitable to be used for subjects 60 years old and over. However, although this is not the scope of this study, the results obtained by us suggest that a higher reference superior value (1.9 ng/dL) should be used for young individuals.

Previous study demonstrated that FT4 remained relatively unchanged with age [36]. These data can be difficult to interpret because evaluation of thyroid function in the elderly is often complicated by the increased prevalence of chronic illness and the use of medication. In the present study, subjects with one or more of these factors were excluded. There is evidence that a low activity of thyroid hormone might be beneficial in the elderly. Low levels of FT4 have been associated with a better survival in elderly subjects [8,33,37,38]. On the other hand, even thyroid hormone levels within the normal range might be associated with thyroid hormone-related endpoints. As an example, in euthyroid subjects, especially the elderly, FT4, regardless of TSH levels is associated with atrial fibrillation, and

Table 3 Comparison of data of TSH (mU/L) obtained regarding RI defined by the manufacturer (without segmentation by age), with the results of this study that redefined RI specific for age range

	Results of TSH below RI (mU/L)			Results of TSH upper RI (mU/L)		
Age ranges (y. old)	**Defined by the manufacturer**	**With segmentation by age in this study**	**Difference***	**Defined by the manufacturer**	**With segmentation by age in this study**	**Difference***
< 60	0.4%	0.8%	+ 0.4%	1.7%	1.5%	- 0.2%
60-79	0.4%	2.1%	+ 1.7%	9.2%	2.7%	- 6.5%
≥ 80	0.4%	0.8%	+ 0.4%	14.5%	2.0%	- 12.5%

*Refers to percentage of subjects detected with TSH levels out of reference interval (*RI*) established by the manufacturer *versus* those where TSH was obtained in this study and *RI* was segmented by age.

lower physical performance [39,40]. One hypothesis is that these lower levels of thyroid hormone could possibly serve as an adaptive mechanism to prevent catabolism in the elderly [41].

We consider relevant the data obtained in this age-related prospective study, once it is very important to distinguish between normal and mildly elevated serum TSH concentrations in elderly subjects. Elevations of TSH in young individuals even light and without decreasing FT4 characterize subclinical hypothyroidism or minimal thyroid dysfunction and are related to comorbidities such as dyslipidemia, adverse obstetric events, impact on cognition, quality of life, cardiovascular events, and evolution to clinical hypothyroidism [42]. These effects have no correspondence in the elderly, since there is no evidence of these effects in this age group [43,44]. There is a consensus that subjects with TSH concentrations above 10.0 mU/L should be treated. However, according to Garber et al., in the Clinical Practice Guidelines for Hypothyroidism, very mild TSH elevations in older individuals, under this level, may not reflect subclinical thyroid dysfunction, but rather be a normal manifestation of aging. While the normal TSH reference may need to be narrowed range for some subpopulations [27,45], the normal RI may widen with aging [24]. This confirms that not all patients who have mild TSH elevations are hypothyroid and therefore would not require thyroid hormone therapy. These data are also relevant for the monitoring of subjects with hypothyroidism, since the target for TSH in levothyroxine treated subjects should be higher in elderly people. Pitfalls in the interpretation of TSH were carefully excluded in this study. Abnormal levels are observed in various non-thyroidal diseases and other conditions, but the effect of possible changes secondary to thyroid diseases were preventable excluding subjects who had used medication containing iodine during the previous 6 months, had had hospitalization, smokers, as well as those not using any medication that may alter minimally TSH or thyroid hormones.

Concluding, this data shows that prevalence of subclinical hypothyroidism is overestimated in the elderly, in almost 20% of subjects, unless age-specific RI is used. This might improve diagnostic accuracy and reduce the need of confirmatory unnecessary tests.

Competing interests

The author's declare that they have no competing interests.

Authors' contributions

RF did the study design, conducted the field study, made the final selection of study participants; computed the data and wrote the text. CRC made the initial guidance on the statistical requirements for the study, led and oversaw all statistical work. FA did the statistical field study under the supervision of CRC, being assisted during the course of the study also by the statistical mentioned in the acknowledgments. MV was the general supervisor of the study. He had discussions with the staff and the necessary modifications to the original design of the study; he revised, and made necessary adaptions to the final text and made the final approval of the text submitted to the journal. All authors read and approved the final manuscript.

Acknowledgments

We appreciate the statistical assistance of Dr. Martha Mutis, MD, PhD, and the revision by Angelo Pereira, teacher and translator of English language.

Author details

[1]Hospital Clementino Fraga Filho, Universidade Federal do Rio de Janeiro, Rua Prof. Rodolpho Paulo Rocco 255, Cidade Universitária, CEP 21941-913, Rio de Janeiro-RJ, Brazil. [2]Diagnósticos da América SA, Rio de Janeiro, Brazil. [3]Núcleo de Estudos de Saúde Coletiva, Universidade Federal do Rio de Janeiro, Rio de Janeiro, Brazil.

References

1. United Nations publication: **The Sex and Age distribution of the world populations.** *Sex and Age Popul Div, United Nations Secretariat, the 1998 Revis* 1998, **I**:2–6. No. E.99.XIII.8.
2. Chiovato L, Mariotti S, Pinchera A: **Thyroid diseases in the elderly.** *Baillieres Clin Endocrinol Metab* 1997, **11**:251–270.
3. Canaris GJ, Manowitz NR, Mayor G, Ridgway EC: **The Colorado thyroid disease prevalence study.** *Arch Intern Med* 2000, **160**:526–534.
4. Hollowell JG, Staehling NW, Flanders WD, Hannon WH, Gunter EW, Spencer CA, Braverman LE: **Serum TSH, T_4, and Thyroid Antibodies in the United States Population (1988 to 1994): National Health and Nutrition Examination Survey (NHANES III).** *J Clin Endocrinol Metab* 2002, **87**:489–499.
5. Ceriotti F: **Prerequisites for use of common reference intervals.** *Clin Biochem Rev* 2007, **28**:115–121.
6. Horowitz GL, Altaie S, Boyd JC, Ceriotti F, Garg U, Horn P, Pesce A, Sine HE, Zakovski J: **Defining, Establishing, and Verifying Reference Intervals in the Clinical Laboratory; Approved Guideline – Third Edition.** *Clin Lab Stand Inst* 2008, **28**:C28–A3.
7. Kahapola-Arachchige KM, Hadlow N, Wardrop R, Lim EM, Walsh JP: **Age-specific TSH reference ranges have minimal impact on the diagnosis of thyroid dysfunction.** *Clin Endocrinol* 2012, **77**:773–779.
8. Vadiveloo T, Donnan PT, Murphy MJ, Leese GP: **Age- and gender-specific TSH reference intervals in People with no obvious Thyroid disease in Tayside, Scotland: the Thyroid Epidemiology, Audit, and Research Study (TEARS).** *J Clin Endocrinol Metab* 2013, **98**:1147–1153.
9. Lei 1944/53 | Lei nº 1.944, de 14 de agosto de 1953 (Law 1944/53 | Law No. 1,944, of August 14, 1953) [http://presrepublica.jusbrasil.com.br/legislacao/128787/lei-1944-53]
10. Netto LS, Coeli CM, Micmacher E, Mamede SC, Nazar LO, Correa EK, Arrastia M, Galvão D, Buescu A, Vaisman M: **Longitudinal study of pituitary-thyroid axis in pregnancy.** *Arq Bras Endocrinol Metab* 2004, **48**:493–498.
11. Resultado do Monitoramento do Teor de Iodo no Sal: **Results of monitoring of iodine in salt.** 2011 [http://portal.anvisa.gov.br/wps/wcm/connect/7d7bb4804be9dbf18c50ddbc0f9d5b29/Relat%C3%B3rio+Pro.Iodo+2011.pdf?MOD=AJPERES]
12. Surks MI, Ortiz E, Daniels GH, Sawin CT, Col NF, Cobin RH, Franklin JA, Hershman JM, Burman KD, Denke MA, Gorman C, Cooper RS, Weissman NJ: **Subclinical thyroid disease: scientific review and guidelines for diagnosis and management.** *JAMA* 2004, **291**:228–238.
13. Oppenheimer JH, Schwartz HL, Dillman W, Surks MI: **Effect of thyroid hormone analogues on the displacement of ^{125}I-L-triiodothyronine from hepatic and heart nuclei in vivo: possible relationship to hormonal activity.** *Bioch Bioph Res Commun* 1973, **55**:544–550.
14. Liewendahl K, Majuri H, Helenius T: **Thyroid function tests in patients on long-term treatment with various anticonvulsivant drugs.** *Clin Endocrinol* 1978, **8**:185–191.
15. Smith PJ, Surks MI: **Multiple effects of 5,5'-diphenylhydantoin on the thyroid hormone system.** *Endocr Rev* 1984, **5**:514–524.
16. Spencer C, Eigen A, Shen D, Duda M, Qualls S, Weiss S, Nicoloff J: **Specificity of sensitive assays of thyrotropin (TSH) used to screen for thyroid disease in hospitalized patients.** *Clin Chem* 1987, **33**:1391–1396.
17. Larkin JG, Macphee GJA, Beastall GH, Brodie MJ: **Thyroid hormone concentrations in epileptic patients.** *Eur J Clin Pharmacol* 1989, **36**:213–216.

18. Davies PH, Franklyn JA: **The effects of drugs on tests of thyroid function.** *Eur J Clin Pharmacol* 1991, **40:**439–451.
19. Stockigt JR: **ree thyroid hormone measurement.** *A Crit appraisal 2001 Endocrinol Metab Clin North Am* 2001, **30:**265–289.
20. Steele BW, Wang E, Klee GG, Thienpont LM, Soldin SJ, Sokoll LJ, Winter WE, Fuhrman SA, Elin RJ: **Analytic bias of thyroid function tests: analysis of a college of American Pathologists fresh frozen serum pool by 3900 clinical laboratories.** *Arch Pathol Lab Med* 2005, **129:**310–317.
21. Crofton KM: **Thyroid disrupting chemicals: mechanisms and mixtures.** *Int J Androl* 2008, **31:**209–223.
22. Stockigt JR, Lim CF: **Medications that distort in vitro tests of thyroid function, with particular reference to estimates of serum free thyroxine.** *Best Pract Clin Endocrinol Metab* 2009, **23:**753–767.
23. Beckett GJ: **Mechanisms behind the non-thyroidal illness syndrome: an update.** *J Endocrinol* 2010, **205:**1–13.
24. Garber JR, Cobin RH, Gharib H, Hennessey JV, Klein I, Mechanick JI, Pessah-Pollack R, Singer PA, Woeber KA: **Clinical practice guidelines for hypothyroidism in adults: Cosponsored by the American Association of Clinical Endocrinologists and the American Thyroid Association.** *Thyroid* 2012, **22:**1200–1235.
25. Dixon WJ: **Processing data for outliers.** *Biometrics* 1953, **9:**74–89.
26. Harris EK, Boyd JC: **On dividing reference data into subgroups to produce reference ranges.** *Clin Chem* 1990, **36:**265–270.
27. Baloch Z, Carayon P, Conte-Devolx B, Demers LM, Feldt-Rasmussen U, Henry JF, LiVosli VA, Niccoli-Sire P, John R, Ruf J, Smyth PP, Spencer CA, Stockigt JR: **Laboratory medicine practice guidelines. Laboratory support for the diagnosis and monitoring of thyroid disease.** *Thyroid* 2003, **13:**3–126.
28. Benhaldi N, Fliers E, Visser TJ, Reitsma JB, Wiersinga WM: **Pilot study on the assessment of the setpoint on the hypothalamus-pituitary-tryroid axis in healthy volunteers.** *Eur J Endocrinol* 2010, **162:**323–329.
29. Kratzsch J, Fiedler GM, Leichtle A, Brügel M, Buchbinder S, Otto L, Sabri O, Matthes G, Thiery J: **New reference intervals for thyrotropin and thyroid hormones based on national academy of clinical biochemistry criteria and regular ultrasonography of the thyroid.** *Clin Chem* 2005, **51:**1480–1486.
30. D'Herbomez M, Jarrige V, Darte C: **Reference intervals for serum thyrotropin (TSH) and free thyroxine (FT4) in adults using the Access Immunoassay System.** *Clin Chem Lab Med* 2005, **43:**102–105.
31. Brochmann H, Bjøro T, Gaarder PI, Hanson F, Frey HM: **Prevalence of thyroid dysfunction in elderly subjects. A randomized study in a Norwegian rural community (Naerøy).** *Acta Endocrinol (Copenh) 1988,* **117:**7–12.
32. Boucai L, Hollowell JG, Surks MI: **An approach for development of age-, gender-, and ethnicity-specific thyrotropin reference limits.** *Thyroid* 2011, **21:**5–11.
33. Atzmon G, Barzilai N, Hollowell JG, Surks MI, Gabriely I: **Extreme longevity is associated with increased serum thyrotropin.** *J Clin Endocrinol Metab* 2009, **94:**1251–1254.
34. Surks MI, Boucai L: **Age- and race- based serum thyrotropin reference limits.** *J Clin Endocrinol Metab* 2010, **95:**496–502.
35. Estrada JM, Soldin D, Buckey TM, Burman KD, Soldin OP: **Thyrotropin isoforms – implications for TSH analysis and clinical practice.** *Thyroid* 2013. in press.
36. Mariotti S, Franceschi C, Cossarizza A, Pinchera A: **The aging thyroid.** *Endocr Rev* 1995, **16:**686–715.
37. Gussekloo J, van Exel E, de Craen AJ, Meinders AE, Frölich M, Westendorp RG: **Thyroid status, disability and cognitive function, and survival in old age.** *JAMA* 2004, **292:**2591–2599.
38. Van Den Beld AW, Visser TJ, Feelders RA, Grobbee DE, Lamberts SWJ: **Thyroid hormone concentrations, disease, physical function, and mortality in elderly Men.** *J Clin Endocrinol Metab* 2005, **90:**6403–6409.
39. Gammage MD, Parle JV, Holder RL, Roberts LM, Hobbs FD, Wilson S, Sheppard MC, Franklyn JA: **Association between serum free thyroxine concentration and atrial fibrillation.** *Arch Intern Med* 2007, **167:**928–934.
40. Heeringa J, Hoogendoorn EH, von der Deure WM, Hofman A, Peeters RP, Hop WCJ, den Heijer M, Visser TJ, Witterman JCM: **High-normal thyroid function and risk of atrial fibrillation. The rotterdam study.** *Arch intern Med* 2008, **168:**2219–2224.
41. Peeters RP: **Thyroid function and longevity: New insights into an Old dilemma.** *J Clin Endocrinol Metab* 2009, **94:**4658–4660.
42. Biondi B, Cooper DS: **The clinical significance of subclinical thyroid dysfunction.** *Endocr Rev* 2008, **29:**76–131.
43. Laurberg P, Andersen S, Carle A, Karmisholt J, Knudsen N, Pedersen IB: **The TSH upper reference limit: where are we at?** *Nat Rev Endocrinol* 2011, **7:**232–239.
44. Tseng F-Y, Lin W-Y, Lin C-C, Lee L-T, Li T-C, Sung P-K, Huang K-C: **Subclinical hypothyroidism is associated with increased risk for All-cause and cardiovascular mortality in adults.** *J Am col Cardiol* 2012, **60:**730–737.
45. Wartofsky L, Dickey RA: **The evidence for a narrower thyrotropin reference range is compelling 2005.** *J Clin Endocrinol Metab* 2005, **90:**5483–5488.

3

Association between genetic mutations and the development of autoimmune thyroiditis in patients with chronic hepatitis C treated with interferon alpha

Janina Krupińska[1], Waldemar Urbanowicz[2^], Mariusz Kaczmarczyk[3], Grzegorz Kulig[1], Elżbieta Sowińska-Przepiera[1], Elżbieta Andrysiak-Mamos[1] and Anhelli Syrenicz[1*]

Abstract

Background: Considerable progress was made by the introduction of interferon to the treatment of chronic hepatitis C virus infection. This treatment, however, is associated with the risk of developing or exacerbating autoimmune diseases, with chronic autoimmune thyroiditis being one of them. The aim of our study was to evaluate the predisposition to autoimmune thyroiditis in patients with chronic hepatitis C virus during IFN-alpha therapy, depending on the presence of polymorphisms in the promoter region of CTLA-4C (−318)T gene and in exon 1 of A49G gene as well as C1858T transition of PTPN22 gene.

Methods: The study was conducted in 149 patients aged between 18 and 70 years (mean of 43.9 years), including 82 men and 67 women. Control group for the assessment of the distribution of analyzed polymorphism of genotypes consisted of 200 neonates, from whom umbilical blood was drawn for the tests. The patients were divided into three groups: group 1 consisted of 114 patients without thyroid impairment before and during IFN-alpha therapy, group 2 contained 9 patients with AT with the onset prior to IFN-alpha treatment, and group 3 comprised 26 patients with AT starting after the beginning of IFN-alpha therapy.

Results: The frequency of C1858Tand C(−318)T genotypes observed in the study group did not differ significantly from control group. A significant difference, however, was found for A49G polymorphism.

Conclusions: No association was demonstrated between the occurrence of autoimmune thyroiditis with the onset during IFN-alpha therapy and the presence of polymorphisms within CTLA-4 C(−318)T gene in the promoter region and A49G in exon 1, as well as C1858T transition of PTPN22 gene.

Keywords: Genetic mutations, Hepatitis C virus, Interferon alpha, Thyroiditis

Background

The development of autoimmune diseases is determined by the coexistence of autoimmune, environmental, and genetic factors. Genetic predisposition to autoimmune diseases depends on many genetic loci, of which three play a key role: alleles of major histocompatibility complex genes (human leukocyte antigen- HLA), mainly class II HLA-DR3; alleles of a gene coding cytotoxic T lymphocyte associated antigen-4 (CTLA-4), and alleles of PTPN22 gene coding for lymphoid-specific tyrosine phosphatase (LYP) [1].

CTLA-4 gene, located on chromosome 2q33, codes for membrane protein (cytotoxic lymphocyte antigen 4), which is important for the regulatory functions of T lymphocytes. Some variants of this gene predispose to autoimmune thyroiditis, including Graves' disease, as well as to type 1 diabetes, Addison's disease; also, such non-endocrine conditions as rheumatoid arthritis or coeliac disease [2-7]. In order for the autoimmune response to

* Correspondence: anhelli@asymed.ifg.pl
^Deceased
[1]Department of Endocrinology, Metabolic Diseases and Internal Diseases, Pomeranian Medical University, Szczecin, Poland
Full list of author information is available at the end of the article

take place, thyroid autoantigens must be presented to immunocompetent cells; class II HLA antigens participate in this process. Many proteins are involved in the activation of T cell dependent on antigen presentation, including CTLA-4, which inhibits this activation. Mutations of CTLA-4 occur spontaneously as a result of DNA copying error during replication or they may be induced by exposure to DNA-damaging chemical factors or viruses incorporated into the genome DNA during the life cycle. The mutation most likely to occur is the erroneous incorporation of a purine or pyrimidine (i.e. A↔G or T↔C substitution) [8]. Three CTLA-4-related polymorphisms have been described to date: substitution of adenine with guanine in exon 1 position 49 codon 17 (CTLA-4 A49G), substitution of thymine with cytosine at position 318 of CTLA-4(T318C) gene promoter, and elongation of AT sequence of microsatellite marker in 3' untranslated region (3'UTR(AT)n [6,7,9]. The majority of studies focus on the association between exon 1 CTLA-4 gene polymorphism (A49G) and the risk of developing diseases with autoimmune background [10,11].

The inhibition of T cell activation by CTLA-4 is governed by two mechanisms. In the first, activation is inhibited by the signal that constitutes a response to the activation of lymphocyte T receptor. It occurs at the early stage of immune response, when the expression of CTLA-4 and B7 receptor is restricted. Consequently, the inhibition of T cell proliferation and IL-2 secretion also take place. The second mechanism comprises surface competition between CTLA-4 and CD28 for B7 ligand on the antigen presenting cell. This mechanism depends on the expression of CTLA-4 on the surface of T lymphocyte and is known to join immune response at a later stage, when B7 and CTLA-4 expression increases. The consequence of B7 and CTLA-4 binding is the termination of response through restriction of signal from CD28, anergy of activated T lymphocytes, and their subsequent apoptosis. The impairment of CTLA-4 expression and/or function results in abnormal regulation of autoimmune response [12-14].

In 2004, Bottini et al. published the results of a study demonstrating that substitution of cytosine with thymidine at position 1858 of PTPN22 gene is associated with type 1 diabetes in patients from North America and Sardinia [15]. PTPN22 gene is located on chromosome 1p13.3-p13.1 [16]. A 1858T>C polymorphism leads to the substitution of arginine (R) with tryptophan (W) at position 620 (R620W), which makes it impossible for the PTPN22 gene-coded phosphatase to properly bind with Csk signaling molecules [16-18]. Under normal conditions, LYP-Csk complex causes the gradual inhibition of activation signal for T lymphocytes. Apart from polymorphisms within the major histocompatibility complex (MHC) and CTLA-4, a 1858 T>C polymorphism of PTPN22 gene is currently a recognized risk factor for autoimmune diseases [17-20].

The aim of this study was to assess the predisposition to autoimmune thyroiditis in patients with chronic hepatitis C virus treated with IFN-α, depending on the presence of CTLA-4 C(−318)T polymorphism in gene promoter region and exon 1 CTLA-4 gene A49G polymorphism, as well as C1858T transition of PTPN22 gene.

Methods

Characteristics of study subjects

The study was approved by the Ethics Committee at Pomeranian Medical University in Szczecin (decision no. KB-0080/88/09).

The study group consisted of 149 patients aged between 18 and 70 years (mean of 43.9 years), including 82 men and 67 women. All subjects were HCV positive and remained under the care of Hepatology Outpatient Clinic at Regional Polyclinical State Hospital in Szczecin between 2003 and 2007. To assess genetic predisposition to autoimmune thyroiditis during IFN-α therapy, C (−318)T polymorphism in gene promoter region and exon 1 CTLA-4 gene A49G polymorphism, as well as C1858T transition of PTPN22 gene were analyzed. Molecular investigations were conducted at the Institute of Clinical Biochemistry and Molecular Diagnostics at Pomeranian Medical University in Szczecin.

The patients were divided into three groups: 1) Group 1 – 114 subjects without impairment of thyroid function before and during IFN-α therapy, 2) Group 2 – 9 subjects with the onset of autoimmune thyroiditis before IFN-α therapy, and 3) Group 3 – 26 patients with the onset of autoimmune thyroiditis after IFN-α therapy.

Detailed clinical characteristics of study subjects can be found in our earlier publication [21].

DNA isolation

To detect CTLA-4 polymorphisms and PTPN22 transition, 5 ml of venous blood was drawn into Vacutainer test tubes containing 0.1 ml 5% EDTA. The study material consisted of DNA isolated from peripheral blood leukocytes with the use of QIAMP® DNA Mini Kit (Qiagen).

The distribution of analyzed polymorphisms was also assessed in umbilical blood obtained from 200 neonates, who constituted the control group.

Sequence of starters

Selected polymorphisms of genes: CTLA-4 [rs 231775 A/G (A49G), rs5742909 C/T(C(−318)T)], and PTPN22 [rs2476601 C/T (C1858T)] were identified with PCR-RFLP (polymerase chain reaction-restriction fragment length polymorphism) with the use of specific starter pairs (Table 1).

Amplification of CTLA-4 and PTPN22 sequences

Optimal PCR conditions for individual starter pairs were established in preliminary experiments (Table 2).

All amplifications were performed in Mastercycler Gradient thermal cycler (Eppendorf).

Amplifications of CTLA4 sequences were performed in 20 µl of reaction mixture containing the following ingredients: 40 ng of genome DNA, PCR buffer [10 mM of Tris–HCl, 50 mM of KCl, and 0.08% of Nonidet P40] (MBI Fermentas), dNTP [200 µM](MBI Fermentas), MgCl2 [1,5 mM](MBI Fermentas), upstream and downstream primer, 4 pmol each (synt. TIB MOLBIOL, Poznań), and 0.5 U of Taq polymerase (MBI Fermentas).

Amplifications of PTPN22 gene sequences were performed in 20 µl of reaction mixture containing: 40 ng of genome DNA, 1 x PCR buffer (QIAGEN), 1 x Q-Solution(QIAGEN), dNTP [200 µM] (MBI Fermentas), upstream and downstream primer, 4 pmol each (synt. TIB MOLBIOL, Poznań), and 1 U of Hot Star Taq polymerase (QIAGEN).

The following temperature-time profile was used in PCR: 1) phase I: preliminary denaturation 94°C – 5 min, 2) phase II (36–37 cycles; Table 2): denaturation: 94°C – 20 sec, annealing: 52-60°C (Table 2) – 40 sec, elongation: 72°C, 3) phase III: final elongation 72°C – 8 min.

Amplification products were subject to restriction analysis with appropriate enzymes (Table 3).

PCR products and restriction fragments were separated by electrophoresis in agarose gel of appropriate concentration and stained with ethidium bromide. The separation was conducted in 1 x TBE buffer (0.089 M of Tris, 0.089 M of boric acid, 2 mM of EDTA), at the temperature of 20°C and voltage of 80V. The length of restriction fragments was estimated on the basis of length marker DNA-pUC Mix Marker 8 (MBI Fermentas). The final stage consisted of photographing the obtained results with Polaroid camera (DS-34 Direct Screen Camera) under UV light (Transiluminator 4000, Stratagene). The photos were scanned and saved as jpeg files (Figures 1, 2, 3).

Table 1 Sequence of starters

Gene	Polymorphism	Sequence of starters
CTLA4	rs231775	5'-GCTCTACTTCTTGAAGACCT-3'
		5'-AGTCTCACTCACCTTTGCAG-3'
	rs5742909	5'-GGATGCCCAGAAGATTGA -3'
		5'-AAGGAAGCCGTGGGTTTA -3'
PTPN22	rs2476601	5'-ACCGCGCCCAGCCCTACTTTTG-3'
		5'-AGCCACCATGCCCATCCCACACT-3'

Table 2 Amplification conditions

Gene	Polymorphism	$T_{annealing}$ [°C]	No. of cycles	Amplicon [bp]
CTLA4	rs231775	58	37	162
	rs5742909	54	36	215
PTPN22	rs2476601	60	37	392

Statistical analysis

The conformity of genotype frequency with Hardy-Weinberg law was evaluated with an exact test using R "genetic" module (version 2.9.0; http://cran.r-project.org).

The analysis of polymorphisms was performed with $\chi 2$ test and logistic regression model for the calculation of odds ratio (OR) with 95% CI (confidence interval). Allele frequency was calculated on the basis of genotype frequency.

The compliance of genotype frequency with Hardy-Weinberg distribution was analyzed separately for the study group and in the control group, as well as for both of these groups together.

Results

Distribution of C1858T, A49G and C(–318)T genotypes in study and control groups

With the exception of A49G polymorphism, genotype frequency did not differ significantly from the theoretical distribution. In the case of A49G polymorphism, the deviations from Hardy-Weinberg equilibrium were found as following for each of the three groups analyzed groups: study group - $p<0.0001$, control group – $p<0.05$, study and control groups together - $p<0.00001$.

The distribution of genotypes of C1858T, A49G, and C(–318)T polymorphisms in the study group and in control group are presented in Table 4. The frequency of C1858T and C(–318)T genotypes in the study group did not differ significantly from that in the control group. A significant difference, however, was observed for A49G polymorphism; moreover, no GG homozygote was detected in the study group, while there were 14 GG

Table 3 Conditions of restriction analysis

Gene	Polymorphism	Restriction enzyme	Restriction fragments [bp]
CTLA4	rs 231775 A/G	Sat I [10 U, 37°C, 12 h]	allele A: 99 + 63
			allele G: 74 + 25 + 63
	rs5742909	Mse I [5 U, 65°C , 12 h]	allele C: 215
			allele T: 124 + 91
PTPN22	rs2476601 C/T	Rsa I [5 U, 37°C, 12 h]	allele C: 228 + 74 + 46 + 44
			allele T: 272 + 74 + 46

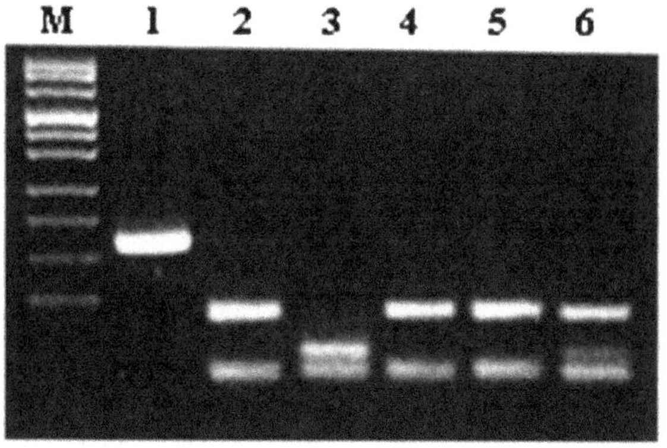

Figure 1 Identification of RS 231775 polymorphism of CTLA4 gene. Lanes: M – DNA length marker (Puc Mix Marker 8, MBI Fermentas), 1 – amplicon (162 bp) not subject to restriction, 2, 4, 5 – AA homozygotes, 3 – GG homozygote, 6 – AG heterozygote.

homozygotes in the control group, being equal to 7% of all genotypes in this group.

Predisposition to chronic viral hepatitis

The results of analysis in relations to different inheritance modes for minor alleles (dominant and recessive) of the mutated gene and to patient's gender are presented in Table 5. Dominant mode was defined as the presence of at least one minor allele in comparison to the absence of this allele, resulting in the following three sets of comparisons: TT+CT vs. CC (minor allele T), GG +AG vs. AA (minor allele G) and TT+CT vs. CC (minor allele T), for C1858T, A49G and C(−318)T polymorphisms, respectively. In the case of the recessive mode, homozygotes for minor alleles were compared with the carriers of major alleles, producing the following sets of comparisons: TT vs. CT+CC, GG vs. AG+AA and TT vs. CT+CC for C1858T, A49G, and C(−318)T, respectively.

Following gender adjustments, C1858T and C(−318)T polymorphisms, irrespective of the analyzed inheritance mode and A49G polymorphism in the dominant mode (GG+AG vs. AA), did not demonstrate any relationship with the predisposition to chronic viral hepatitis. Odds ratio for A49G in the recessive mode (GG vs. AG+AA) could not be obtained due to the absence of GG homozygotes in the study group, but the observed difference in the frequency of GG homozygotes (0% of patients treated with interferon and 7% of the control group) and allele A carriers (100% of patients treated with interferon and 96% of the control group) was significant (p=0.00334, two-tailed Fisher's test).

Distribution of genotypes in patients with autoimmune thyroiditis and in patients without thyroid impairment

Table 6 presents the number and frequency of genotypes of C1858T, A49G, and C(−318)T polymorphisms in patients with autoimmune thyroiditis (AT, n=18) and in patients without impairment of thyroid function during treatment (n=62). The comparison of genotype frequencies in these two groups did not show any significant differences with regards to any of analyzed polymorphisms. It is worth noticing that there were no GG homozygotes of A49G polymorphism, both in AT group and in patients without thyroid impairment.

Predisposition to AT during IFN-α therapy

Our study attempted to assess the predisposition to AT depending on the possessed genotype in relation to two inheritance modes and the gender of the patient (Table 7). Since AT group lacked homozygotes of mutated TT C1858T, GG A49G, and TT C(−318)T alleles, the assessment of predisposition to AT in the carriers of these genotypes as compared to the carriers of wild-type (major) alleles (recessive mode) proved impossible. Additionally, A49G GG homozygotes were not detected in patients without thyroid impairment. Conversely, the carriers of mutated (minor) alleles (TT+CT C1858T, GG+AG A49G, and TT+CT C(−318)T) did not

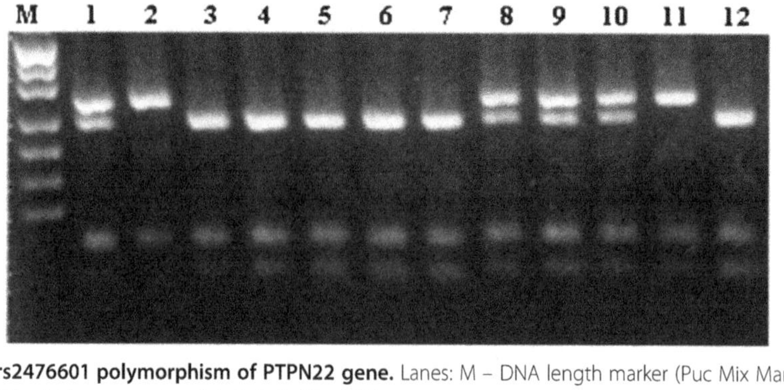

Figure 2 Identification of rs2476601 polymorphism of PTPN22 gene. Lanes: M – DNA length marker (Puc Mix Marker 8, MBI Fermentas), 1, 8, 9, 10 – CT heterozygotes, 2, 11 – TT homozygotes, 3, 4, 5, 6, 7, 12 – CC homozygotes.

show a greater predisposition to AT as compared to wild-type homozygotes (dominant mode).

OR was not obtained in three cases (recessive inheritance): C1858T – absence of TT homozygotes in the study group vs. one (1.6%) TT homozygote in the control group (p=1.0, two-tailed Fisher's test); A49G – no GG homozygotes in both groups; C(−318)T – no TT homozygotes in the study group as compared to 2 TT homozygotes (3.2%) in the control group (p=1.0, two-tailed Fisher's test).

Discussion

At present, genetic studies are being employed with increasing frequency for the assessment of predisposition to many diseases, especially those that are genetically determined (monogenic and polygenic) as well as those that involve the chromosomes. Diagnostic assessments have become markedly easier to carry out as a result of considerable progress in the investigational methods of molecular biology following the discovery of polymerase chain reaction (PCR) in early 1990s, allowing for the replication of selected DNA fragments in billions of copies. Approximately 80 monogenic diseases have a direct influence on body's endocrine function; although, polygenic factors are also known to play a role [2].

Genetic polymorphism is the consequence of two types of structural changes in gene sequence, i.e. single nucleotide polymorphism (SNP) and major structural changes such as simple sequence length polymorphism (SSLP), i.e. a variable number of tandem repeats-VNTR (147). According to current genetic research, a common genetic background of autoimmune diseases seems to comprise the following components: C1858T polymorphism of a single nucleotide of PTPN22 gene coding for lymphocyte-specific phosphatase and A/G polymorphism at position 49 of CTLA-4 gene, acting as a negative regulator of lymphocyte T activation, The first results in excessive activation of T lymphocytes, while the second modifies post-translation processes in endoplasmic reticulum through the substitution of threonine with alanine in a signal peptide and this, in turn, causes less effective glycosylation and reduced surface expression of CTLA-4 peptide [22-24]. In 2007, Lee et al. conducted a meta-analysis showing the association between C1858T polymorphism of PTPN22 gene and Graves' (G) disease, type 1 diabetes, rheumatoid arthritis, and lupus erythematosus [16,22]. Another study published in 2007 demonstrated a very strong causal relationship between 49A/G polymorphism of CTLA-4 gene and the development of Hashimoto Thyroiditis (HT) and the presence of anti-thyroid antibodies in Graves' disease and HT [25]. A solid correlation between autoimmune thyroid diseases and CTLA-4 polymorphism on chromosome 2q33 was proved by Bicek et al. in 2009, namely two A>G polymorphisms of a single nucleotide of CTLA-4 gene at position +49 of exon 1 (49A/G) and +6230 (CT60) in 3'UTR [26]. We analyzed the distribution of genotypes of C1858T, A49G, and C(−318)T polymorphisms in the study subjects and in the control group. A significant difference was found for A49G polymorphism in the study group vs. control group, while the frequency of C1858T and C(−318)T genotypes did not differ significantly in both groups. The aim of our study was to assess the occurrence of C(−318)T polymorphism of CTLA-4 gene within the promoter region. Additionally, we aimed to evaluate A49G polymorphism in exon 1 and C1858T transition of PTPN22 gene in a group of patients with the onset of AT during INF-α therapy for HCV as compared to subjects without any impairment of thyroid function during treatment. The comparison of genotype frequency between these groups conducted in our study showed no significant differences for all polymorphisms. This result differs from that reported by Kula et al. in 2003, who found the strongest association between CTLA-4 polymorphism and the development and clinical picture of HT in a group of 89 Polish subjects [27]. 49A/G polymorphism associated with the activation of T lymphocytes influences the high level of anti-thyroid antibody production in G-B disease and HT [23,28]. Kula et al. [27] did not find any significant differences in mean TPOAb level for CTLA-4 gene in relation to the genotype with demonstrated association with the exacerbation of hypothyroidism and thyroid volume. Slovenian investigators examined 328 Caucasian patients with G-B disease and Postpartum Thyroiditis (PPT), and compared the results with those obtained in a control group of 117 healthy subjects. The distribution of genotypes of both polymorphisms was similar in these two groups. The frequency of GG genotype in G-B disease was 13.8% for 49A/G polymorphism as compared to 5.1% in the control group; the corresponding values for CT60 polymorphism were 40.7% in the study group and 25.6% in the control group. The frequencies of GG genotype for HT and PPT were comparable and were found to equal to 12.9% for 49AG polymorphism and 34.4% for CT60 polymorphism. A comparison of G allele vs. A allele for both polymorphisms within CTLA-4 gene was also performed and showed that the likelihood of developing G-B disease is 1.6 times greater for individuals with G allele in 49A/G or CT60 polymorphism of CTLA-4 gene. It was demonstrated that 49A/G and CT60 polymorphisms of CTLA-4 gene display strong causal relationship with autoimmune thyroid diseases (AITD) in Slovenian population [26]. Additionally, a correlation between the presence of GG genotype and the development of HT and PPT were also showed [11,26]. We evaluated the frequencies of genotypes in patients treated with INF-α and in the control group and, as mentioned before, a

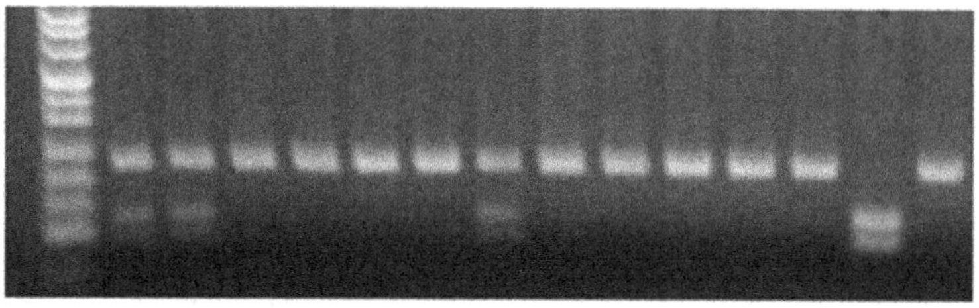

Figure 3 Identification of rs5742909 polymorphism of CTLA4 gene. Lanes: M – DNA length marker (pUC Mix Marker 8, MBI Fermentas), 1, 2, 7 – CT heterozygotes, 3, 4, 5, 6, 8, 9, 10, 11, 12, 14 – CC homozygotes, 13 – TT homozygote.

significant difference was observed for A49G polymorphism in both groups. Namely, no GG homozygotes were detected in the study group as compared to the control group with 14 GG homozygotes, constituting 7% of all genotypes in this group. Furthermore, A49G GG homozygotes were not found in patients without thyroid impairment. Conversely, in a meta-analysis published by Roycroft et al. in 2009, which examined C1858T polymorphism of PTPN22 gene in the population of Caucasian patients with Addison's disease living in Britain and in Poland [29], sixty-one out of 502 (12.2%) British patients were the carriers of T allele in PTPN22 C1858T(R620W)SNP. This allele was detected in 67 (7.8%) of 858 healthy subjects from the control group. In the Polish population of 174 patients, 1858T alleles were found in 34 (19.5%) subjects compared with 11.7% in the control group. The authors performed another comparison within this study, namely, they compared the frequency of 1858T allele in control groups originating from different parts of Europe and obtained the following results: Newcastle (England) – 7.8%, Sheffield (England) – 10.5%, and Norway – 10.8%. Therefore, it is our opinion that the correlation between the polymorphism of PTPN22 gene and the occurrence of Addison's disease in European population cannot be confirmed beyond a reasonable doubt as authors claim [29].

Table 4 Distribution of C1858T, A49G, and C(−318)T genotypes in the study group and control group

SNP	Genotypes	Study group (n=101)	Control group (n=200)
C1858T	CC	74 (73.2%)	147 (73.5%)
	CT	25 (24.8%)	50 (25.0%)
	TT	2 (2.0%)	3 (1.5%)
	p=0.95347		
A49G	AA	43 (42.6%)	81 (40.5%)
	AG	58 (57.4%)	105 (52.5%)
	GG	0 (0.0%)	14 (7.0%)
	p=0.02423		
C(−318)T	CC	79 (78.2%)	151 (75.5%)
	CT	20 (19.8%)	48 (24.0%)
	TT	2 (1.98%)	1 (0.5%)
	p=0.35636		

Ever since the relationship between CTLA-4 polymorphisms and G-B disease and type 1 diabetes in southern European countries was demonstrated for the first time, numerous studies have been conducted to link a given polymorphism with a specific disease. So far, many authors have stressed a strong association between G-B disease and the polymorphism of CTLA-4 gene; however, a considerable controversy has arisen as to the site of polymorphism. For example, Bicek et al., state that CT60 polymorphism shows the strongest correlation only with G-B disease and that its association with HT and PPT is weaker [26]. Petrone et al. demonstrated that in Italian population A49G polymorphism was correlated with G-B disease, especially when G allele was present [30]. Ban et al. observed a much greater frequency of G allele SNP CT60 associated with G-B disease in Japanese subjects than in Caucasian population: 72.6% vs. 52.3%, respectively [31]. In Japanese population, the presence of G allele CT60 was more common in patients with G-B disease than in the control group: 84.0% and 72.6%, respectively; just as it was in the whole group of patients with autoimmune thyroid diseases: 80.1% and 72.6%, respectively. A dominant genotype model among AITD patients was GG+GA vs. AA, while a recessive genotype model was found to be GG vs. AG+AA [32]. We tried to analyze the various modes of inheritance of mutated allele, i.e. dominant inheritance (a necessary condition was the presence of at least one mutated allele versus the absence of this allele), producing three sets of comparisons: TT+CT vs. CC (mutated T allele), GG +AG vs. AA

Table 5 Predisposition to chronic viral hepatitis

SNP	Variable	OR (95% CI)	p*
C1858T	TT+CT vs. CC	0.96 (0.56-1.67)	0.895
	TT vs. CT+CC	1.34 (0.22-8.26)	0.749
A49G	GG+AG vs. AA	0.94 (0.57-1.53)	0.799
	GG vs. AG+AA	—	—
C(−318)T	TT+CT vs. CC	0.87 (0.49-1.54)	0.630
	TT vs. CT+CC	3.82 (0.34-43.3)	0.278

*gender-adjusted p values.

Table 6 Distribution of genotypes in patients with AT and in patients without thyroid impairment

SNP	Genotypes	AT (n=18)	No thyroid impairment (n=62)
C1858T	CC	12 (66.7%)	49 (79.0%)
	CT	6 (33.3%)	12 (19.4%)
	TT	0 (0.0%)	1 (1.6%)
	p=0.41034		
A49G	AA	7 (38.9%)	26 (41.9%)
	AG	11 (61.1%)	36 (58.1%)
	GG	0 (0.0%)	0 (0.0%)
	p=0.81720		
C(−318)T	CC	14 (77.8%)	47 (75.8%)
	CT	4 (22.2%)	13 (21.0%)
	TT	0 (0.0%)	2 (3.2%)
	p=0.74153		

(mutated G allele), and TT+CT vs. CC (mutated T allele) for C1858T, A49Gm and C(−318)T polymorphisms, respectively. Recessive inheritance (the presence of both mutated alleles was necessary) resulting in the following genotypes: TT vs. CT+CC, GG vs. AG+AA, and TT vs. CT+CC for C1858T, A49G, and (C-318T) polymorphisms, respectively, was also analyzed. We found that the carriers of mutated alleles (TT+CT C1858T, GG +AG A49G, and TT+CT C(−318t)) did not have a higher predisposition to autoimmune thyroiditis (AT) as compared to homozygotes of dominant mode. We also tried to assess the predisposition to AT depending on the genotype possessed, taking into consideration two different modes of inheritance and patient's gender. However, since AT group lacked homozygotes of mutated alleles: TT C1858T, GG A49G, and TT C(−318)T, the evaluation of predisposition to AT in the carriers of these genotypes as compared to the carriers of wild-type alleles (recessive mode) was not feasible in our study. Kucharska et al. reports that among 68 HT patients, G allele and homozygotes with rare G/G allele were significantly more frequent. These authors found no significant difference in the occurrence of homozygotes with common A/A allele

Table 7 Predisposition to AT during IFN-α therapy

SNP	Variable	OR (95% CI)	p*
C1858T	TT+CT vs. CC	1.92 (0.57-6.44)	0.282
	TT vs. CT+CC	—	—
A49G	GG+AG vs. AA	1.26 (0.41-3.89)	0.678
	GG vs. AG+AA	—	—
C(−318)T	TT+CT vs. CC	1.02 (0.27-3.83)	0.971
	TT vs. CT+CC	—	—

*gender-adjusted p values.

and heterozygotes [9]. Kinjo et al. demonstrated that in a group of 144 patients with G-B disease, the frequency of AA, AG, and GG genotypes at position 49 of CTLA-4 gene was significantly higher than in the control group [28]. The frequency of GG genotype was significantly greater, while the frequency of AA genotype was significantly lower in patients with G-B disease as compared to the control. In 1997, Witas et al. analyzed the occurrence of polymorphic alleles of CTLA-4 gene in Polish population of 122 children and found C(−318)T polymorphism in 20.5% of analyzed subjects. Their data indicates that the frequency of T allele was 0.107 and estimated occurrence of heterozygotes 19.1% [33]. The study conducted in Germany by Deichmann et al. in a group of 239 patients with G-B disease demonstrated that C(−318)T polymorphism was found in 13.4% of patients, and heterozygotes were detected in 23.2% of cases [17]. The studies of genetic predisposition to autoimmune endocrine diseases, including autoimmune thyroiditis, focus on the search for polymorphisms within candidate gene's responsible for autoimmune diseases. In Hashimoto autoimmune thyroiditis, apart from known genetic liability related to the presence of histocompatibility antigens class II DR 3, 4 and 5, and the recognized effect of such environmental factors as the excess of iodine or medications (e.g. interferon), the presence of polymorphisms within CTLA-4 gene and PTPN22 gene must also be taken into account. The results of studies conducted to date are inconclusive; therefore, further research is necessary to explain the etiopathogenesis of autoimmune thyroid diseases.

Conclusions

No association was found between the occurrence of autoimmune thyroiditis during interferon therapy and the presence of polymorphisms within CTLA-4 C(−318) T gene in the promoter region and A49G in exon 1, as well as C1858T transition of PTPN22 gene.

Competing interests
The authors declare that they have no competing interests.

Authors' contributions
JK and AS conceived of the study, participated in its design and coordination, and helped to draft the manuscript. WU, GK, ESP and EAM conceived of the study and helped to draft the manuscript. MK carried out the molecular genetic studies and participated in the design and coordination of the study. All authors read and approved the final manuscript.

Author details
[1]Department of Endocrinology, Metabolic Diseases and Internal Diseases, Pomeranian Medical University, Szczecin, Poland. [2]Department of Infectious Diseases and Hepatology, Pomeranian Medical University, Szczecin, Poland. [3]Institute of Clinical Biochemistry and Molecular Diagnostics, Pomeranian Medical University, Szczecin, Poland.

References

1. Syrenicz A, Syrenicz M: **Hyperthyroidism.** In *Endocrinology in clinical practice.* Edited by Syrenicz A. Szczecin: Pomeranian Medical University; 2011:170–181.
2. Ciechanowicz A, Kokot F: *Genetyka molekularna w chorobach wewnętrznych.* Warszawa: PZWL; 2009.
3. Dittmar M, Kahaly GJ: **Immunoregulatory and susceptibility genes in thyroid and polyglandular autoimmunity.** *Thyroid* 2005, **15**:239–250.
4. Donner H, Braun J, Seidl C, Rau H, Finke R, Ventz M, Walfish PG, Usadel KH, Badenhoop K: **Codon 17 polymorphism of the cytotoxic T lymphocyte antigen 4 gene in Hashimoto's thyroiditis and Addison's diseases.** *J Clin Endocrinol Metab* 1997, **82**:4130–4132.
5. Kavvoura FK, Akamizu T, Awata T, Ban Y, Chistiakov DA, Frydecka I, Ghaderi A, Gough SC, Hiromatsu Y, Ploski R, Wang PW, Ban Y, Bednarczuk T, Chistiakova EI, Chojm M, Heward JM, Hiratani H, Juo SH, Karabon L, Katayama S, Kurihara S, Liu RT, Miyake I, Omrani GH, Pawlak E, Taniyama M, Tozaki T, Ioannidis JP: **Cytotoxic T-lymphocyte associated antigen 4 gene polymorphism and autoimmune thyroid disease: a meta-analysis.** *J Clin Endocrinol Metab* 2007, **92**:3162–3170.
6. Vaidya B, Kendall-Taylor P, Pearce SHS: **The genetics of autoimmune thyroid disease.** *J Clin Endocrinol Metab* 2002, **87**:5385–5397.
7. Yeşilkaya E, Koç A, Bideci A, Camurdan O, Boyraz M, Erkal O, Ergun MA, Cinaz P: **CTLA-4 gene polymorphism in children and adolescents with autoimmune thyroid diseases.** *Genet Test* 2008, **12**:461–464.
8. Bradley JR, Johnson DR, Pober BR: *Genetyka medyczna.* Warszawa: PZWL; 2009.
9. Kucharska AM, Wiśniewska A, Rymkiewicz-Kluczyńska B: **Występowanie polimorfizmu w pozycji 49 eksonie 1 genu CTLA-4 u dzieci z chorobą Hashimoto.** *Endokrynol Diabetol Chor Przemiany Materii Wieku Rozw* 2006, **12**:163–166.
10. Suwalska K, Tutak A, Frydecka I: **Polimorfizm genu kodującego antygen supresorowy - ryzyko autoimmunizacji.** *Postępy Biologii Komórki* 2003, **30**:549–562.
11. Yang J, Qin Q, Yan N, Zhu YF, Li C, Yang XJ, Wang X, Pandey M, Hou P, Zhang JA: **CD40 C/T(−1) and CTLA-4 A/G(49) SNPs are associated with autoimmune thyroid diseases in the Chinese population.** *Endocrine* 2012, **41**:111–115.
12. Kosmaczewska A, Ciszak L, Boćko D, Frydecka I: **Expression and functional significance of CTLA-4, a negative regulator of T cell activation.** *Arch Immunol Ther Exp (Warsz)* 2001, **49**:39–46.
13. Benhatchi K, Jochmanová I, Habalová V, Wagnerová H, Lazúrová I: **CTLA-4 exon A49G polymorphism in Slovak patients with rheumatoid arthritis and Hashimoto thyroiditis – results and the review of the literature.** *Clin Rheumatol* 2011, **30**:1319–1324.
14. Kucharska AM, Górska E, Popka K, Wąsik M, Rymkiewicz-Kluczyńska B: **Ekspresja powierzchniowa CD 152(CTLA-4) na limfocytach krwi obwodowej u dzieci z chorobą Hashimoto.** *Endokrynol Diabetol Chor Przemiany Materii Wieku Rozw* 2006, **12**:167–170.
15. Bottini N, Musumeci L, Alonso A, Rahmouni S, Nika K, Rostamkhani M, MacMurray J, Meloni GF, Lucarelli P, Pellecchia M, Eisenbarth GS, Comings D, Mustelin T: **A functional variant of lymphoid tyrosine phosphatase is associated with type I diabetes.** *Nat Genet* 2004, **36**:337–338.
16. Lee YH, Rho YH, Choi SJ, Ji JD, Song GG, Nath SK, Harley JB: **The PTPN22 C1858T functional polymorphism and autoimmune diseases – a meta-analysis.** *Rheumatology (Oxford)* 2007, **46**:49–56.
17. Deichmann K, Heinzmann A, Brüggenolte E, Forster J, Kuehr J: **An Mse I RELP in the human CTLA-4 promotor.** *Biochem Biophys Res Commun* 1996, **225**:817–818.
18. Skórka A: **Cukrzyca typu 1 – aspekty genetyczne. Klinika Pediatryczna.** *Szkoła Pediatrii* 2009, **12**:5131–5134.
19. Eschler DC, Hasham A, Tomer Y: **Cutting edge: the etiology of autoimmune thyroid diseases.** *Clin Rev Allerg Immunol* 2011, **41**:190–197.
20. Yu X, Sun JP, He Y, Guo X, Liu S, Zhou B, Hudmon A, Zhang ZY: **Structure, inhibitor, and regulatory mechanism of Lyp, a lymphoid-specific tyrosine phosphatase implicated in autoimmune diseases.** *Proc Natl Acad Sci USA* 2007, **104**:19767–19772.
21. Krupińska J, Wawrzynowicz-Syczewska M, Urbanowicz W, Pobłocki J, Syrenicz A: **The influence of interferon alpha on the induction of autoimmune thyroiditis in patients treated for chronic viral hepatitis type C.** *Endokrynol Pol* 2011, **62**:517–522.
22. Wojewoda E: **Czynniki genetyczne w patogenezie i współwystępowaniu chorób autoimmunologicznych, ze szczególnym uwzględnieniem chorób reumatycznych wieku dziecięcego.** *Reumatologia* 2009, **47**:39–43.
23. Pastuszak-Lewandowska D, Sewerynek E, Domańska D, Gładyś A, Skrzypczak R, Brzezińska E: **Basic research CTLA-4 gene polymorphism and their influence on predisposition to autoimmune thyroid diseases (Graves' disease and Hashimoto's thyroiditis).** *Arch Med Sci* 2012, **3**:415–421.
24. Kucharska AM, Rogozińska I, Pyrżak B, Miszkurka G, Wiśniewska A: **Polimorfizm A/G w pozycji 49 eksonu 1 genu CTLA-4 u dzieci z cukrzycą typu 1 – doniesienie wstepne.** *Endokrynologia Pediatryczna* 2009, **8**:27–32.
25. Zalatel K: **Determinants of thyroid autoantibody production in Hashimoto's thyroiditis.** *Expert Rev Clin Immunol* 2007, **3**:217–222.
26. Bicek A, Zaletel K, Gaberscek S, Pirnat E, Krhin B, Stopar TG, Hojker S: **49A/G and CT60 polymorphisms of the cytotoxic T-lymphocyte-associated antigen 4 gene associated with autoimmune thyroid disease.** *Hum Immunol* 2009, **70**:820–824.
27. Kula D, Stęchły D, Jurecka-Lubieniecka B, Hasse-Lazar K, Krawczyk A, Szpak S, Jarząb M, Pawelczak A, Gubała E: **Predyspozycja genetyczna do choroby Hashimoto w populacji polskiej:związek z polimorfizmem genów TNF i CTLA-4.** *Endokrynol Pol* 2003, **54**:495–496.
28. Kinjo Y, Takasu N, Komiya I, Tomoyose T, Takara M, Kouki T, Shimajiri Y, Yabiku K, Yoshimura H: **Remission of Graves hyperthyroidism and A/G polymorphism at position 49 in exon 1 of cytotoxic T lymphocyte-associated molecule-4 gene.** *J Clin Endocrinol Metab* 2002, **87**:2593–2596.
29. Roycroft M, Fichna M, McDonald D, Owen K, Zurawek M, Gryczyńska M, Januszkiewicz-Lewandowska D, Fichna P, Cordell H, Donaldson P, Nowak J, Pearce S: **The tryptophan 620 allele of the lymphoid tyrosine phosphatase (PTPN22) gene predisposes to autoimmue Addison's disease.** *Clin Endocrinol (Oxf)* 2009, **70**:358–362.
30. Petrone A, Giorgi G, Galgani A, Alemanno I, Corsello SM, Signore A, Di Mario U, Nisticò L, Cascino I, Buzzetti R: **CT60 single nucleotide polymorphism of the cytotoxic T-lymphocyte-associated antigen-4 gene region is associated with Graves' disease in an Italian population.** *Thyroid* 2005, **15**:232–238.
31. Ban Y, Tozaki T, Taniyama M, Tomita M, Ban Y: **Association of a CTLA-4 3' untranslated region (CT60) single nucleotide polymorphism with autoimmune thyroid disease in the Japanese population.** *Autoimmunity* 2005, **38**:151–153.
32. Chopra IJ, Hershman JM, William M, Pardridge WM, Nicoloff JT: **Thyroid function in nonthyroidal illnesses.** *Ann Intern Med* 1983, **98**:946–957.
33. Witas HW, Różalski M, Młynarski W, Sychowski R, Bodalski J: **Polymorphism of CTLA-4 gene in Polish population.** *Przegl Pediatr* 1997, **27**:246–248.

4

Thyroid heterogeneity, as indicated by the CV of ultrasonographic intensities, correlates with anti-thyroid peroxidase antibodies in euthyroid Hashimoto's thyroiditis

Yosuke Wakita, Toshiki Nagasaki*, Yuki Nagata, Yasuo Imanishi, Shinsuke Yamada, Koichiro Yoda, Masanori Emoto, Eiji Ishimura and Masaaki Inaba

Abstract

Objective: To prospectively evaluate the heterogeneous appearance of the thyroid gland, reflecting inflammation and destruction in euthyroid Hashimoto's thyroiditis (HT), we investigated the clinical utilities of the heterogeneity index (HI) [the coefficient of variance (CV) of the ultrasonographic (US) intensities], focusing on anti-thyroid peroxidase antibodies (TPO-Ab), which represent not only disease activity but also subsequent thyroid destruction of HT.

Methods: Forty-four consecutive patients with euthyroid HT [60.5 ± 2.7 years old (mean ± SE)] and 30 age-matched normal controls were studied. HI was calculated as the CV (SD/mean) of US intensities of either four points per lobe of the thyroid gland along a horizontal line at the depth of the right common carotid artery. Evaluation included serum levels of free thyroxine (FT4), free triiodothyronine (FT3), thyroid stimulating hormone (TSH), anti-thyroid peroxidase antibodies (TPO-Ab), anti-thyroglobulin antibodies (Tg-Ab), thyroglobulin and thyroid volume.

Results: While no differences were observed for TSH, FT_4 and FT_3, thyroglobulin and thyroid volume between the two groups, HI exhibited a tendency towards a significant difference (3.59 ± 0.20% in HT patients *vs* 3.23 ± 0.19% in normal group, $p = 0.089$). In HT patients, there was a significant and positive correlation of HI with TPO-Ab ($r = 0.396$, $p = 0.034$), whereas such a correlation was absent in normal controls. In both groups, there were no significant correlations of HI with Tg-Ab, FT_3, FT_4 or TSH.

Conclusions: This is the first report of the close relation between heterogeneity of US of the thyroid gland and TPO-Ab in euthyroid HT patients before the heterogeneity becomes distinguishable from normal thyroid glands. Furthermore, at this stage, subsequent thyroid destruction in HT might be already be predicted through the heterogeniety of the thyroid tissue.

Keywords: Hashimoto's thyroiditis, Heterogeneity, Ultrasonography, Anti-thyroid peroxidase antibodies

Introduction

Ultrasonographic (US) examination is a very accurate and highly sensitive method for assessing thyroid gland lesions, especially thyroid nodules, that can be performed quickly even in out-patient clinics [1]. Nevertheless, few studies have reported the use of US to estimate inflammation and destruction of thyroid parenchymal tissue. While hypoechogenicity has been reported in untreated and levothyroxine-treated overt hypothyroid Hashimoto's thyroiditis (HT) patients [2,3], the clinical utility of measuring US intensities remains unknown in euthyroid HT without apparent hypoechogenicity.

In the current report, we used a newly-designed sensitive US method that was able to distinguish from the hypoechogenicity [2,3] and enabled to assess and quantify heterogeneity in the euthyroid state, as the heterogeneity index (HI) [CV of the US intensities of eight points of thyroid gland on horizontal line between bilateral common

* Correspondence: toshi-n@jg7.so-net.ne.jp
Department of Metabolism, Endocrinology and Molecular Medicine, Osaka City University Graduate School of Medicine, 1-4-3, Asahi-machi, Abeno-ku, Osaka-city 545-8585, Japan

carotid arteries]. This method was not affected by depth of the thyroid gland and weakening of ultrasound because it was based on the CV (SD/mean) of the US intensities along a horizontal line.

For patients with HT, a highly sensitive radioimmunoassay system for anti-thyroid antibodies [anti-thyroglobulin antibodies (Tg-Ab) and anti-thyroid peroxidase antibodies (TPO-Ab)] has proven to be essential for diagnosis [4]. In particular, TPO-Ab has been established to represent the current activity of HT and subsequent thyroid destruction, because the TPO-antigen is closely involved with cell-mediated cytotoxicity, whereas the Tg-Ab is not [5].

Therefore, we investigated the clinical meaning of HI in euthyroid HT patients, and attempted to correlate HI with a variety of thyroid markers, such as thyroid hormones, thyroglobulin and thyroid volume, and autoimmune anti-thyroid antibodies.

Patients and methods

Subjects

The study was approved by the ethical review committee of Osaka City University Hospital. Written informed consent was obtained from each patient. Newly detected 56 HT patients in a euthyroid state (M/F, 10/40) were enrolled consecutively during the 7-month period from January to July, 2011.

The diagnosis of HT was made based on the elevation of either Tg-Ab or TPO-Ab above the normal upper limit. To confirm sustained euthyroidism, thus excluding patients with a temporary condition, i.e., during the recovery from painless thyroiditis or occult subacute thyroiditis, measurement of TSH was conducted at least twice over 6 months. Moreover, to avoid confounding factors known to affect thyroid hormones, patients who were pregnant or post-partum [6], patients receiving other hormone-replacement therapy or taking any drugs that could affect thyroid hormones, such as amiodarone hydrochloride, interferon and Interleukin-2, lithium carbonate, gonadotropin releasing hormone, raloxifene hydrochloride, anti-convulsion drugs, and rifampicin, and those with autoimmune antibodies, were excluded from the study [7,8].

Normal control subjects who joined the Health-Check Program at Osaka City University Hospital were enrolled consecutively as age-matched controls (M/F, 10/40). Normal controls had no history of thyroid disease, had neither goiter nor an autoimmune-antibody titer, and were in a euthyroid state.

The smoking index (the daily number of cigarettes multiplied by the number of years of smoking) was similar between the HT patients and normal controls and individual smoking habits did not change during this study.

Serum parameters

Blood was drawn just before ultrasonography after overnight fasting. Commercially available electrochemiluminescent immunoassay (ECLIA) kits were used for the thyroid hormone assay. TSH was measured by sandwich Elecsys®, and FT4 and FT3 levels were determined by competitive Elecsys® (Roche Diagnostics K.K., Tokyo, Japan) [9]. Anti-thyroglobulin (Cosmic Co., Tokyo, Japan) and anti-thyroid peroxidase antibodies (Cosmic Co., Tokyo, Japan) were also determined using highly-sensitive, commercially available, radioimmunoassay kits [10]. In this system, highly purified thyroglobulin and thyroid peroxidase were used as antigens. Serum concentrations of anti-thyroglobulin and anti-thyroid peroxidase antibodies greater than 0.4 and 0.3 U/ml, respectively, were considered positive. Serum thyroglobulin levels were measured using an ECLIA kit, Elecsys® (Roche Diagnostics K.K., Tokyo, Japan) [11].

Quantitative ultrasonographic measurements of heterogeneity index and thyroid volume

Thyroid HI was determined using an US apparatus (LOGIQ 7PRO, GE healthcare, Princeton, NJ, USA) with a 10-MHz linear array probe operating in B-mode (Figure 1). Four open-circle cursors (2 mm in diameter) per half lobe were positioned along a horizontal line at the depth of the right common carotid artery adjacent to the thyroid gland. US intensity within each circle was automatically calculated immediately after one cursor was set. HI was defined as the CV (SD/mean) of eight US intensities. All measurements were performed by the same examiner (Y.N.), who was blinded to the characteristics of the subjects.

Thyroid volume was also determined by ultrasonography, based on a calculation using an ellipsoid model (width × length × thickness × 0.7 for each lobe) [12].

Statistical analysis

Data are expressed as the mean ± SE unless otherwise indicated. Statistical analyses were performed using StatView (version 5.0, SAS Institute, Cary, NC). Differences in clinical factors between HT patients and normal controls were examined using the Mann–Whitney *U* test for assessment of the median values. The difference in the male/female ratio between the two groups was analyzed using the chi-square test. Simple regression analysis was used to examine the relationships between the two factors. *P*-values less than 0.05 were considered to be statistically significant.

Results

Clinical variables in normal controls and HT patients

A comparison of the variables between normal controls and HT patients is presented in Table 1. In addition to

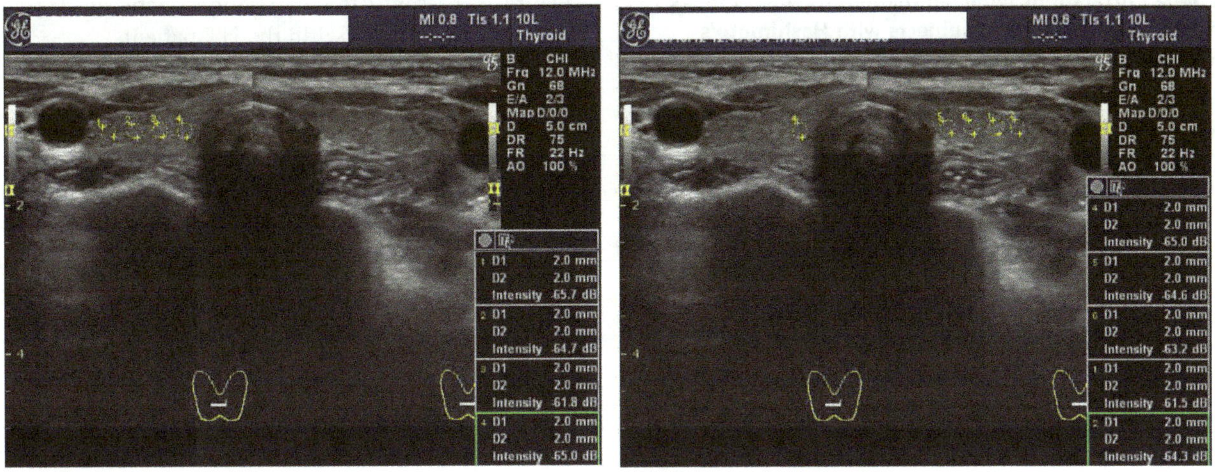

Figure 1 Recording of the ultrasonographic intensities and calculation of the thyroid heterogeneity index (HI). The appropriate sampling points were first determined for measuring. Four open-circle cursors (2 mm in diameter) per half lobe were positioned straight along a horizontal line at the depth of the right common carotid artery adjacent to the thyroid gland. US intensity within each circle was automatically calculated immediately after the cursor was set. HI was defined as the CV (i.e., SD/mean) of eight US intensities.

common biochemical markers, such as liver enzymes, renal function and lipid profiles, no significant differences were found in age, male/female ratio, BMI, smoking index, the serum level of TSH, FT_3 and FT_4, thyroglobulin, or thyroid volume between normal controls and HT patients (data not shown).

HI in normal controls and HT patients

As shown in Table 1, HI exhibited a tendency towards a significant difference between normal controls and HT patients (3.23 ± 0.19% in the normal group vs. 3.59 ± 0.20% in the HT patients, p = 0.089).

Correlations between HI and clinical variables in normal controls and HT patients

The correlations between HI and the clinical variables in normal controls and HT patients are presented in Table 2. In the HT patients there was a significant and positive correlation between HI and TPO-Ab (r = 0.396, p = 0.034) but not Tg-Ab (r = −0.014, p = 0.941) or TSH (r = −0.012, p = 0.953). In normal controls HI did not correlate with these factors. There were no significant correlations between HI and age, BMI, smoking index, serum level of FT_3, FT_4, thyroglobulin or thyroid volume in either group (data not shown).

Table 1 Baseline characteristics of the subjects with Hashimoto's thyroiditis and the controls

	Subjects with Hashimoto's thyroiditis	Normal controls	P
Number of subjects	44	44	
Gender (female/male)	32/12	32/12	ns
Age (years)	60.5 ± 2.7	58.7 ± 1.9	ns
Body mass index (kg/m^2)	21.7 ± 0.48	21.4 ± 0.58	ns
Smoking index	74 ± 59	67 ± 72	ns
Tg-Ab (U/ml) [<0.4]	8.37 ± 2.55	<0.4	
TPO-Ab (U/ml) [<0.3]	15.3 ± 6.13	<0.3	
FT_4 (pmol/l) [11.6-21.9]	14.5 ± 0.37	14.6 ± 0.57	ns
FT_3 (pmol/l) [3.54-6.16]	4.17 ± 0.11	3.95 ± 0.15	ns
TSH (mIU/l) [0.5-5]	2.40 ± 0.33	2.53 ± 0.28	ns
Thyroglobulin (mg/l) [0.0-30.0]	43.4 ± 20.6	40.6 ± 11.5	ns
Thyroid volume (mm^3)	14687.1 ± 1494.3	15757.2 ± 1984.4	ns
HI (%)	3.23 ± 0.19	3.59 ± 0.20	ns(0.089)

Data are expressed as the mean ± SE. The differences between two groups were examined using the Mann-Whitney *U* test for assessment of the medians.
ns: not significant, *Systolic BP*: systolic blood pressure, *Diastolic BP*: diastolic blood pressure, *Tg-Ab*; anti-thyroglobulin antibody, *TPO-Ab*; antithyroid peroxidase antibody, *HI*: heterogeneity index.

Table 2 Correlations between the heterogeneity index and other parameters in subjects with Hashimoto's thyroiditis and controls

	Subjects with Hashimoto's thyroiditis		Normal controls	
	r	P	r	P
Age (years)	0.077	ns	0.082	ns
Body mass index	0.253	ns	0.201	ns
Smoking index	0.292	ns	0.201	ns
Systolic BP	0.044	ns	0.153	ns
Diastolic BP	−0.045	ns	0.279	ns
Pulse rate	−0.143	ns	−0.017	ns
Tg-Ab	−0.014	ns		
TPO-Ab	0.396	0.034		
FT_4	−0.045	ns	0.188	ns
FT_3	−0.239	ns	−0.048	ns
TSH	−0.125	ns	−0.172	ns
Thyroglobulin	−0175	ns	−0.204	ns
Thyroid volume	0.264	ns	0. 175	ns

Data are expressed as the mean ± SE. Simple regression analysis was used. ns: not significant, Systolic *BP*: systolic blood pressure, Diastolic *BP*: diastolic blood pressure, *Tg-Ab*; anti-thyroglobulin antibody, *TPO-Ab*; antithyroid peroxidase antibody, *HI*: heterogeneity index.

Figure 2 presents the correlations between HI and TPO-Ab, Tg-Ab and TSH in the HT patients.

Discussion

The results of the study revealed a significant and positive correlation between HI and TPO-Ab in euthyroid HT patients. In these patients, HI might reflect not only the extent of current inflammation and destruction of the thyroid tissue, but also subsequent destruction in HT, because TPO-Ab is responsible for these changes through an autoimmune reaction in HT [5]. However, in the cases with very mild destruction, this correlation likely suggests the subsequent potential for terminal destruction.

TPO, originally described as thyroid microsomal antigen, is present on the apical surface of thyroid follicular cells and is the antigen most closely involved in cell-mediated cytotoxicity [13]. Hence, among auto-immune antibodies specific for the thyroid gland, the TPO-Ab titer represents the degree of lymphocytic infiltration of the thyroid gland, reflecting the current activity of HT, as well as subsequent stages in the development of HT [5,13].

Nevertheless, since only a tendency of HI was found between HT patients and normal controls (Table 1), inflammation and destruction of the thyroid tissue would likely be slight or mild in the early phase of HT, namely the euthyroid state. Therefore, the clinical interpretation of

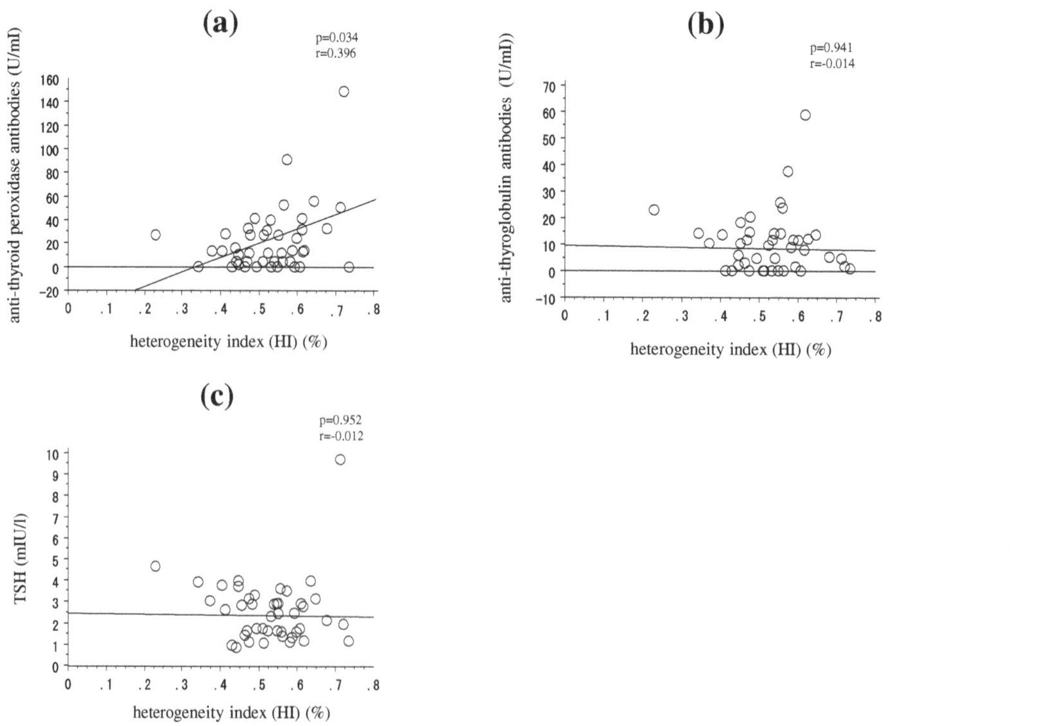

Figure 2 Simple regression analysis to determine the correlation of the heterogeneity index (HI) with anti-thyroid peroxidase antibody (TPO-Ab) (a), anti-thyroglobulin antibody (Tg-Ab) (b), and TSH (c) in Hashimoto's thyroiditis (HT). HI correlated significantly with TPO-Ab (r = 0.396, p = 0.034), but not with HI and Tg-Ab or TSH (r = −0.014, p = 0.941 and r = −0.012, p = 0.953, respectively).

HI might be not the degree of current inflammation and destruction but more likely a measure of the potential for terminal destruction of the thyroid gland that can be achieved in the early stages of HT.

In a previous report, an interaction between the HLA-DRB4 and cytotoxic T-lymphocyte associated antigen 4 (CTLA-4) genes was shown to determine the thyroid function of TPO-positive Japanese HT patients with goiter [13]. This is consistent with our findings, supporting that terminal destruction of thyroid gland is genetically predisposed.

Meanwhile, Tg-Ab, another auto-immune anti-thyroid antibody [4], did not correlate with HI in HT patients (Figure 2). Multiple antigen configurations of thyroglobulin are produced when it becomes iodinated, resulting in functionally active but immunologically distinct molecules [13]. Therefore, changes in Tg-Ab could occur independent of immune responses or the consequent inflammation and destruction in HT.

The lack of correlation of HI with FT_3, FT_4 and TSH in HT patients (Table 2) might be explained by similar degrees of heterogeneity and thyroid hormones between HT patients and normal controls. Thus, in the euthyroid state of early HT inflammation, the simultaneous destruction of thyroid tissue had not progressed sufficiently to affect these factors. If measured in a stage of overt hypothyroidism, a correlation might be observed between HI and thyroid hormones, as was reported previously, with respect to hypoechogenicity in HT [2,3]. This is the subject of ongoing and future investigations by our group.

Serum thyroglobulin did not correlate with HI in this study (Table 2). Possible explanations for this are as follows: although thyroglobulin is intimately associated with the thyroid, it is a normal component of the blood, as some thyroglobulin is invariably secreted, during normal thyroid hormone release [14]. Therefore, the elevation of serum thyroglobulin in HT could be due to increased leak in response to TSH stimulation or the excessive production by the associated cancer. Moreover, problems include variable sensitivity and reproducibility of the assays and interference by thyroglobulin autoantibodies [15]. Hence, in the euthyroid state the existence of Tg-Ab thyroglobulin may be of less clinical importance.

HI did not correlate with thyroid volume (Table 2), likely due to the same reason of the early stage of HT; i.e., in the presence of a very mild inflammation and early destruction of thyroid tissue in the euthyroid state of HT, the changes in thyroid volume did not reach statistical significance. In another previous investigation of overt autoimmune hypothyroidism, thyroid volume correlated negatively with echogenicity [16].

HI is easily and reproducibly obtained using ultrasonography, and is not affected by the depth of the thyroid gland and weakening of ultrasound, because it represents the CV (SD/mean) of US intensities along a horizontal line.

Thus, computerized grey-scale analysis using US was previously reported to be useful in quantifying thyroid hypoechogenicity in untreated and levothyroxine-treated overt hypothyroid HT patients [7]. The marked difference from our method is not in the assessment of heterogeneity but in the quantification of hypoechogenicity, which would be affected by the depth of the thyroid gland and weakening of the ultrasound. Furthermore, while their subjects included untreated and levothyroxine-treated overt hypothyroid HT patients, our method was applied to euthyroid and subclinical hypothyroid patients with visually indistinguishable heterogeneity.

Further, computerized grey-scale analysis allows for significant correlations between hypoechogenicity and indices of the thyroid gland, namely serum TSH, FT4 and TPO-Ab values. Interestingly, even in overt hypothyroidism echogenicity did not correlate with Tg-Ab, but rather correlated with TPO-Ab, possibly due to the same underlying reasons noted above.

One limitation of HI is obstruction by the tumor or cyst along the horizontal line for sampling, which interferes with positioning of the four open-circle cursors for each half lobe. Another limitation occurs when the thyroid gland is too small or atrophic, and cursors cannot be positioned properly. Since each open-circle is 2 mm in diameter, a straight line more than 8 mm in length is needed for each lobe.

In summary, our results demonstrate the close relation between heterogeneity of the thyroid gland and TPO-Ab in euthyroid and subclinical hypothyroid patients with Hashimoto's thyroiditis. It was suggested that even in such hormonal states, without distinguishable inflammation or destruction of thyroid tissue compared with normal subjects, subsequent thyroid destruction of HT might already be indicated through heterogeniety of the thyroid tissue.

Competing interests

We declare that there is no competing interests that could be perceived as prejudicing the impartiality of the research reported.

Authors' contributions

YW carried out the ultrasonographic measurements and analyzed the data. TN drafted the protocol and manuscript, analyzed the data. YN assisted ultrasonographic measurements and analysis of the data. YI, SY, KY, ME, EI and MI participated in the logical composition of manuscript. All authors read and approved the final manuscript.

Acknowledgement

This research project was not supported by any specific grant from any funding agency in the public, commercial or not-for-profit sectors.

References

1. Ross DS: **Nonpalpable thyroid nodules: managing an epidemic.** *J Clin Endocrinol Metab* 2002, **87**:1938–1940.
2. Mazziotti G, Sorvillo F, Iorio S, Carbone A, Romeo A, Piscopo M, Capuano S, Capuano E, Amato G, Carella C: **Grey-scale analysis allows a quantitative evaluation of thyroid echogenicity in the patients with Hashimoto's thyroiditis.** *Clin Endocrinol (Oxf)* 2003, **59**:223–229.
3. Schiemann U, Avenhaus W, Konturek JW, Gellner R, Hengst K, Gross M: **Relationship of clinical features and laboratory parameters to thyroid echogenicity measured by standardized grey scale ultrasonography in patients with Hashimoto's thyroiditis.** *Med Sci Monit* 2003, **9**:13–17.
4. Engler H, Riesen WF, Keller B: **Anti-thyroid peroxidase (anti-TPO) antibodies in thyroid diseases, non-thyroidal illness and controls. Clinical validity of a new commercial method for detection of anti-TPO (thyroid microsomal) autoantibodies.** *Clin Chim Acta* 1994, **225**:123–136.
5. Sinclair D: **Clinical and laboratory aspects of thyroid autoantibodies.** *Ann Clin Biochem* 2006, **43**:173–183.
6. Chiovato L, Lapi P, Fiore E, Tonacchera M, Pinchera A: **Thyroid autoimmunity and female gender.** *J Endocrinol Investig* 1993, **16**:384–391.
7. Bindra A, Braunstein GD: **Thyroiditis.** *Am Fam Physician* 2006, **15**:1769–1776.
8. Kasayama S, Miyake S, Samejima Y: **Transient thyrotoxicosis and hypothyroidism following administration of the GnRH agonist leuprolide acetate.** *Endocr J* 2000, **47**:83–785.
9. Kulmala S, Suomi J: **Current status of modernanalytical luminescence methods.** *Anal Chim Acta* 2003, **500**:21–69.
10. Arai T, Kurashima C, Utsuyama M, Sawabe M, Ito H: **Measurement of anti-thyroglobulin and anti-thyroid peroxidase antibodies using highly sensitive radioimmunoassay: an effective method for detecting asymptomatic focal lymphocytic thyroiditis in the elderly.** *Endocr J* 2000, **47**:575–582.
11. Algeciras-Schimnich A, Lasho MA, Ness KM, Cheryk LA, Grebe SK: **The Roche elecsys and Siemens-centaur thyroglobulin autoantibody assays show comparable clinical performance to the recently unavailable Beckman-coulter access thyroglobulin autoantibody assay in identifying samples with potentially false-low thyroglobulin measurements due to thyroglobulin autoantibody interference.** *Thyroid* 2011, **21**:813–814.
12. Urakami Y, Takamatsu J, Sakane S, Kuma K, Ohsawa N: **Changes in thyroid volume in response to radioactive iodine for Graves' hyperthyroidism correlated with activity of thyroid-stimulating antibody and treatment outcome.** *J Clin Endocrinol Metab* 1996, **81**:3257–3260.
13. Terauchi M, Yanagawa T, Ishikawa N, Ito K, Fukazawa T, Maruyama H, Saruta T: **Interactions of HLA-DRB4 and CTLA-4 genes influence thyroid function in Hashimoto's thyroiditis in Japanese population.** *J Endocrinol Invest* 2003, **26**:1208–1212.
14. Lerman J: **Iodine components of the blood. Circulating thyroglobulin in normal persons and in persons with thyroid disease.** *J Clin Invest* 1940, **19**:555–560.
15. Pacini F, Pinchera A: **Serum and tissue thyroglobulin measurement: clinical applications in thyroid disease.** *Biochimie* 1999, **81**:463–467.
16. Carlé A, Pedersen IB, Knudsen N, Perrild H, Ovesen L, Jørgensen T, Laurberg P: **Thyroid volume in hypothyroidism due to autoimmune disease follows a unimodal distribution: evidence against primary thyroid atrophy and autoimmune thyroiditis being distinct diseases.** *J Clin Endocrinol Metab* 2009, **94**:833–839.

5

TSH receptor antibodies have predictive value for breast cancer

Paweł Szychta[1,4], Wojciech Szychta[1,5], Adam Gesing[1], Andrzej Lewiński[2,3] and Małgorzata Karbownik-Lewińska[1,3*]

Abstract

Background: Associations between breast cancer and thyroid disorders are reported in numerous studies. Relationships between thyroperoxidase antibodies (TPOAb), thyroglobulin antibodies (TgAb) and breast cancer have been previously demonstrated. However, no analysis has been performed concerning an association between thyrotropin (TSH) receptor antibodies (TSHRAb) and breast cancer. The aim of the study was to evaluate the prevalence of breast cancer or benign breast tumors in patients with Graves' disease and to analyze a possible relationship between Graves' disease and these two groups of breast diseases with emphasis to epidemiology and laboratory findings.

Patients and methods: Clinical and laboratory details of 2003 women hospitalized for endocrine disorders were retrospectively analyzed, using an unpaired Student's *t*-test, logistic regression analysis, χ^2 test of independence or the two-sided ratio comparison test.

Results: The coexistence of Graves' disease and breast cancer was statistically significant. We observed TSHRAb and TgAb more frequently in patients with breast cancer. We found that TSHRAb is the only variable possessing predictive value for breast cancer.

Conclusions: The strong relationship between Graves' disease and breast cancer is proposed. We suggest that TSHRAb could be described as a positive determinant of breast cancer. The present data call attention to the usefulness of screening for breast cancer in long-term follow-up of patients with autoimmune thyroid disorders, especially of those with Graves' disease. Similarly, screening for autoimmune thyroid disorders should be performed in patients with nodular breast disease. Additionally, the article draws ideas for further research in order to develop targeted treatment for more successful outcome in patients with breast cancer.

Keywords: Breast cancer, Thyroid, Autoimmune disease, Graves' disease, TSH receptor antibody, TSH, Thyroglobulin antibody, Thyroperoxidase antibody

Introduction

Breast cancer is a hormone dependent malignancy. Thyroid hormone receptors affect both the normal breast cell differentiation and breast cancer cell proliferation, with effects of thyroid hormones similar to those caused by estrogens [1,2]. Relationship between thyroid diseases, such as nodular hyperplasia, hyperthyroidism and thyroid cancer, with breast cancer was demonstrated in several studies [3-6]. However, ambiguous results concerning the above association have been recently summarized [7]. In contrast, hypothyroidism due to Hashimoto's thyroiditis was documented as a protective factor against breast cancer [8-10], but also this observation was not confirmed in other sources [11].

Graves' disease, one of the thyroid autoimmune diseases, is characterized – in its typical form – by hyperthyroidism with laboratory results of decreased thyrotropin (TSH) level, increased free thyroxine (FT_4) and/or free triiodothyronine (FT_3) levels, detectable TSH receptor (TSHR) stimulating antibodies (TSHRAb), usually positive thyroid peroxidase antibodies (TPOAb) and thyroglobulin antibodies (TgAb) [12]. An exclusive diagnostic feature of Graves' disease is the presence of TSHRAb. The ligand

* Correspondence: MKarbownik@hotmail.com
[1]Department of Oncological Endocrinology, Medical University of Lodz, 7/9 Zeligowski St., 90-752, Lodz, Poland
[3]Department of Endocrinology and Metabolic Diseases, Polish Mother's Memorial Hospital, Research Institute, Lodz, Poland
Full list of author information is available at the end of the article

for TSHRAb, i.e. TSHR, is also present in breast cancer tissue [13].

Only limited aspects of potential association between Graves' disease and breast cancer have been postulated [14,15], whereas the exact mechanism has not been identified [16]. Genetic, environmental and molecular pathways of both female predominant diseases have been described, and integrated analysis of the above entities provides opportunity to identify the potential relevant common etiological mechanisms [17]. The potential relationship between antithyroid autoantibodies and breast cancer has not been clearly documented, as the elevated serum levels of TPOAb and TgAb in patients with breast cancer, detected in some studies [18-21], have not been confirmed elsewhere [22,23]. Moreover, no conclusive research has been undertaken concerning significance of TSHRAb in patients with breast cancer [24].

The aim of the study was to evaluate the prevalence of breast cancer or benign breast tumors in patients with Graves' disease and to analyze a possible relationship between Graves' disease and these two groups of breast diseases with emphasis to epidemiology and laboratory findings.

Patients and methods

Retrospective clinical details of 2003 women, who were hospitalized for endocrine disorders in the Department of Endocrinology and Metabolic Diseases at the Polish Mother's Memorial Hospital – Research Institute in Lodz within a 3-year period between 2002 and 2005, were retrieved from the hospital records following the internal audit approval. Inclusion criteria were female adults. Exclusion criteria were all oncological conditions other than breast neoplasia and thyroid disorders other than Graves' disease, such as nodular goiter, thyroid cancer, autoimmune thyroiditis (AIT), etc.

After exclusion, 1686 women aged 36.48 ± 15.95 years were enrolled to the study (Table 1). Two studied groups consisted of 47 patients with benign breast tumors (BBT), aged 46.27 ± 14.18 years and 9 patients with breast cancer (BC), aged 54.55 ± 9.60 years. Therefore, 1630 women hospitalized for several non-oncological diseases and without thyroid diseases other than Graves' disease (polycystic ovary syndrome, primary infertility, osteopenia, osteoporosis, obesity, dwarfism, anorexia, atherosclerosis, cardiomyopathy, dyslipidemia, hirsutism, hypertension, ischemic heart disease, gastric ulcer, metabolic syndrome or diabetes of any type) were considered as a control group (C) with an average age of 36.10 ± 15.89 years.

Because of the relatively high age range of women with breast cancer and to analyze the cause-effect relation, age-matched groups of patients and healthy women could not be investigated in all stages of the analysis. Therefore, the predictors of breast cancer were analyzed in the age-matched group of 499 patients, including 9 patients with BC aged 54.55 ± 9.60 years and 490 control individuals (C) aged 53.86 ± 8.88 years ($p > 0.05$).

The following parameters were recorded with the use of the data analysis program, designed by one of co-authors of the study (P.S.): age and laboratory parameters, i.e. TSH, FT_4, FT_3, TSHRAb, TgAb and TPOAb. The following diagnoses were considered: Graves' disease, benign breast tumors (BBT) and breast cancer (BC). The normal ranges of the laboratory tests in our hospital are: TSH (0.27–4.2 mIU/L), FT_4 (0.93–1.7 ng/dL), FT_3 (1.8–4.6 pg/mL), TPOAb (<35 IU/mL), TgAb (<115 IU/mL) and TSHRAb (<1.8 IU/mL).

The data were statistically analyzed using an unpaired Student's *t*-test – for continuous variables. The two-sided ratio comparison test was used to evaluate the frequency of events. Univariate logistic regression analysis, followed by multivariate logistic regression analysis, was used to determine which continuous variable might have predicted breast cancer or benign breast tumors. The $\chi 2$ test of independence was used to determine, which dichotomized variable might have predicted breast cancer or benign breast tumors. The results are presented as mean ± standard deviation (SD). Statistical significance was determined at the level of $p < 0.05$.

Results

Statistically significant differences were found in age distribution between patients with breast cancer (BC) and control group (C), as well as between women with benign breast tumors (BBT) and control group (C) (Table 1). However, there were no statistical differences

Table 1 Clinical characteristics of patients with breast cancer, benign breast tumors, Graves' disease and in controls

Parameter	Clinical characteristics				Statistical analysis		
	BC	BBT	C	All patients	p (BC vs. BBT)	p (BC vs. C)	p (BBT vs. C)
Patients – No (%)	9 (0.53%)	47 (2.78%)	1630 (96.6%)	1686 (100%)	ns	<0.0001	<0.0001
Age – yr (mean ± SD)	54.55 ± 9.60	46.27 ± 14.18	36.10 ± 15.89	36.48 ± 15.95	ns	0.0005	<0.0001
Graves' disease – No (%)	3 (33.3%)	6 (12.7%)	111 (6.8%)	120 (7.1%)	ns	0.0025	ns

Clinical characteristics of patients with breast cancer (BC), patients with benign breast tumors (BBT) and controls (C) and the occurrence of Graves' disease. Statistical evaluation was done by an unpaired Student's *t*-test (for age) or by the two-sided ratio comparison test (for no. of patients and for Graves' disease occurrence); ns, non-significant.

Table 2 Graves' disease as the dichotomized determinant of breast cancer or benign breast tumors

Dichotomized determinant	Association with BC (n = 9)		Association with BBT (n = 47)	
	χ^2	p	χ^2	p
Graves' disease (n = 120)	9.41	0.0021	2.33	ns

χ^2 test of independence analysis of the dichotomized determinant (i.e. Graves' disease occurrence) of breast cancer (BC) or of benign breast tumors (BBT), performed in all patients; ns, non-significant in all patients.

in age distribution between patients with benign breast tumors (BBT) and patients with breast cancer (BC).

Graves' disease was diagnosed on the basis of clinical findings and the presence of TSHRAb in 120 (7.11%) female patients aged 41.65 ± 15.19 years. Graves' disease coexisted more frequently with breast cancer ($p = 0.0021$), but not with benign breast tumors ($p > 0.05$) (Table 2).

In breast cancer patients, the mean values for TSH were 1.724 ± 3.629 mU/L and they did not differ significantly from those in controls (2.12 ± 5.41 mU/L) and from those in patients with benign breast tumors (1.35 ± 0.89 mU/L) (Figure 1). In turn, FT_4 was 1.283 ± 0.427 ng/dL in patients with breast cancer and did not differ significantly from levels found either in controls (1.34 ± 1.93 ng/dL) or in women with benign breast tumors (1.30 ± 0.67 ng/dL). In patients with breast cancer, FT_3 was 2.882 ± 1.617 pg/mL and was similar to controls (3.33 ± 1.91 pg/mL) and to patients with benign breast tumors (3.54 ± 1.65 pg/mL).

When levels of thyroid antibodies were compared among three groups of patients, the following differences were found. The mean values of serum TSHRAb were 25.65 ± 20.29 IU/ml in breast cancer patients, they were significantly lower in controls (4.83 ± 8.19 IU/ml, $p = 0.0006$), and were lower in patients with benign breast tumors (8.52 ± 14.04 IU/ml), but the differences between BC and BBT or between BBT and controls did not reach statistical significance (Figure 2). Serum concentrations of TgAb in patients with breast cancer were 1120.8 ± 1914.9 IU/ml and were considerably higher than in controls (241.4 ± 565.0 IU/ml, $p = 0.0100$) and markedly higher than in patients with benign breast tumors (191.7 ± 267.1 IU/ml, $p = 0.0443$) (Figure 3). In turn, TPOAb in patients with breast cancer were at level of 157.8 ± 294.8 IU/ml and were similar to control group (135.7 ± 206.0 IU/ml, $p > 0.05$) and to benign breast tumors (178.9 ± 221.9, $p > 0.05$).

Several parameters, such as hormones and antibodies concentrations were submitted to a univariate and a multivariate logistic regression model. The purpose of the model was to determine which of those continuous variables might predict breast cancer or benign breast tumors either in the entire group of female patients or in age-matched groups. No predictive value for any of the examined hormones and for TPOAb was documented at univariate regression analysis in the entire group of patients (Table 3). In opposite, breast cancer predictive value for TSHRAb (OR = 1.10, 95% CI = 1.01-1.20, $p = 0.0222$) and TgAb (OR = 1.00, 95% CI = 1.00-1.01, $p = 0.0377$) was found at univariate regression analysis in the entire group of patients. Thus, TSHRAb and TgAb could be theoretically considered as positive risk factors for breast cancer. However, both above determinants lost their predictive value at multivariate analysis. In turn, meticulous logistic regression analysis, based on the age-matched

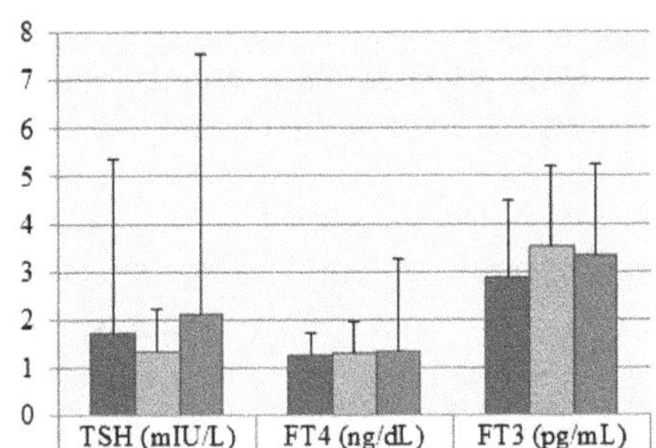

	TSH (mIU/L)	FT4 (ng/dL)	FT3 (pg/mL)
BC vs. C (p)	ns	ns	ns
BBT vs. C (p)	ns	ns	ns
BC vs. BBT (p)	ns	ns	ns

■ Breast cancer ■ Benign breast tumor ■ Controls

Figure 1 Levels of hormones in patients with breast cancer, with benign breast tumors and in controls. Levels of hormones in: patients with breast cancer (BC), patients with benign breast tumors (BBT) or controls (C), expressed as mean ± SD; Statistical analysis with Student's unpaired *t*-test; ns, non-significant.

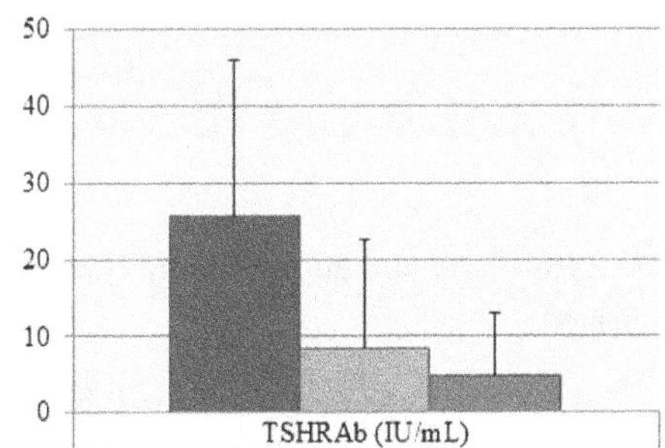

	TSHRAb (IU/mL)
BC vs. C (p)	0.0006
BBT vs. C (p)	ns
BC vs. BBT (p)	ns

■ Breast cancer ■ Benign breast tumor ■ Controls

Figure 2 Levels of TSHRAb in patients with breast cancer, with benign breast tumors and in controls. Levels of TSHRAb in: patients with breast cancer (BC), patients with benign breast tumors (BBT) or controls (C), expressed as mean ± SD; Statistical analysis with Student's unpaired *t*-test; ns, non-significant.

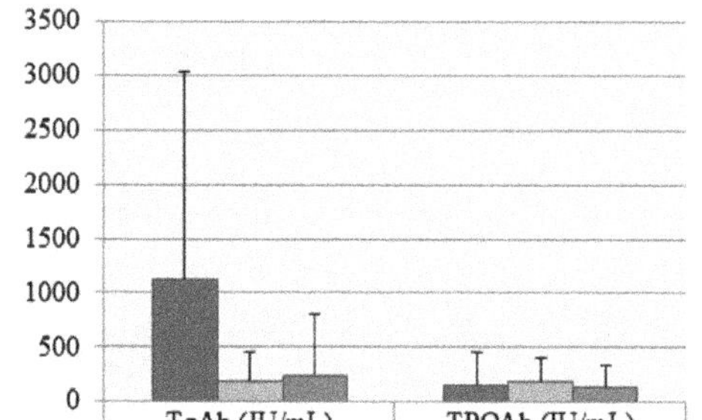

	TgAb (IU/mL)	TPOAb (IU/mL)
BC vs. C (p)	0.01	ns
BBT vs. C (p)	ns	ns
BC vs. BBT (p)	0.0443	ns

■ Breast cancer ■ Benign breast tumor ■ Controls

Figure 3 TgAb and TPOAb levels in patients with breast cancer, benign breast tumors and in controls. Levels of TgAb and TPOAb in: patients with breast cancer (BC), patients with benign breast tumors (BBT) or controls (C), expressed as mean ± SD; Statistical analysis with Student's unpaired *t*-test; ns, non-significant.

groups of patients with breast cancer and controls, revealed that TSHRAb is the only variable possessing predictive value for breast cancer (OR = 1.09, 95% CI = 1.00-1.20, p = 0.0368) (Table 4). No other predictors of breast cancer or benign breast tumors were documented in our series.

Distribution of breast tumors in relation to age intervals and in comparison to Graves' disease is presented in Figure 4. A shift between diagnosis of Graves' disease and breast cancer was observed. Peak incidence of Graves' disease was seen in patients at age of about 35 years and the lowest frequency was observed at age of about 45 years, whereas peak level of breast cancer diagnosis were noted at about 65 years, and the lowest frequency at about 75 years. In contrast, we observed no similar distribution trends in relation to age intervals between benign breast tumors and breast cancers or between benign breast tumors and Graves' disease.

Discussion

Mammary gland is derived from iodide-concentrating ectoderm [17]. Breast functions are similar to the thyroid gland in relation to the absorption capacity of iodide for use as a milk ingredient during lactation [4,25]. Altered thyroid hormonal function due to abnormal iodine uptake has an impact on incidence of iodine deficiency disorders (IDD) [25], autoimmune diseases and could possibly affect cancer development. Increased intake of iodine is considered as a protective factor against the occurrence of breast cancer [26]. In conformity, low levels of iodine were described in the breast cancer tissues as compared to normal breast tissue or benign breast tumors [27].

Uptake of serum iodide into the breast alveolar and ductular cells happens in the mechanism of active transport via the glycoprotein – Na+/I-symporter (NIS) [28]. The expression of NIS occurs in 80% to 90% of breast cancer cases and, thus, symporter could be potentially used in the radioisotope breast imaging with ^{125}I (alternatively ^{99}mTc) and in the breast cancer treatment with ^{131}I (alternatively ^{188}Re) [13], following administration of stimulants enhancing NIS expression [29,30].

Assessment of hormonal thyroid function in breast cancer patients was assessed in our study with measurement of TSH, FT_4 and FT_3 levels and we found no differences among breast cancer patients, women with benign breast tumors and female controls. However, limited short-term hormone observations cannot be interpreted in relation to the long-term cancer development because of the changeable thyroid activity affected by several extrinsic and intrinsic factors. In turn, concerning the impact of autoimmune diseases on breast cancer incidence, we confirmed the high prevalence of breast cancer in patients with Graves' disease (Table 2).

Thyroid antibodies in the autoimmune thyroid disorders could interact with the receptors on breast tumors and thus they were previously designated as precursors for the coincidence of mammary and thyroid disorders [31]. Autoantigens, TPO in the thyroid and lactoperoxidases in

Table 3 Hormone and autoantibody concentrations as determinants of breast cancer or benign breast tumors

Parameter	Association with BC (n = 9)						Association with BBT (n = 47)		
	Univariate logistic regression			Multivariate logistic regression			Univariate logistic regression		
	OR	95% CI	p	OR	95% CI	p	OR	95% CI	p
TSH (mIU/L)	0.97	0.75-1.26	ns		-		1.20	0.92-1.55	ns
FT_4 (ng/dL)	0.96	0.42-2.21	ns				1.01	0.78-1.31	ns
FT_3 (pg/mL)	0.48	0.71-1.82	ns				0.95	0.81-1.11	ns
TSHRAb (IU/mL)	1.10	1.01-1.20	0.0222	0.92	0.66-1.28	ns	0.97	0.91-1.03	ns
TgAb (IU/mL)	1.00	1.00-1.01	0.0377	0.99	0.99-1.00	ns	1.00	0.99-1.00	ns
TPOAb (IU/mL)	1.00	0.99-1.01	ns		-		1.00	0.99-1.00	ns

Univariate and multivariate logistic regression analysis of the univariate determinants (such as hormone and autoantibody concentrations) of breast cancer (BC) or breast benign tumor (BBT), performed in all patients (n = 1686); OR, odds ratio; CI, confidence interval; ns, non-significant.

Table 4 Hormone and autoantibody concentrations as breast cancer or benign breast tumors determinants, in age-matched groups

Parameter	Association with BC (n = 9)		
	OR	95% CI	p
TSH (mIU/L)	0.96	0.77-1.21	ns
FT_4 (ng/dL)	0.92	0.32-2.67	ns
FT_3 (pg/mL)	0.69	0.29-1.62	ns
TSHRAb (IU/mL)	1.09	1.00-1.20	0.0368
TgAb (IU/mL)	1.00	0.99-1.00	ns
TPOAb (IU/mL)	0.99	0.99-1.00	ns

Univariate logistic regression analysis of the univariate determinants (such as hormone and autoantibody concentrations) of breast cancer (BC) or breast benign tumor (BBT), performed in the age-matched groups of patients (n = 499); OR, odds ratio; CI, confidence interval; ns, non-significant.

the breast, are required for organification of iodine to produce iodoproteins [32], as they catalyze H_2O_2 production to oxidize I^- [33]. Previously reported potential association between TPOAb or TgAb and breast cancer was arguable and the results were summarized in Table 5 [4,18,34-36]. The presence of TPOAb was previously described as a prognostic index of a more favorable outcome in patients with breast cancer, with similar importance to the tumor size and to the axillary nodal status [37]. In our study, TPOAb levels were similar among the three analyzed groups. In turn, TgAb levels were higher in our series in patients with breast cancer comparing to controls and to patients with benign breast tumors. However, the ligand for TgAb, thyroglobulin (Tg), has antigenicity affected by the iodine content within the protein [18,38], and thus TgAb are present non-specifically in different diseases coexisting with the altered iodine intake [39]. More importantly, TgAb can be also found in patients with chronic disorders not involving thyroid [40] or even in healthy patients without any thyroid disease [41]. Thus, clinical impact of the elevated concentrations of TgAb is unreliable, as they were detected non-specifically to thyroid diseases or breast cancer.

Relationship between incidence of benign breast tumors and thyroid diseases with the increased levels of TgAb and TPOAb in serum has been also proposed [42]. Previous report documented the increased level of TPOAb in 28% of women with benign fibrocystic mastopathies and 80% had thyroid hypertrophy [21,43]. In contrary, we did not observe any association between Graves' disease, hormones or antibodies concentrations and occurrence of benign breast tumors.

Interaction between thyroid and breast cancer can occur in the mechanism involving TSHR, common in the adipose breast tissue [35]. Under physiological conditions, TSH via TSHR stimulates growth, differentiation and function of the thyroid cells [4,44]. This receptor is a target for THSRAb in Graves' disease. It should be stressed that TSHR expression is common in breast cancer, with higher prevalence in low-grade breast cancer [13]. The clinical significance of the serum TSHRAb in relation to breast cancer and Graves' disease was unresolved in the previous observations [6,15]. In our study, TSHRAb levels were significantly higher in breast cancer comparing to controls. They were positive determinants of breast cancer in the univariate logistic regression analysis, which did not reach statistical significance in multivariate logistic regression analysis. However, in the analysis of the age-matched groups of patients, TSHRAb was found to be the only positive determinant of breast cancer. Therefore, we suggest that TSHRAb can be called a positive predictor for the subsequent development of breast cancer. However,

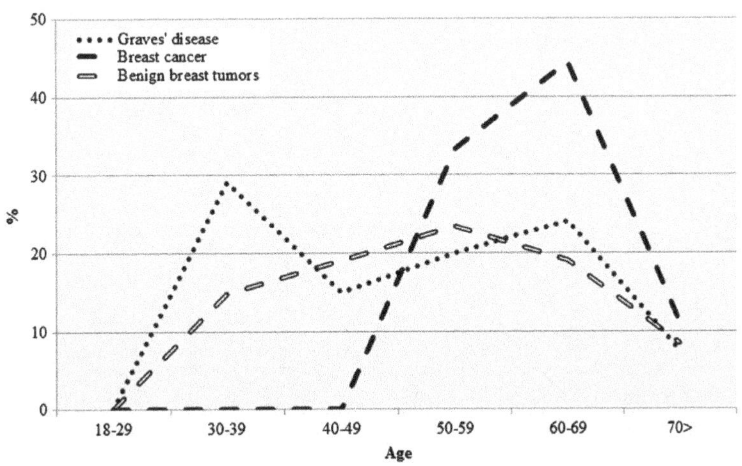

Figure 4 Trends in occurrence of breast cancer, benign breast tumors and Graves' disease. Distribution of breast cancer (BC) or benign breast tumors (BBT) in relation to age intervals and in comparison to Graves' disease, expressed as linear trends.

Table 5 Summarized previous reports concerning relationship between thyroid diseases and breast cancer or benign breast tumors

Parameter	[Previously reported data] (n = number of patients enrolled to study)														
	[3] (n = 150)			[18] (n = 115)			[34] (n = 61)			[35] (n = 175)			[36] (n = 48)		
	BC	C	p	BC	C	p	BC	C	p	BC	C	p	BC	C	p
n	150	100	-	66	49	-	36	100	-	100	75	-	26	22	-
Age-yr means ± SD (min-max)	63 (38–80)	age-matched	-	63.5 ± 11.8	68.4 ± 12.8	ns	52.8 ± 10.2	age-matched	-	63 (38–80)	-	-	(30–85)	age-matched	-
TSH	3.12 ± 1.40	1.46 ± 0.82	ns	1.77 (0.15-47.9)	1.52 (0.45-14.56)	ns	1.9 ± 0.7	1.8 ± 1.4	ns	4.12 ± 1.40	1.39 ± 0.79	**0.030**	1.36 ± 0.63	2.41 ± 0.35	<0.05
units	*μIU/ml*			*mIU/dl*			*μIU/ml*			*μIU/ml*			*μU/ml*		
FT_4	2.64 ± 0.91	1.42 ± 0.31	ns	15.70 (7.38-22.63)	15.19 (10.5-21.5)	ns	9.76 ± 2.73	9.9 ± 2.4	ns	2.93 ± 0.57	1.39 ± 0.21	**0.030**	1.40 ± 1.64	1.10 ± 0.83	<0.05
units	*ng/dl*			*pmol/dl*			*pg/ml*			*ng/dl*			*ng/dl*		
FT_3	8.47 ± 0.75	4.48 ± 0.75	ns	-			3.58 ± 0.7	3.2 ± 0.6	ns	7.25 ± 0. 75	3.42 ± 0.91	**0.030**	3.56 ± 3.14	2.87 ± 3.12	<0.001
units	*pmol/l*						*pg/ml*			*pmol/l*			*pmol/ml*		
TgAb	140.92 ± 21.52	27.75 ± 7.60	ns	35.80 (26.1-6000.0)	27.70 (18.5-298.0)	**<0.001**	12/36	12/100	**p < 0.01**	-			-		
units	*IU/ml*			*kIU/dl*			*Patients' ratio with positive TgAb*								
TPOAb	105.82 ± 21.46	23.08 ± 4.16	**0.030**	6.10 (6.1-871.0)	6.10 (6.1-1621.6)	ns	12/36	8/100	**p < 0.01**	104.57 ± 19.39-	24.81 ± 5.16	**0.030**	-		
units	*IU/ml*			*kIU/dl*			*Patients' ratio with positive TPOAb*			*IU/ml*					
Diagnosis	**BC**	**C**	**p**	**BC**	**C**	**p**				**-**					
Graves' disease	-			0/66	0/49	-									
AITD	57/150	17/100	**0.001**	16/66	8/49	-									

Summary of the previously reported endocrine and immunological laboratory status in patients with breast cancer (BC) and controls (C); ns, non-significant.

further prospective research is required on a larger group of patients to determine unquestionably the significance of the above association.

Consequently, neutral TSHR antagonists (ligands inhibiting receptor activation by agonists), such as NIDDK-CEB-52, NCGC00242595 and NCGC00229600, could play a potential role in the breast cancer prophylaxis, acting as precursors of drugs preventing from TSHRAb activation in patients with Graves' disease [45]. Monoclonal antibodies, currently used in experimental studies on the medical therapeutic intervention in Graves' disease by vaccination with chemically altered autoantigens, could selectively deplete specific T lymphocytes subsets and block the T-cell receptor MHC interaction [46]. Additionally, no reports were found assessing the theoretical suppressive effect of blocking subtype of TSHRAb (causing hypothyroidism) on breast cancer and thus such clinical research would be advisable.

As discussed above, reduced iodide concentration, elevated levels of the thyroid hormones and antibodies contributed to an increased risk of breast cancer in previous reports and in our study. However, some authors suggested also the possible impact of breast cancer on the thyroid with the resulting increased level of thyroid hormones and the autoimmune response with the detectable thyroid antibodies [5]. In our series we found shift of about 15–20 years between the primary peak of the diagnosed Graves' disease and the secondary maximal incidence of breast cancer (Figure 4). However, the observed long shift is partially affected by the fact that participants in our study were younger than the general population of patients with Graves' disease, as they were hospitalized due to the more prominent symptoms. Older patients with usually more subtle clinical course of Graves' disease are treated as outpatients [47]. Despite some possible level of bias, we claim that it is the Graves' disease which could contribute to the subsequently observed development of breast cancer.

In conclusion, the strong relationship between Graves' disease and breast cancer is proposed. We suggest that TSHRAb could be described as a positive determinant of breast cancer. The present data call attention to the usefulness of screening for breast cancer in long-term follow-up of patients with autoimmune thyroid disorders, especially of those with Graves' disease. Similarly, screening for autoimmune thyroid disorders should be performed in patients with nodular breast disease. Additionally, the article draws ideas for further research in order to develop targeted treatment for more successful outcome in patients with breast cancer.

Competing interests
The authors declare that they have no competing interests.

Authors' contributions
PS, WS, AL & MKL have made substantial contributions to conception and design of the study. PS and WS were involved in the acquisition of data. PS designed the data analysis program. All authors (PS, WS, AG, AL & MKL) performed analysis and interpretation of data. PS was involved in drafting the manuscript. MKL revised the draft critically for important intellectual content. AL & MKL supervised and guided all the steps of preparing the manuscript and gave final approval of the version to be published. All authors read and approved the final manuscript.

Acknowledgements
The study was supported by the statutory funds No. 503/1-107-03/503-01 and No. 503/1-107-05/503-01 from the Medical University of Lodz.

Author details
[1]Department of Oncological Endocrinology, Medical University of Lodz, 7/9 Zeligowski St., 90-752, Lodz, Poland. [2]Department of Endocrinology and Metabolic Diseases, Medical University of Lodz, Lodz, Poland. [3]Department of Endocrinology and Metabolic Diseases, Polish Mother's Memorial Hospital, Research Institute, Lodz, Poland. [4]Current address: Department of Oncological Surgery and Breast Diseases, Polish Mother's Memorial Hospital, Research Institute, Lodz, Poland. [5]Current address: 1st Department of Cardiology, Medical University of Warsaw, Warsaw, Poland.

References
1. Dinda S, Sanchez A, Moudgil V: **Estrogen-like effects of thyroid hormone on the regulation of tumor suppressor proteins, p53 and retinoblastoma, in breast cancer cells.** *Oncogene* 2002, **21**:761–768.
2. Conde I, Paniagua R, Zamora J, Blanquez MJ, Fraile B, Ruiz A, Arenas MI: **Influence of thyroid hormone receptors on breast cancer cell proliferation.** *Ann Oncol* 2006, **17**:60–64.
3. Turken O, Narln Y, Demlrbas S, Onde ME, Sayan O, Kandemlr EG, Yaylacl M, Ozturk A: **Breast cancer in association with thyroid disorders.** *Breast Cancer Res* 2003, **5**:R110–R113.
4. Hellevik AI, Asvold BO, Bjøro T, Romundstad PR, Nilsen TI, Vatten LJ: **Thyroid function and cancer risk: a prospective population study.** *Cancer Epidemiol Biomarkers Prev* 2009, **18**:570–574.
5. Tosovic A, Bondeson AG, Bondeson L, Ericsson UB, Malm J, Manjer J: **Prospectively measured triiodothyronine levels are positively associated with breast cancer risk in postmenopausal women.** *Breast Cancer Res* 2010, **12**:R33.
6. Siegler JE, Li X, Jones SD, Kandil E: **Early-onset breast cancer in a woman with Graves' disease.** *Int J Clin Exp Med* 2012, **5**:358–362.
7. Angelousi AG, Anagnostou VK, Stamatakos MK, Georgiopoulos GA, Kontzoglou KC: **Mechanisms in endocrinology: primary HT and risk for breast cancer: a systematic review and meta-analysis.** *Eur J Endocrinol* 2012, **166**:373–381.
8. Ito K, Maruchi N: **Breast cancer in patients with Hashimoto's thyroiditis.** *Lancet* 1975, **2**:1119–1121.
9. Kapdi JJ, Wolfe JN: **Breast cancer relationship to thyroid supplements for hypothyroidism.** *JAMA* 1976, **236**:1124–1127.
10. Nelson M, Hercbergs A, Rybicki L, Strome M: **Association between development of hypothyroidism and improved survival in patients with head and neck cancer.** *Arch Otolaryngol Head Neck Surg* 2006, **132**:1041–1046.
11. Maruchi N, Annegers JF, Kurland LT: **Hashimoto's thyroiditis and breast cancer.** *Mayo Clin Proc* 1976, **51**:263–265.
12. Hamasaki H, Yoshimi T, Yanai H: **A patient with Graves' disease showing only psychiatric symptoms and negativity for both TSH receptor autoantibody and thyroid stimulating antibody.** *Thyroid Res* 2012, **5**:19.
13. Oh HJ, Chung JK, Kang JH, Kang WJ, Noh DY, Park IA, Jeong JM, Lee DS, Lee MC: **The relationship between expression of the sodium/iodide symporter gene and the status of hormonal receptors in human breast cancer tissue.** *Cancer Res Treat* 2005, **37**:247–250.
14. Munoz JM, Gorman CA, Elveback LR, Wentz JR: **Incidence of malignant neoplasms of all types of patients with Graves' disease.** *Arch Intern Med* 1978, **138**:944–947.

15. Chen YK, Lin CL, Chang YJ, Cheng FT, Peng CL, Sung FC, Cheng YH, Kao CH: **Cancer risk in patients with Graves' disease: A nationwide cohort study.** *Thyroid.* in press.
16. Hardefeldt PJ, Eslick GD, Edirimanne S: **Benign thyroid disease is associated with breast cancer: a meta-analysis.** *Breast Cancer Res Treat* 2012, **133:**1169–1177.
17. Venturi S: **Is there a role for iodine in breast diseases?** *Breast* 2001, **10:**379–382.
18. Jiskra J, Límanová Z, Barkmanová J, Smutek D, Friedmannová Z: **Autoimmune thyroid diseases in women with breast cancer and colorectal cancer.** *Physiol Res* 2004, **53:**693–702.
19. Smyth PP: **The thyroid, iodine and breast cancer.** *Breast Cancer Res* 2003, **5:**235–238.
20. Giani C, Fierabracci P, Bonacci R, Gigliotti A, Campani D, De Negri F, Cecchetti D, Martino E, Pinchera A: **Relationship between breast cancer and thyroid disease: relevance of autoimmune thyroid disorders in breast malignancy.** *J Clin Endocrinol Metab* 1996, **81:**990–994.
21. Smyth PPA, Shering S, Kilbane MT, Murray MJ, McDermott EWM, Smith DF, O'Higgins NJ: **Serum thyroid peroxidase autoantibodies, thyroid volume and outcome in breast cancer.** *J Clin Endocrinol Metab* 1998, **83:**2711–2716.
22. Kuijpens JL, Nyklíctek I, Louwman MW, Weetman TA, Pop VJ, Coebergh JW: **Hypothyroidism might be related to breast cancer in post-menopausal women.** *Thyroid* 2005, **15:**1253–1259.
23. Simon MS, Tang MT, Bernstein L, Norman SA, Weiss L, Burkman RT, Daling JR, Deapen D, Folger SG, Malone K, Marchbanks PA, McDonald JA, Strom BL, Wilson HG, Spirtas R: **Do thyroid disorders increase the risk of breast cancer?** *Cancer Epidemiol Biomarkers Prev* 2002, **11:**1574–1578.
24. Latif R, Morshed SA, Zaidi M, Davies TF: **The thyroid-stimulating hormone receptor: impact of thyroid-stimulating hormone and thyroid-stimulating hormone receptor antibodies on multimerization, cleavage, and signaling.** *Endocrinol Metab Clin North Am* 2009, **38:**319–341.
25. Zygmunt A, Adamczewski Z, Wojciechowska-Durczyńska K, Cyniak-Magierska A, Krawczyk-Rusiecka K, Zygmunt A, Karbownik-Lewińska M, Lewiński A: **Evaluation of efficacy of iodine prophylaxis in Poland based on the examination of schoolchildren living in Opoczno Town (Lodz Voivodship).** *Thyroid Res* 2012, **5:**23.
26. Mittra I, Perrin J, Kumaoka S: **Thyroid and other autoantibodies in British and Japanese women: an epidemiological study of breast cancer.** *BMJ* 1976, **1:**257–259.
27. Kilbane MT, Ajjan RA, Weetman AP, Dwyer R, McDermott EW, O'Higgins NJ, Smyth PP: **Tissue iodine content and serum-mediated 125I uptake-blocking activity in breast cancer.** *J Clin Endocrinol Metab* 2000, **85:**1245–1250.
28. Beyer SJ, Jimenez RE, Shapiro CL, Cho JY, Jhiang SM: **Do cell surface trafficking impairments account for variable cell surface sodium iodide symporter levels in breast cancer?** *Breast Cancer Res Treat* 2009, **115:**205–212.
29. Daniels GH, Haber DA: **Will radioiodine be useful in treatment of breast cancer?** *Nat Med* 2000, **6:**859–860.
30. Boelaert K, Franklyn JA: **Sodium iodide symporter: a novel strategy to target breast, prostate, and other cancers?** *Lancet* 2003, **361:**796–797.
31. Dumont JE, Maenhaut C: **Growth factors controlling the thyroid gland.** *Baillieres Clin Endocrinol Metabol* 1991, **5:**727–753.
32. Fernández-Soto ML, Jovanovic LG, González-Jiménez A, Lobón-Hernández JA, Escobar-Jiménez F, López-Cózar LN, Barredo-Acedo F, Campos-Pastor MM, López-Medina JA: **Thyroid function during pregnancy and the postpartum period: iodine metabolism and disease states.** *Endocr Pract* 1998, **4:**97–105.
33. Karbownik-Lewińska M, Kokoszko-Bilska A: **Oxidative damage to macromolecules in the thyroid - experimental evidence.** *Thyroid Res* 2012, **5:**25.
34. Giustarini E, Pinchera A, Fierabracci P, Roncella M, Fustaino L, Mammoli C, Giani C: **Thyroid autoimmunity in patients with malignant and benign breast diseases before surgery.** *Eur J Endocrinol* 2006, **154:**645–649.
35. Ali A, Mir MR, Bashir S, Hassan T, Bhat SA: **Relationship between the levels of Serum Thyroid Hormones and the Risk of Breast Cancer.** *J Biol Agr Healthc* 2011, **2:**56–60.
36. Saraiva PP, Figueiredo NB, Padovani CR, Brentani MM, Nogueira CR: **Profile of thyroid hormones in breast cancer patients.** *Braz J Med Biol Res* 2005, **38:**761–765.
37. Smyth PPA: **Autoimmune thyroid disease and breast cancer: a chance association.** *J Endocrinol Invest* 2000, **23:**42–43.
38. Belkadi A, Jacques C, Savagner F, Malthièry Y: **Phylogenetic analysis of the human thyroglobulin regions.** *Thyroid Res* 2012, **5:**3.
39. Cahoon EK, Rozhko A, Hatch M, Polyanskaya O, Ostroumova E, Tang M, Nadirov E, Yauseyenka V, Savasteeva I, McConnell RJ, Pfeiffer RM, Brenner AV: **Factors associated with serum thyroglobulin levels in a population living in Belarus.** *Clin Endocrinol (Oxf)* 2012. in press.
40. Molleston JP, Mellman W, Narkewicz MR, Balistreri WF, Gonzalez-Peralta RP, Jonas MM, Lobritto SJ, Mohan P, Murray KF, Njoku D, Rosenthal P, Barton BA, Talor MV, Cheng I, Schwarz KB, Haber BA, for the PEDS-C Clinical Research Network: **Autoantibodies and Autoimmune Disease During Treatment of Children With Chronic Hepatitis C.** *J Pediatr Gastroenterol Nutr* 2013, **56:**304–310.
41. Hill OW: **Thyroglobulin antibodies in 1,297 patients without thyroid disease.** *Br Med J* 1961, **5242:**1793–1796.
42. Tunbridge WM, Vanderpump MP: **Population screening for autoimmune thyroid disease.** *Endocrinol Metab Clin North Am* 2000, **29:**239–253.
43. Mizia-Stec K, Zych F, Widala E: **Mastopathy and simple goiter–mutual relationships.** *Przegl Lek* 1998, **55:**250–258.
44. Kopp P: **The TSH receptor and its role in thyroid disease.** *Cell Mol Life Sci* 2001, **58:**1301–1322.
45. Gershengorn MC, Neumann S: **Update in TSH receptor agonists and antagonists.** *J Clin Endocrinol Metab* 2012, **97:**4287–4292.
46. Swain M, Swain T, Mohanty BK: **Autoimmune thyroid disorders-An update.** *Indian J Clin Biochem* 2005, **20:**9–17.
47. Gesing A, Lewiński A, Karbownik-Lewińska M: **The thyroid gland and the process of aging; what is new?** *Thyroid Res* 2012, **5:**16.

6

Eye findings and immunological markers in probands and their euthyroid relatives from a single family with multiple cases of thyroid autoimmunity

Melissa Ardley[1], Thomas McCorquodale[1], Hooshang Lahooti[1], Bernard Champion[1] and Jack R Wall[1,2*]

Abstract

Background: Ophthalmopathy is a common manifestation of Graves' disease (GD) occurring in up to 50% of patients. Mild eye signs are also common in patients with Hashimoto's thyroiditis. Whilst a genetic predisposition to GD has been demonstrated this is not the case for the ophthalmopathy which often runs a separate course.

Objective: We determined the prevalences of eye and eyelid signs and positive thyroid and orbital antibody tests in first and second degree relatives from a single family with multiple cases of Graves' disease, ophthalmopathy and Hashimoto's thyroiditis.

Design: The study cohort comprised 16 subjects from the same family, 4 probands namely, 3 with GD and one with Hashimoto's thyroiditis and hypothyroidism and 12 of their euthyroid first or second degree relatives. We measured antibodies against calsequestrin (CASQ1) and collagen XIII in an enzyme-linked-immunosorbent assays and TSH-Receptor (TSH-R) antibodies as i) TSH-R binding inhibiting immunoglobulin (TBII) and ii) thyroid stimulating immunoglobulin (TSI). Eye signs were classified and quantified using the clinical activity score (CAS), NOSPECS classes, Nunery types 1 and 2 and the margin-reflex-distance (MRD) as a measure of upper eyelid retraction (UER).

Main outcomes: Whilst significant ophthalmopathy was uncommon in the relatives, mild eye signs, in particular UER, were demonstrated in about a third of them. The presence of eye signs was moderately, but not significantly, associated with the detection of CASQ1 and collagen XIII antibodies, but not TSH-R antibodies.

Conclusion: Our study demonstrates a significant prevalence of positive orbital antibody tests and ophthalmopathy in probands with thyroid autoimmunity and their euthyroid relatives, favouring a role of genetic factors in the development of ophthalmopathy in patients with thyroid autoimmunity.

Keywords: Thyroid autoimmunity, Ophthalmopathy, Graves' disease, Genetics, Euthyroid relatives, Calsequestrin

Introduction

Graves' disease (GD) is the most common form of hyperthyroidism, affecting up to 1% of the population [1]. There is a marked gender differences in prevalence with a 5–10 fold excess in females and a significant clustering of disease in families, with 40-50% of patients reporting at least one family member with a thyroid disorder [2]. GD is considered to be a heterogeneous autoimmune disorder affecting, with varying degrees of severity, the thyroid, eyes and skin [3]. McKenzie [4] has defined GD as "a multi system disorder of unknown aetiology, characterized by one or more of three clinical entities; 1) hyperthyroidism associated with diffuse hyperplasia of the thyroid gland 2) infiltrative ophthalmology and 3) infiltrative dermopathy (localized pretibial myxedema)".

GD is a classical autoimmune disorder in which targeting of thyroid antigens, in particular the thyroid stimulating hormone (TSH) receptor (TSH-R), by antibodies and sensitized T lymphocytes leads to proliferation of

* Correspondence: jackw@med.usyd.edu.au
[1]The Department of Medicine, The University of Sydney, Nepean Hospital, PO Box 63, Penrith, NSW 2751, Australia
[2]University of Sydney, Western Clinical School, Nepean Hospital, PO Box 63, Penrith, NSW 2751, Australia

thyrocytes and overproduction of thyroid hormone. There is a genetic susceptibility to autoimmunity which is triggered by unknown environmental factors [5,6]. Recent studies have identified several genetic susceptibility loci including human leukocyte antigen (HLA, 6p21.3) and cytotoxic T-lymphocyte antigen-4 (CTLA-4, 2q33) [7]. Several environmental factors have also been elucidated including cigarette smoking, psychosocial stress, iodine intake, intrauterine growth, bacterial and viral infections and drugs such as interferon [8].

Ophthalmopathy is a common manifestation of autoimmune thyroid disease occurring in about 50% of patients with GD where it is called Graves' ophthalmopathy (GO) [9], and in about 25% of patients with Hashimoto's thyroiditis [10]. Ophthalmopathy may develop as a result of cross-reaction against a thyroid and orbital tissue antigen(s) in orbital connective tissue and eye muscle. Candidate orbital connective tissue antigen include the TSH-R, which is also expressed in the orbital fat and pre adipocytes [11-14] and possibly eye muscle as well [15], and the fibroblast cell membrane antigen collagen type XIII [16,17]. Of the several eye and eyelid muscle antigens identified [3] the skeletal muscle calcium binding protein calsequestrin (CASQ1) is the best candidate [17-19]. In order to further study the role of orbital antibodies in the pathogenesis of ophthalmopathy, and to address a possible genetic role, we have determined the prevalences of eye and eyelid signs and positive thyroid and orbital antibody tests in first and second degree relatives from a single family with multiple cases of thyroid autoimmunity.

Materials and methods

Clinical Subjects

The study involved 16 subjects, 10 females and 6 males aged 13–76 (mean age 40 years) from the same family in Melbourne, Victoria (Figure 1). Within this branch of the family there are three cases of confirmed GD, both male, one case of Hashimoto's thyroiditis and hypothyroidism and 12 first or second degree relatives of whom 6, 4 females and 2 males had a history of thyroid disease of unknown aetiology. Diagnosis of thyroid disease was based on standard clinical criteria and confirmed by thyroid function testing and thyroid antibody measurements. The grade, severity and activity of any ophthalmopathy were classified as; 1) Nunery types 1 (without restrictive myopathy) or 2 (with restrictive myopathy) [20] (2) as the clinical activity score (CAS) (0–10) of Mourits *et al.* [21] which is a measure of disease activity 3) Werner's NOSPECS class [22] and 4) the upper eyelid margin-reflex distance (MRD) which is the distance between the centre of the pupillary light reflex and the upper eyelid margin with the eye in primary gaze, as a measure of upper eyelid retraction (UER). An MRD of > 5 mm, which correlates with an UER score of > + using our assessment protocol, is taken as significant UER. Local Ethical Committee approval was received for the study and informed consent of participating subjects was obtained.

Serum antibody measurement

The presence and level of serum orbital antibodies in probands and their relatives were determined using an enzyme-linked immunosorbent assay (ELISA). This procedure has been described in previous publications by this laboratory [10,17-19] and is standard. The antigens used were i) highly purified rabbit skeletal muscle CASQ1 which shares 97% homology with human calsequestrin and ii) recombinant human collagen XIII. Results were expressed as optical density (OD) at 405 nM. A positive test was taken as an OD > the upper limit of the reference range, which was 194 for CASQ1 and 193 for collagen XIII. Serum TSH-R antibodies were measured as i) TSH-R binding inhibiting immunoglobulin (TBII) where a positive test was taken as a level of > 1.5 IU/L and ii) thyroid stimulating immunoglobulin (TSI) using fresh human thyroid cells as source of cyclic AMP (cAMP) following stimulation with test serum and a cAMP ELISA kit where a positive test was, taken as a %B/BO > 19%, following the manufacturers instructions and reference ranges.

Statistical analysis

Differences in prevalences of orbital and TSH-R antibodies were determined using the Mann–Whitney test for a non parametric data. A P value of <0.5 was taken as significant in all assessments.

Results

The study cohort comprised 16 subjects from a single family, 4 probands of whom 3 had GD and one had Hashimoto's thyroiditis and hypothyroidism and 12 first or second degree relatives. We measured antibodies against CASQ1 and collagen XIII in an ELISA, and TSH-R antibodies in two assays, and eye signs were classified and quantified as described in methods.

Prevalence of thyroid dysfunction

At the time of study, all patients and relatives were clinically well and euthyroid. Sera were available from 16 subjects namely, the 4 probands [WH-18, WH-25 and WH-30 who had GD] and WH-15 who had hypothyroidism due to Hashimoto's thyroiditis], and 11 first or second degree relatives. Of these, 3 subjects had abnormal TSH levels namely, two probands; WH-15 with a high TSH, and WH-18 with a low TSH both of whom were receiving thyroxine replacement, and one of the untreated relatives, WH-28, who had a low TSH

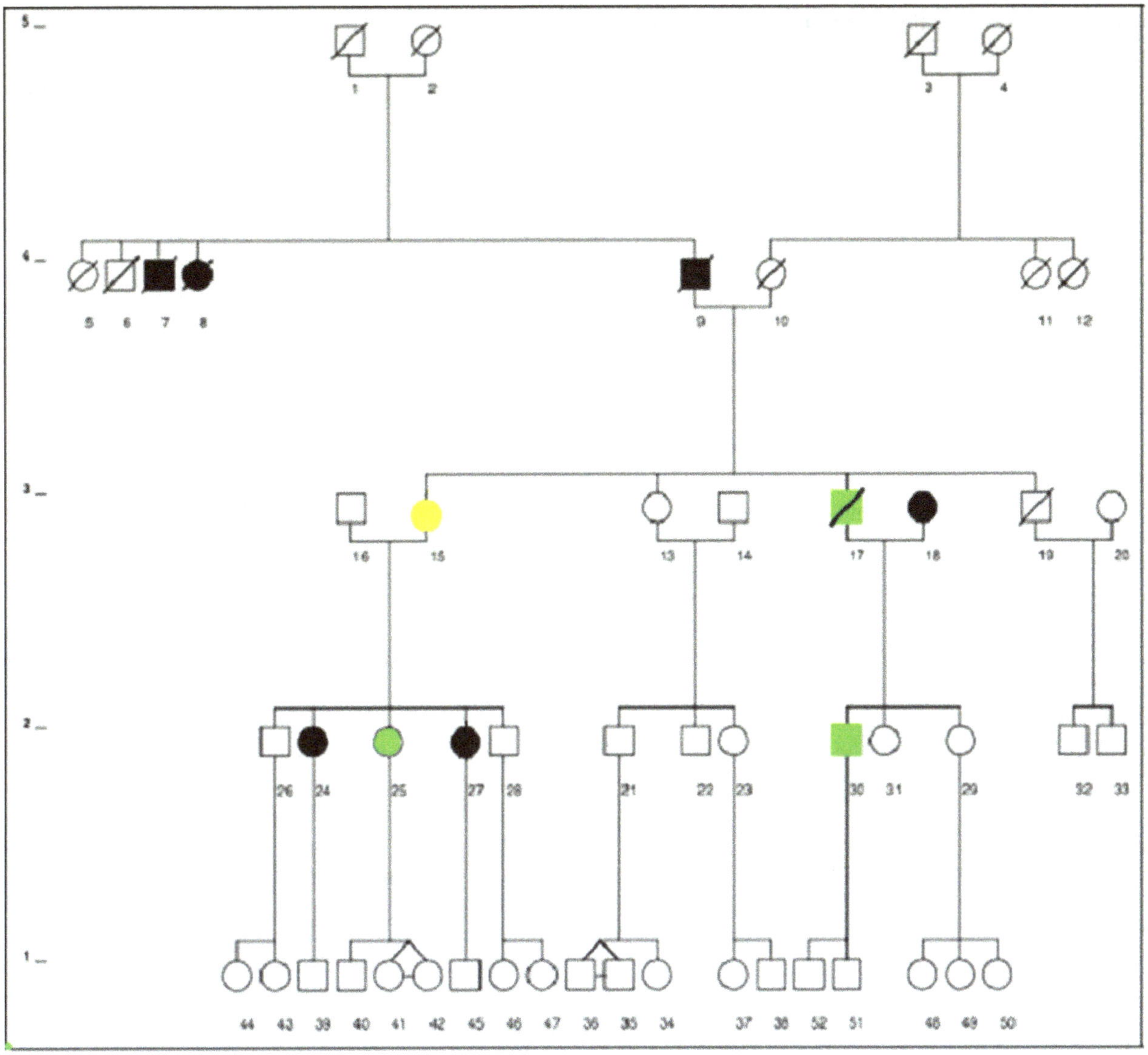

Figure 1 Family Tree showing probands with Graves' disease or Hashimoto's thyroiditis and their euthyroid relatives, 6 of whom had "thyroid disease of unknown aetiology".

(Table 1). The other probands and relatives were biochemically and clinically euthyroid at the time of testing.

Thyroid antibodies

Serum from two of the three probands with previously documented GD namely, WH-25 and WH-30, and from the hypothyroid subject WH-15, was positive for TPO antibodies. It is interesting to note that WH-15 has a daughter (not tested) with Hashimoto's thyroiditis. Although none of the relatives were clinically or biochemically hyperthyroid, two, WH-29 and WH-31, the daughters and sisters of two of the Graves' probands (see Figure 1), were positive for TPO antibodies (Table 1).

TSH-R antibodies, as TBII and TSI, were measured in most of the subjects. Positive TBII tests were demonstrated in two probands with GD, WH-30, and WH-25 and TSI tests were borderline positive in one apparently normal first degree relative, WH-26. The prevalences of positive TSH-R antibodies in probands vs relatives with and without ophthalmopathy were not significantly different (Mann–Whitney tests, P = NS).

Ophthalmopathy

Next, we examined the 16 probands and relatives for eye and upper eyelid abnormalities. The overall prevalence of any eye signs was 37.5%. Three (20%) of the subjects

Table 1 Demographic data, biochemical and immunological findings and treatment of probands with thyroid autoimmunity and their first or second degree relatives

Subjects		Age (range yr)	Sex (F/M)	Mean serum TSH[1] (mIU/L)	Positive TPO[2] antibodies	TSH-R Ab[3]		Treatment[4]		
						TBII	TSI	L-T_4	RAI	ATD
Probands	GD[5] with ophthalmopathy (n = 3)	52-75	2/1	1.84	2	2	0	3	3	1
	Other thyroid disorders (n = 1)	77	1/0	6.52	1	0	0	1	0	0
Relatives	No documented thyroid disorders (n = 11)	13-54	7/5	1.26	2	0	1	0	0	0

[1] TSH = thyroid stimulating hormone (normal range 0.3-4.0 mIU/L).
[2] TPO = thyroid peroxidase (cut-off titre 100).
[3] A positive test for thyroid stimulating antibodies (TSI) was taken as a % B/BO >19%, a positive test for TSH-R binding inhibitory immunoglobulin (TBII) was taken as >1.5 IU/Litre.
[4] Number of patients treated with thyroxine (L-T_4), ^{131}I or antithyroid drugs (ATD).
[5] GD = Graves' disease.

were current smokers. In more detail, two probands (WH-18, WH-21) and two second-degree relatives (WH-49, WH-50) had mild ophthalmopathy (CAS = 1) and one proband (WH-30) had severe ophthalmopathy (CAS = 5) of many years duration which required corrective eye muscle surgery. Four of the probands (all 3 probands with GD and WH-15 with Hashimoto's thyroiditis) also had mild UER and WH-30 had moderate ocular muscle dysfunction with restricted lateral gaze of the left eye. The duration of eye signs in these subjects was difficult to determine as they did not recognize any particular eye symptoms. All 4 probands with autoimmune thyroid disease, WH-15 with hypothyroidism and WH-18, WH-25 and WH-30 with GD, had eye signs. The other relatives were normal (Table 2).

Table 2 Prevalence of eye signs in probands and first or second degree relatives from a single family with multiple cases of thyroid autoimmunity

Subject	CAS[1]	UER[2]	Nunery types 1, 2[3]	NOSPECS classes[4]
WH-15	1	Yes	1	1
WH-18	2	0	1	2
WH-25	2	0	1	2
WH-26	0	0		0
WH-28	0	0		0
WH-29	0	0		0
WH-30	5	Yes	2	4
WH-31	0	0		0
WH-32	0	0		0
WH-41	0	0		0
WH-42	0	0		0
WH-48	0	0		0
WH-49	1	2	1	1
WH-50	1	0	1	2
WH-51	0	0		0
WH-52	0	0		0

[1] CAS = Clinical activity score (CAS) (0–10) as described by Mourits *et al* (see ref no. 21).
[2] UER = Upper eyelid retraction, taken as a MRD >5 mm which corresponds to an UER score of > +.
[3] see ref no [20].
[4] see ref. no [22].

Orbital antibodies

We measured CASQ1 and collagen XIII antibodies in serum from all 16 subjects; namely, 4 probands and 12 euthyroid first or second degree relatives. Two of the three probands with GD, WH-18 and WH-30 who was also positive for TBII (but not for TSI), were positive for CASQ1 antibodies and one, WH-30, for collagen XIII antibodies (Table 3). The subject who tested positive for both antibodies was WH-30, the proband with severe ophthalmopathy (see Table 2). Of the four euthyroid relatives with positive eye muscle antibody tests only two (one with reactivity against CASQ1, WH-41, and one with reactivity against collagen XIII, WH-29) were first-degree relatives of probands with autoimmune thyroid disease. The other two euthyroid subjects with positive antibody results, WH-49 and WH-50, were the children of WH-29, i.e. second-degree relatives of probands with GD (see Figure 1). One of the second-degree relatives WH-49, had positive CASQ1 and collagen XIII antibody tests while another, WH-50, had a positive collagen XIII antibody test only. There was a modest overall correlation between any eye signs and positive antibody reactivity against CASQ1 and/or collagen XII, I although this did not reach statistical significance for ether antibody (Mann-Witney test P = NS, P = NS respectively) (Table 3).

Finally, all subjects with Graves' disease and two first-degree relatives reported the presence of other autoimmune disorders (results not shown).

Discussion

Graves' ophthalmopathy is a common disorder which can present with either hyperthyroidism or hypothyroidism or in the apparent absence of thyroid autoimmunity, so called euthyroid Graves' disease [9]. The ophthalmopathy

Table 3 Prevalence of CASQ1 and collagen XIII antibodies in probands and first or second degree relatives from a single family with multiple cases of thyroid autoimmunity

Subjects	Subjects	Prevalence (%) of positive antibody reactivity	
		CASQ1[1]	Collagen XIII
Probands	GD[2] with ophthalmopathy (*n* = 3)	2 (66%)	1 (33%)
	Other disorders (*n* = 1)	0	0
Relatives	No documented thyroid disorders (*n* = 12)	2 (16%)	3 (25%)

[1] CASQ1 = skeletal muscle calsequestrin.
[2] GD = Graves' disease.

associated with Graves' hyperthyroidism and, less often, Hashimoto's thyroiditis [10] is presumed to be an autoimmune disorder of the extraocular muscles and orbital connective tissue. There is substantial evidence that the eye muscles are targets of the autoimmune reactions of "thyroid-associated ophthalmopathy" because more than 90% of Graves' patients with or without clinical signs of ophthalmopathy have extraocular muscle enlargement by orbital imaging techniques [23].

In the present study we determined the prevalence of CASQ1 and collagen XIII antibodies in serum from probands and first or second degree relatives of a single family with multiple cases of thyroid autoimmunity. We observed a fairly close relationship between CASQ1 and collagen XIII antibodies and ophthalmopathy, eye signs including stare and lid lag being demonstrated in all but one subject with positive eye muscle antibodies, although this was not significant, possibly because of the small numbers of subjects studied. Two thirds of those with positive eye muscle antibodies and eye signs had documented thyroid disease, 3 with GD and one with hypothyroidism, whilst two of the six subjects with eye signs were second-degree relatives of three probands with GD. It is interesting to note that WH-49 had a TSH result at the upper limit of normal and detectable antibodies against CASQ1 and collagen XIII, making her an interesting subject for long term follow-up at risk to develop thyroid dysfunction and/or ophthalmopathy in the future.

Several groups [24-26] have shown that relatives of patients with Graves' disease have an increased prevalence of thyroid antibodies compared with controls, as well as an increased tendency to develop other autoimmune diseases. The notion that autoimmunity against the TSH-R is involved in the development of GD and GO and evidence for increased thyroid antibodies in euthyroid relatives of patients with GD makes a strong case for the familial inheritance of orbital antibodies as well. While significant ophthalmopathy is uncommon in relatives of subjects with GD, mild eye signs, in particular upper eyelid abnormalities, associated with eye muscle antibodies against CASQ1 and collagen XIII, were seen in about 33% of euthyroid relatives in a single family in the present study. This raises the possibility of a role for genetic factors in the development of ophthalmopathy.

In conclusion, it seems likely that the development of ophthalmopathy in patients with Graves' hyperthyroidism and Hashimoto's thyroiditis results from the concurrence of several environmental and genetic factors. Because individual families are small, the best approach to understanding the "genetic factor" would be to study large numbers of patients with thyroid autoimmunity with and without ophthalmopathy, for example looking for linkages between eye signs and selected polymorphisms (SNPs) of the CASQ1 and collagen XIII genes.

Competing interests
All the authors declare that they have no competing interests.

Authors' contributions
MA participated in study design, collection of clinical data in primary writing of the manuscript. TM and HL carried out the laboratory assays and contributed to manuscript revision. BC contributed to project design and manuscript writing and revision. JW contributed to study design, collection of clinical data, manuscript writing and revisions and overall study supervision. All authors read and approved the final manuscript.

Acknowledgements
We thank Dr. Nicole Beard (ANU, Canberra, Australia) for suppling rabbit skeletal muscle calsequestrin, and Dr. Tania Pihlajaniemi (Oulu University, Finland) for suppling recombinant human collagen XIII. We thank Barratt and Smith Pathology for testing subjects' sera for biochemical markers of thyroid disease and Gary Ma, for the measurement of TSH-R antibodies.

References
1. Tunbridge WM, Evered DC, Hall R, Appleton D, Brewis M, Clark F, *et al*: **The spectrum of thyroid disease in a community; the Whickham survey.** *Clin Endocrinol* 1977, 7:481–493.
2. Manji N, Carr-Smith JD, Boelaert K, Allahabadia A, Armitage M, Chatterjee VK, *et al*: **Influences of Age, Gender, Smoking, and family History on Autoimmune Thyroid Disease Phenotype.** *J Clin Endocrinol Metab* 2006, 91:4873–4880.
3. Lahooti H, Parmar K, Wall JR: **Pathogenesis of Thyroid Eye Disease: important role of autoimmunity against calsequestrin and collagen XIII.**

Pathogenesis of Thyroid Eye Disease: important role of autoimmunity against calsequestrin and collagen XIII. *Clin Ophthalmol* 2010, **4**:417–425.
4. McKenzie JM: **Humoral factors in the pathogenesis of Grave's disease.** *Physiol Rev* 1968, **48**:252–310.
5. Bednarczuk T, Gopinath B, Ploski R, Wall JR: **Susceptibility genes in Grave's ophthalmopathy: searching for a needle in a haystack?** *Clin Endocrinol* 2007, **67**:3–19.
6. Brix TH, Christensen K, Holm NV, Harvald B, Hegedus L: **What is the evidence of genetic factors in the etiology of Grave's disease? A brief review.** *Thyroid* 1998, **8**:627–634.
7. Kim N, Hatton MP: **The Role of genetics in Graves' disease and thyroid orbitopathy.** *Semin Ophthalmol* 2008, **23**:67–72.
8. Prummel MF, Strieder T, Wiersinga WM: **The Environment and autoimmune thyroid diseases.** *Eur J Endocrinol* 2004, **150**:605–618.
9. Burch HB, Wartofsky L: **Graves' ophthalmopathy: current concepts regarding pathogenesis and management.** *Endocr Rev* 1993, **14**:747–793.
10. Tjiang H, Lahooti H, McCorquodale T, Wall JR: **Eye and eyelid abnormalities are common in patients with Hashimoto's thyroiditis.** *Thyroid* 2010, **20**:287–290.
11. Hagg P, Rehn M, Huhtala P, Vaisanen T, Tamminen M, Pihlajaniemi T: **1998 Type XIII collagen is identified as a plasma membrane protein.** *J Biol Chem* 1998, **273**:15590–15597.
12. Bahn RS: **Clinical review 157: Pathophysiology of Graves' ophthalmopathy: the cycle of disease.** *J Clin Endocrinol Metab* 2003, **88**:1939–1946.
13. Paschke R, Vassart G, Ludgate M: **Current evidence for and against the TSH receptor being the common antigen in Graves' disease and thyroid associated ophthalmopathy.** *Clin Endocrinol (Oxf)* 1995, **42**:565–569.
14. Wakelkamp IM, Bakker O, Baldeschi L, Wiersinga WM, Prummel MF: **TSH-R expression and cytokine profile in orbital tissue of active vs. inactive Graves' ophthalmopathy patients.** *Clin Endocrinol (Oxf)* 2003, **58**:280–287.
15. Hiromatsu Y, Sato M, Inoue Y, Koga M, Miyake I, Kameo J, *et al*: **Localization and clinical significance of thyrotropin receptor mRNA expression in orbital fat and eye muscle tissues from patients with thyroid-associated ophthalmopathy.** *Thyroid* 1996, **6**:553–562.
16. De Bellis A, Bizzarro A, Conte M, Coronella C, Solimeno S, Perrino S, *et al*: **Relationship between longitudinal behaviour of some markers of eye autoimmunity and changes in ocular findings in patients with Graves' ophthalmopathy receiving corticosteroid therapy.** *Clin Endocrinol* 2003, **59**:388–395.
17. Gopinath B, Musselman R, Adams C, Tani J, Beard N, Wall JR: **Study of serum antibodies against three eye muscle antigens and the connective tissue antigen collagen XIII in patients with Graves' disease with and without ophthalmopathy: Correlation with clinical features.** *Thyroid* 2006, **16**:967–974.
18. Gopinath B, Musselman R, Beard N, Tani J, Adams C, Wall JR: **Antibodies targeting the calcium binding skeletal muscle protein calsequestrin are sensitive and specific markers of ocular myopathy in patients with Graves' disease.** *Clin Exp Immunol* 2006, **145**:56–62.
19. Gopinath B, Gary M, Wall JR: **Eye Signs and serum eye muscle and collagen XIII antibodies in patients with transient and progressive thyroiditis.** *Thyroid* 2007, **17**:1123–1128.
20. Nunery WR, Martin RT, Hinz GW, Gavin TJ: **The association of cigarette smoking with clinical subtypes of ophthalmic Graves' disease.** *Ophthal Plast Reconstr Surg* 1993, **9**:77–82.
21. Mourits MP, Koornneef L, Wiersinga WM, Prummel MF, Berghout A, van der Gaag R: **Clinical criteria for the assessment of disease activity in Grave's ophthalmopathy: a novel approach.** *Br J Ophthalmol* 1989, **73**:639–644.
22. Werner SC: **Classification of the eye changes of Graves' disease.** *Am J Ophthalmol* 1969, **68**:646–648.
23. Villadolid MC, Yokoyama N, Izumi M, Nishikawa T, Kimura H, Ashizawa K, *et al*: **Untreated Graves' disease patients without clinical ophthalmopathy demonstrate a high frequency of extraocular muscle (EOM) enlargements by magnetic resonance.** *J Clin Endocrinol Metab* 1995, **80**:2830–2833.
24. Campbell PN, Doniach D, Hudson RV, Roitt IM: **Auto-antibodies in Hashimoto's disease (lymphadenoid goitre).** *Lancet* 1956, **271**:820–821.
25. Hall R, Owen SG, Smart GA: **Evidence for genetic predisposition to formation of thyroid autoantibodies.** *Lancet* 1960, **2**:187–188.
26. Wall JR, Good BF, Hetzel BS: **Long-acting thyroid stimulator in euthyroid relatives of thyrotoxic patients.** *Lancet* 1969, **2**:1024–1026.

7

Treatment related morbidity in differentiated thyroid cancer–a survey of clinicians

Ovie Edafe[1*], Jonathan Wadsley[2], Barney J Harrison[3] and Sabapathy P Balasubramanian[1,3]

Abstracts

Background: Differentiated thyroid cancer (DTC) has excellent long term survival in most patients. Long-term treatment related morbidity is therefore important, but may not be well characterised. The aim of this study was to conduct an electronic survey of clinicians involved in the care of patients with DTC to determine their views on treatment related morbidity.

Methods: A nine item questionnaire was developed, piloted locally and sent by email to members of three United Kingdom (UK) medical organisations (Thyroid Cancer Forum, British Association of Endocrine and Thyroid Surgeons, British Thyroid Association).

Results: 125 responses were received. Less than 5% of respondents had a formal protocol to detect morbidity associated with TSH suppression. Over 50% agreed that morbidity from TSH suppression is not well defined. The majority of responders also agreed that the long-term morbidity of hypocalcaemia, significant voice change and TSH suppression in DTC are not well characterised. Physicians perceived treatment related morbidity to be a bigger problem than surgeons (P = 0.019).

Conclusion: Clinicians treating thyroid cancer agree that long-term treatment related morbidity from DTC is not well characterised. A study of the prevalence and severity of treatment related morbidity and its impact on health of patients with DTC is warranted.

Keywords: Thyroid cancer, Treatment, Hypocalcaemia, Voice change, TSH suppression, Morbidity, Survey

Introduction

The standard treatment regimen in most patients with differentiated thyroid cancer (DTC) includes thyroidectomy, radio-iodine (RAI) ablation and thyroid stimulating hormone (TSH) suppression therapy [1]. Diagnosis of DTC is associated with an excellent 10 and 20 year survival [2]. Long term treatment related morbidity is therefore important and includes post-thyroidectomy hypocalcaemia, the effects of TSH suppression therapy and significant voice change.

A retrospective study of 316 patients who underwent thyroidectomy for DTC found rates of transient and permanent hypocalcaemia to be 27.5% and 5.1% respectively [3]. Hypocalcaemia commonly presents with paraesthesia, muscle twitching and spasms. In more severe cases, patients may develop tetany, seizure and cardiac arrhythmias [4]. Long term hypoparathyroidism is associated with renal impairment, basal ganglia calcifications and damage to bone health [5,6].

Recurrent laryngeal nerve palsy is another potential complication following thyroid surgery and can significantly affect voice, swallowing and predispose to aspiration. Temporary and permanent recurrent laryngeal nerve palsy can occur in up to 8% and 3% of patients respectively [7]. Bilateral nerve palsy is rare and may occasionally necessitate a tracheostomy. In addition to recurrent laryngeal nerve injury, other factors affecting the quality of voice postoperatively include injury/damage to the superior laryngeal nerves, strap muscle injury and irritation or oedema of the airways [8]. Postoperative voice change after thyroidectomy can have a significant impact on an individual's personal and professional life [9].

Although traditional practice was to continue lifelong TSH suppression treatment for all patients with thyroid cancer, recent guidelines from the American Thyroid

* Correspondence: ovieedafe@hotmail.co.uk
[1]Department of Oncology, University of Sheffield, Beech Hill Road, Sheffield S10 2RX, UK
Full list of author information is available at the end of the article

Table 1 Do you see patients with the following problems following treatment for DTC?

Complication (number of responders)	Never/NA	Rarely (≤1/year)	Occasionally (≤1/month)	Commonly (≤6/month)	Frequently (>6/month)
Temporary hypocalcaemia (118)	9 (7.6%)	18 (15.3%)	63 (53.4%)	28 (23.7%)	0 (0.0%)
Long term hypocalcaemia (118)	10 (8.5%)	51 (43.2%)	43 (36.4%)	14 (11.9%)	0 (0.0%)
Significant voice change (117)	6 (5.1%)	70 (59.8%)	36 (30.8%)	5 (4.3%)	0 (0.0%)
Symptoms/poor quality of life from TSH suppression (118)	19 (16.1%)	57 (48.3%)	30 (25.4%)	12 (10.2%)	0 (0.0%)
Bone/CVS complications from TSH suppression (118)	41 (34.7%)	58 (49.2%)	19 (16.1%)	0 (0.0%)	0 (0.0%)

NA, not applicable; CVS, cardiovascular; TSH, thyroid stimulating hormone.

Association (ATA) recommended that TSH suppression to less than 0.1 mU/l for initial management for DTC in high risk patients and a lower degree of TSH suppression (to between 0.1-0.5 mU/l) for low risk patients [10]. The guideline also recommended the TSH level be suppressed long term in patients with persistent disease. It is also suggested that TSH be kept at the lower limit of normal for 5-10 years in patients who were high risk at presentation and subsequently show no residual disease. Recent European guidelines suggest that patients who are free of thyroid cancer following treatment may be shifted from suppression to replacement, regardless of their initial risk [1]. There are no recommendations regarding TSH suppression in DTC patients with pre-existing bone and cardiovascular disease. Here, clinicians must balance risk from thyroid cancer recurrence and risk of bone and cardiac morbidity from TSH suppression [11].

A prospective study found that TSH suppression following thyroidectomy for PTC in women aged 50 or over was associated with a significant reduction in bone mineral density (BMD) one year after surgery [12]. In a multicentre prospective study, Bauer et al. evaluated the associated between low TSH and fracture risk in women aged 65 or over. They found that a suppressed TSH level (0.1 mU/L) increased the risk of hip and vertebrae fracture by threefold and fourfold respectively in multivariable analysis [13]. A systematic review evaluating the effects on bone metabolism of long term TSH suppression found postmenopausal women to be at increased risk of low BMD [14]. The authors recommended measurements of BMD in postmenopausal women with DTC starting TSH suppression therapy. A prospective study examined BMD in 26 pre-menopausal women having long term TSH suppression therapy for DTC [15]. They found significant reduction in BMD of femoral neck, femoral trochanter and Ward's triangle at one-year and four-years following treatment.

The long term effect of TSH suppression on BMD, including low impact fracture rate in males has also been studied [16]. Authors found no difference in BMD or fracture rates between men on long term TSH suppressive therapy (mean ± SD duration of treatment; 15 ± 5 years) and controls. However, the study group was limited by a small sample size of 33; large sample size is required to adequately study the effect on TSH suppression on fracture rates as frequency of fractures are low in the population [16].

Adverse cardiovascular effects and symptoms associated with long term TSH suppression for DTC have been reported by various studies [17-19]. Patients receiving TSH suppression scored higher for symptoms mimicking increased adrenergic activity including palpitations and increased heart rate compared to controls [17]. One study found a significant reduction in exercise tolerance in patients with long term TSH suppression for DTC compared to matched controls [18]. This study also found significant changes in cardiac morphology including greater intraventricular thickness and left ventricular posterior wall thickness in patients with long term TSH suppression for DTC compared to controls. An increase in ventricular

Table 2 Do you have a locally agreed protocol for the detection of the following problems following treatment for DTC?

Complication (number of responders)	NA/Not involved	Don't know	No agreed arrangements	Informal arrangements	Formal protocol
Temporary hypocalcaemia (118)	1 (0.8%)	1 (0.8)	7(5.9%)	32 (21.7%)	77 (65.3%)
Long term hypocalcaemia (117)	2 (1.7%)	0 (0.0%)	13 (11.1%)	51 (43.6%)	51 (43.6%)
Significant voice change (118)	2 (1.7%)	2 (1.7%)	20 (16.9%)	61 (51.7%)	33 (28.0%)
Symptoms/poor quality of life from TSH suppression (118)	14 (11.9%)	5 (4.2%)	43 (36.4%)	53 (44.9%)	3 (2.5%)
Bone/CVS complications from TSH suppression (118)	17 (14.4%)	8 (6.8%)	47 (39.8%)	42 (35.6%)	4(3.4%)

NA, not applicable; CVS, cardiovascular; TSH, thyroid stimulating hormone.

Table 3 Treatment related morbidity is a significant clinical problem in patients with DTC

Profession	NA	Strongly disagree	Disagree	Neutral	Agree	Strongly agree
Surgeons	0 (0.0%)	4 (5.0%)	40 (50.0%)	15 (18.8%)	17 (21.2%)	4 (5.0%)
Physicians	0 (0.0%)	0 (0.0%)	12 (31.6%	10 (26.3%)	14 (36.8%)	2 (5.3%)

NA, not applicable.

mass following long term TSH suppression for DTC was also confirmed by another group [19].

Aims and objectives

This project aims to understand perceptions of clinicians involved in the management of DTC on long term treatment related morbidity. The objectives were to conduct an internet based survey of clinicians involved in the care of patients with DTC to understand their perceptions of treatment related morbidity, with particular reference to hypocalcaemia, significant voice change and TSH suppression.

Methods

A questionnaire survey incorporating nine items was designed to address information pertinent to the objectives outlined above. A web based tool (http://www.surveymonkey.com) was used to create the questionnaire. Responses to treatment related morbidities were recorded on a Likert scale.

A pilot version was sent via email (embedded link to the web survey) to consultants involved in the care of patients with DTC. This was done to get feedback on the structure, appropriateness for purpose, design and usability of the web survey. The survey was amended in accordance with feedback received from three consultants.

All nine questions were included on one web page. Responders were able to change their answers during the survey; however, once submitted they were unable to review or change their answers. The survey was sent via email to doctors involved in the treatment of patients with thyroid cancer. These doctors were approached via national organisations in the UK whose members were doctors likely to be involved in thyroid cancer management. An email explaining the study and a link to the online survey was then forwarded by the secretaries of the organisations to their members.

The following UK organisations were contacted: British Association of Thyroid and Endocrine Surgeons (BAETS), Thyroid Cancer Forum (TCF) and the British Thyroid Association (BTA) with approximately 200, 230 and 150 members respectively. Considerable membership overlap exists between the organisations. A reminder email was sent 7-12 weeks after initial contact to all organisations. The survey remained open for at least four weeks after the second reminder.

A combination of IP address, response date and time was used to detect multiple entries being recorded on the electronic survey. In cases where the questionnaires were terminated early, completed questions were included in data analysis. Any unanswered questions/missing values were excluded from data analysis. All responses were downloaded and exported directly into Microsoft Excel 2007 with a Survey Monkey professional account. This avoided errors associated with manual data entry.

Data analysis

Percentages were used to summarise responses. The outcome measure was on a Likert scale (of 4 to 6 points). The Mann-Whitney U test was used to calculate differences in perception of treatment related morbidity between surgeons and physicians (oncologist, endocrinologist and nuclear medicine physician) and between clinicians seeing higher (>12 patients per month with DTC) and lower (≤12 patients per month with DTC) volumes of patients. The significance level was set at 0.05.

Ethical consideration

Ethics approval was obtained from the University of Sheffield Medical School Ethics Committee and the study was conducted in accordance to the submitted protocol [SMBRER244]. An amendment was obtained to send an email reminder to all potential participants.

Table 4 The incidence/prevalence of the following problems are not well defined in patients undergoing treatment for DTC

Complication (number of responders)	Strongly agree	Disagree	Neutral/don't know	Agree	Strongly agree
Temporary hypocalcaemia (118)	16 (13.6%)	47 (39.8%)	8 (6.8%)	42 (35.6%)	5 (4.2%)
Long term hypocalcaemia (118)	16 (13.6%)	50 (42.4%)	9 (7.6%)	37 (31.4%)	6 (5.1%)
Significant voice change (117)	14 (12.0%)	42 (35.9%)	12 (10.3%)	42 (35.9%)	7 (6.0%)
Symptoms/poor quality of life from TSH suppression (118)	6 (5.1%)	10 (8.5%)	24 (20.3%)	62 (52.5%)	16 (13.6%)
Bone/CVS complications from TSH suppression (118)	5 (4.2%)	10 (8.5%)	27 (22.9%)	59 (50.0%)	17 (14.4%)

NA, not applicable; CVS, cardiovascular; TSH, thyroid stimulating hormone.

Results

A total of 77 responses were received following initial contact by email. The total number of responses increased to 125 following the second reminder. Four responders were excluded from analysis as they were from outside the UK. A further three were also excluded from analysis as they were not involved in the management of patients with DTC. A total of 118 responses were analysed.

A response rate was not calculated as significant overlap exists between memberships of the organisation and collection of details that may identify members was not allowed. All responders were assumed to be consultants or senior trainees.

Background of the respondents

The responders included 80 surgeons (67.8%), 19 oncologists (16.1%), 16 endocrinologists (13.6%) and 3 nuclear medicine physicians (2.5%). The approximate number of patients (new and follow up) with DTC (at any stage of treatment) seen each month by responders was as follow: less than one, 11 (9.3%); between one and six, 52 (44.1%); between six and twelve, (17.8%) and more than twelve, 34 (28.8%). Eighty four of 118 (72.2%) and 34/118 (28.8%) of the responders were considered to be seeing lower and higher volumes of patients respectively.

Table 1 shows the number/frequency of patients seen with treatment related morbidity by responders. Table 2 shows responses to the question: 'Do you have a locally agreed protocol for the detection of the following problems following treatment for DTC? The proportion of clinicians who had a formal protocol for detecting temporary hypocalcaemia, long term hypocalcaemia, significant voice change, symptoms/poor quality of life from TSH suppression, and bone and cardiovascular complication of TSH suppression were 65.3%, 43.6%, 28.0%, 2.5% and 3.4% respectively (Table 2).

Table 3 shows clinicians' perceptions of the clinical significance of treatment related morbidity in DTC. Physicians perceived treatment related morbidity to be a bigger problem than surgeons ($P = 0.019$). Table 4 shows clinicians' perceptions on how well the incidence of treatment related morbidity is defined. Clinicians seeing higher volumes of patients with DTC were more likely to agree that the incidence of the following complications is not well defined: temporary hypocalcaemia ($P = 0.014$), long term hypocalcaemia ($P = 0.042$) and significant voice change ($P = 0.028$). Table 5 shows clinicians' perceptions of the characterisation of long term treatment related morbidity in DTC. Most clinicians agreed that the characterisation of long term treatment related morbidity of the following are not well defined: hypocalcaemia (55.1%), significant voice change (50.5%) and TSH suppression (57.7%).

Discussion

To our knowledge this is the first survey evaluating perceptions of clinicians on treatment related morbidity of DTC.

Although almost half of the clinicians perceived morbidity associated with TSH suppression to be *'rarely'* identified in clinic; only 2.5% and 4.0% had a formal protocol for detecting symptoms/poor quality of life from TSH suppression, and bone and cardiovascular complications respectively. It is unclear whether a lack of a formal protocol to detect these complications plays a role in the perception of morbidity. In addition, clinicians seeing higher volumes of patients with DTC perceived a higher frequency of long term hypocalcaemia, significant voice change and morbidity associated with TSH suppression ($P < 0.05$).

The lack of formal protocol to detect treatment related morbidity has also been confirmed by a recent survey of Japanese hospitals. They found most hospital did not perform BMD measurements in patients with TSH suppression for DTC. Less than 30% of hospitals routinely measure BMD in patients receiving TSH suppression for DTC. Of the hospitals that routinely measure BMD, measurements were taken yearly or twice yearly (44%), while 56% had no agreed interval for measurement [20].

Over 50% of clinicians perceived that the incidence of symptoms/poor quality of life from TSH suppression, and bone and cardiovascular complications of TSH suppression are not well defined. The picture was less clear with regards to temporary hypocalcaemia, long term hypocalcaemia and significant voice change: approximately equal numbers of clinicians 'agree' and *'disagree'* with the statement. Further analysis revealed that higher volume clinicians perceived that the incidence of temporary hypocalcaemia, long term hypocalcaemia and significant voice change are not well defined ($P < 0.05$).

Table 5 The long term morbidity of the following are not well characterised

Complication (number of responders)	Strongly agree	Disagree	Neutral/don't know	Agree	Strongly agree
Hypocalcaemia (118)	7 (5.9%)	32 (27.1%)	14 (11.9%)	59 (50.0%)	6 (5.1%)
Significant voice change (117)	12 (10.3%)	34 (29.1%)	12 (10.3%)	54 (46.2%)	5 (4.3%)
TSH suppression (116)	6 (5.2%)	19 (16.4%)	24 (20.7%)	57 (49.1%)	10 (8.6%)

NA, not applicable; CVS, cardiovascular; TSH, thyroid stimulating hormone.

Finally, over 50% of clinicians perceived that the long term morbidity of hypocalcaemia, significant voice change and TSH suppression are not well characterised. This in context of the overall perceptions over the clinical significance of treatment related morbidity (44.1% of clinicians perceived treatment related morbidity not to be a significant clinical problem) is of particular interest. One could postulate that it is difficult to ascertain the scale of a problem that is not well characterised or ill-defined.

One limitation of this survey was the inability to calculate the response rate due to significant overlaps between institutions contacted. The significance of bias due to non-response is therefore unclear. The potential impact of non-responders cannot be ignored as they may not have perceived treatment related morbidity in DTC to be a significant clinical problem. The survey only targeted surgeons and physicians who are members of specific organisations (TCF, BAETS and BTA), the findings may not be applicable to the entire population of thyroid surgeons and physicians.

The results reported are clinicians' perceptions of treatment related morbidity; it may not mirror the reality or true scale of the problem. The results could have been skewed as surgeons represented the majority (67.8%) of the sample given; particularly, given that physicians seemed to perceive greater treatment related morbidity than surgeons. The difference between physicians and surgeons could be attributed to differences in current follow up protocols. The extent to which these groups of clinicians are involved in the follow up management of thyroid cancer patients is unclear and was not investigated in this survey. Another limitation of the survey was the relatively small proportion of clinicians seeing higher volumes of patients with DTC (28.8%); although it could be argued that this is more representative of current practice. This survey did not evaluate perceptions of morbidity associated with radioiodine ablation. Ascertainment of morbidity attributed to radioiodine ablation is important.

Conclusion

There is a lack of formal protocols to detect complications associated with TSH suppression and most clinicians agreed that the incidence of complications associated with TSH suppression is not well defined. Over 50% of clinicians agreed that the long term morbidity of hypocalcaemia, significant voice change and TSH suppression are not well characterised. Physicians perceived treatment related morbidity to be a bigger problem than surgeons; this difference in perception could be related to differences in current follow up practices and differences in medical and surgical literature. A study of the prevalence and severity of treatment related morbidity and its impact on health of patients with DTC is warranted.

Abbreviations

ATA: American Thyroid Association; BAETS: British Association of Endocrine and Thyroid Surgeons; BMD: Bone mineral density; BTA: British Thyroid Association; DTC: Differentiated thyroid cancer; SD: Standard deviation; TCF: Thyroid Cancer Forum; TSH: Thyroid stimulating hormone; UK: United Kingdom.

Competing interests

The authors declare that they have no competing interests.

Authors' contributions

All authors were involved in conception, design and drafting of the manuscript. OE conducted the study and analysed the data. All authors read and approved the final manuscript.

Authors' information

Ovie Edafe, Medical Student.
Jon Wadsley, Consultant Oncologist.
Barney Harrison, Consultant Endocrine Surgeon.
Saba Balasubramanian, Clinical Senior Lecturer.

Acknowledgements

The following organisations and their membership are acknowledged for taking part in this study–Thyroid Cancer Forum (TCF), British Association of Endocrine and Thyroid Surgeons (BAETS) and the British Thyroid Association (BTA).

Author details

[1]Department of Oncology, University of Sheffield, Beech Hill Road, Sheffield S10 2RX, UK. [2]Department of Oncology, Weston Park Hospital, Sheffield, UK. [3]Endocrine Surgical Unit, Sheffield Teaching Hospitals NHS Foundation Trust, Sheffield, UK.

References

1. Pacini F, Castagna MG, Brilli L, Pentheroudakis G: **Thyroid cancer: ESMO clinical practice guidelines for diagnosis, treatment and follow-up.** *Ann Oncol* 2012, **23**(Suppl 7):110–119.
2. Sipos JA, Mazzaferri EL: **Thyroid cancer epidemiology and prognostic variables.** *Clin Oncol (R Coll Radiol)* 2010, **22**:395–404.
3. Goncalves Filho J, Kowalski LP: **Surgical complications after thyroid surgery performed in a cancer hospital.** *Otolaryngol Head Neck Surg* 2005, **132**:490–494.
4. Cooper MS, Gittoes NJ: **Diagnosis and management of hypocalcaemia.** *BMJ* 2008, **336**:1298–1302.
5. Mitchell DM, Regan S, Cooley MR, Lauter KB, Vrla MC, Becker CB, Burnett-Bowie SA, Mannstadt M: **Long-term follow-up of patients with hypoparathyroidism.** *J Clin Endocrinol Metab* 2012, **97**:4507–4514.
6. Rubin MR, Bilezikian JP: **Hypoparathyroidism: clinical features, skeletal microstructure and parathyroid hormone replacement.** *Arq Bras Endocrinol Metabol* 2010, **54**:220–226.
7. Hayward NJ, Grodski S, Yeung M, Johnson WR, Serpell J: **Recurrent laryngeal nerve injury in thyroid surgery: a review.** *ANZ J Surg* 2013, **83**:15–21.
8. Chandrasekhar SS, Randolph GW, Seidman MD, Rosenfeld RM, Angelos P, Barkmeier-Kraemer J, Benninger MS, Blumin JH, Dennis G, Hanks J, Haymart MR, Kloos RT, Seals B, Schreibstein JM, Thomas MA, Waddington C, Warren B, Robertson PJ: **Clinical practice guideline: improving voice outcomes after thyroid surgery.** *Otolaryngol Head Neck Surg* 2013, **148**(6 Suppl):1–37.
9. Kuhn MA, Bloom G, Myssiorek D: **Patient perspectives on dysphonia after thyroidectomy for thyroid cancer.** *J Voice* 2013, **27**:111–114.
10. Cooper DS, Doherty GM, Haugen BR, Kloos RT, Lee SL, Mandel SJ, Mazzaferri EL, McIver B, Pacini F, Schlumberger M, Sherman SI, Steward DL, Tuttle RM: **Revised American Thyroid Association management guidelines for patients with thyroid nodules and differentiated thyroid cancer.** *Thyroid* 2009, **19**:1167–1214.
11. Cooper DS: **TSH suppressive therapy: an overview of long-term clinical consequences.** *Hormones (Athens)* 2010, **9**:57–59.

12. Sugitani I, Fujimoto Y: **Effect of postoperative thyrotropin suppressive therapy on bone mineral density in patients with papillary thyroid carcinoma: a prospective controlled study.** *Surgery* 2011, **150:**1250–1257.
13. Bauer DC, Ettinger B, Nevitt MC, Stone KL: **Risk for fracture in women with low serum levels of thyroid-stimulating hormone.** *Ann Intern Med* 2001, **134:**561–568.
14. Heemstra KA, Hamdy NA, Romijn JA, Smit JW: **The effects of thyrotropin-suppressive therapy on bone metabolism in patients with well-differentiated thyroid carcinoma.** *Thyroid* 2006, **16:**583–591.
15. Mazokopakis EE, Starakis IK, Papadomanolaki MG, Batistakis AG, Papadakis JA: **Changes of bone mineral density in pre-menopausal women with differentiated thyroid cancer receiving L-thyroxine suppressive therapy.** *Curr Med Res Opin* 2006, **22:**1369–1373.
16. Reverter JL, Colome E, Holgado S, Aguilera E, Soldevila B, Mateo L, Sanmarti A: **Bone mineral density and bone fracture in male patients receiving long-term suppressive levothyroxine treatment for differentiated thyroid carcinoma.** *Endocrine* 2010, **37:**467–472.
17. Biondi B, Cooper DS: **The clinical significance of subclinical thyroid dysfunction.** *Endocr Rev* 2008, **29:**76–131.
18. Mercuro G, Panzuto MG, Bina A, Leo M, Cabula R, Petrini L, Pigliaru F, Mariotti S: **Cardiac function, physical exercise capacity, and quality of life during long-term thyrotropin-suppressive therapy with levothyroxine: effect of individual dose tailoring.** *J Clin Endocrinol Metab* 2000, **85:**159–164.
19. Shargorodsky M, Serov S, Gavish D, Leibovitz E, Harpaz D, Zimlichman R: **Long-term thyrotropin-suppressive therapy with levothyroxine impairs small and large artery elasticity and increases left ventricular mass in patients with thyroid carcinoma.** *Thyroid* 2006, **16:**381–386.
20. Tanaka K, Sonoo H: **Current trends in TSH suppression therapy for patients with papillary thyroid carcinoma in Japan: results of a questionnaire distributed to councilors of the Japanese society of thyroid surgery.** *Surg Today* 2012, **42:**633–638.

8

Proposed algorithm for management of patients with thyroid nodules/focal lesions, based on ultrasound (US) and fine-needle aspiration biopsy (FNAB); our own experience

Zbigniew Adamczewski and Andrzej Lewiński*

Abstract

Background: The standard management in patients with thyroid nodules is to assess the risk of malignancy, based on cytological examination. On the other hand, there are thyroid patterns of ultrasound (US) image, associated with an increased risk of malignancy.
The aim of our study was to create a diagnostic algorithm that would employ both data from US examination (expressed by a total score, according to our scoring system) and FNAB results, classified according to Bethesda system (The Bethesda System for Reporting Thyroid Cytopathology - TBSRTC categories).

Material and methods: 100 thyroid cancer foci (94 papillary carcinomas, 4 medullary carcinomas, 2 undifferentiated carcinomas) and 100 benign focal lesions were selected during postoperative histopathological examination of thyroid glands excised during surgery from 111 patients. The corresponding US images of each lesion – performed in the course of preoperative diagnostics – were evaluated for the presence of seven (7) different features in US image, suggesting a malignant character of lesion, viz. vascularity, i.e., the increased central intranodular blood flows, microcalcifications, "taller-than-wide" orientation, solid composition, hypoechogenicity, irregular margin and either absence of peripheral halo or the presence of outer shell of uneven thickness, surrounding the lesion. The sensitivity, specificity, positive predictive values, negative predictive values and odds ratios for each US feature were calculated.

Results: In US image of the analyzed cancer foci, we obtained the following values of odds ratio for each of the above mentioned features suggesting malignancy: "taller-than-wide" orientation - odds ratio - 301.0, microcalcifications - 24.67, increased intranodular vascularity - 20.44, hypoechogenicity - 18.61, irregular margins - 7.81, absence of halo - 5.88, and solid composition - 4.16.
Taking into account our own experience and the present data, in juxtaposition with the opinions of other authors, we propose a division of US features into 3 groups of different prognostic importance, expressed by a total score calculated based on our scoring system. Accordingly, microcalcifications, "taller-than-wide" orientation, the increased intranodular vascularity, and hypoechogenicity constitute one group - each of the features in this group is awarded 1 point. In turn, the characteristics of minor prognostic importance, such as irregular margin, absence of halo, solid composition, and large size (a diameter longer than 3.0 cm) - are associated with the granting 0.5 points each. The most important prognostic features – a rapid growth (enlargement) of nodules/focal lesions and a presence of pathologically altered lymph nodes are associated with the granting 3 points for each.

(Continued on next page)

* Correspondence: alewin@csk.umed.lodz.pl
Department of Endocrinology and Metabolic Diseases, Medical University of Lodz, Polish Mother's Memorial Hospital – Research Institute, Rzgowska 281/289, 93-338, Lodz, Poland

(Continued from previous page)

Our scoring system can be applied in order to better assessment of thyroid US patterns in whole. In patients with a total score ranging from 0 < 4 points there is US pattern of a low risk of malignancy, with ≥ 4 < 7 points - intermediate risk, and in patients with a score ≥ 7 points – a high risk in question.

Conclusion: Complementary use of our scoring system and FNAB TBSRTC categories can help to make optimal clinical decisions as regards the selection of treatment strategy.

Background

Common use of ultrasonography (US) in the diagnostics of thyroid diseases and of other diseases in the neck region caused rapid increase of the number of detected impalpable, asymptomatic lesions in the gland. According to some authors, it allows to visualize 10 times more US lesions than the number of palpable nodules detected during the physical examination [1-3]. It creates diagnostic and therapeutic dilemmas, dominated by the question: what is the most proper medical management – observation and careful monitoring of existing nodule, or – the opposite - referring the patients for surgery. While follow up, the most frequent way to proceed are the repeated US examination and a fine needle aspiration biopsy (FNAB). Even though the biopsy is considered by many doctors as a basis for further monitoring, performing FNAB of any identified lesions may not be prudent [4,5]. It happens that FNAB confirms the benign nature of the lesion and, nevertheless, it is quite frequently repeated (often many times) in spite of the fact that US image pattern does not change during a long-term observation. On the other hand, the surgical treatment in patients with obvious clinical signs and symptoms of malignant neoplastic disease is sometimes delayed because of unnecessary diagnostic procedures (e.g., due to awaiting for recommended time after which FNAB should be performed again). Thus, the endocrinologist - while diagnosing the thyroid nodule - cannot forget a question of fundamental importance – what is a bigger threat to the patients – observation, i.e., monitoring of lesion and live with the existing thyroid nodule or subjecting the patient to surgical treatment of his/her thyroid.

The aim of our study was to create an algorithm that would employ both data from US examination and FNAB results, classified according to Bethesda recommendations (The Bethesda System for Reporting Thyroid Cytopathology - TBSRTC categories), in order to optimise diagnostic and therapeutic management in case of nodules/US focal lesions in the thyroid [6].

Methods

The algorithm was developed on the basis of prospective diagnostics in patients with nodules/US focal lesions of the thyroid, hospitalized in the Department of Endocrinology and Metabolic Diseases, in the time period from January 2008 to June 2012, who – then - were referred for surgery. At the same time, data of other authors on assessing the risk of thyroid malignancy, based on US characteristics, FNAB results, family medical history, and - above all - clinical signs and symptoms were considered.

100 thyroid cancer foci (94 papillary carcinomas, 4 medullary carcinomas, 2 undifferentiated carcinomas) and 100 benign focal lesions were selected during postoperative histopathological examination of thyroid glands excised during surgery carried out in 111 patients, aged 23 to 79 years (mean age – 57.0 years). The corresponding US images of each lesion – obtained in the course of preoperative diagnostics – were evaluated in order to assess seven (7) US characteristics, the most useful in differentiating benign and malignant lesions [7-10]. All examinations were performed by the same diagnostician, with extensive experience in thyroid US, using Toshiba Aplio XG US device with a linear probe PLT 1204 BT 12–18 MHz. An evaluation of focal lesions was carried out in the grey scale (B-mode), also with use of Power-Doppler method.

The following US features were subjected to analysis (for each characteristics - an appearance suggesting a malignant character of lesion is specified, followed by the respective image of the same feature, speaking for its benign nature):

1. Vascularity - defined as the presence of irregular chaotic intranodular hypervascularity; also images of a total absence of blood flow in hypoechogenic, solid lesions were included into that group; in contrast to the peripheral, subcapsular blood flows, suggesting benign lesions [11,12].
2. Calcifications - assessed as the presence of microcalcifications, also their coexistence with other forms of calcifications (e.g., dystrophic); in contrast to the absence of calcifications, the latter suggesting benign nature of lesions.
3. Orientation - "taller than wide" shape of lesion in transverse and/or longitudinal planes; in contrast to all other lesion shapes.
4. Composition - solid lesions, also mixed lesions with cystic component not exceeding 10% of the volume; in contrast to lesions with cystic parts greater than 10% of total volume and/or to solely cystic lesions.

Table 1 Distribution of US characteristics in malignant and benign thyroid lesions; p values indicating a statistical significance are marked by bold

Parameter	No. of cases (%)	Malignant lesions No. of cases (%)	Benign lesions No. of cases (%)	p value
Vascularity				
Intranodular and increased or completely absent	150 (75.0)	96 (64.0)	54 (46.0)	**<0.0001**
Peripheral, subcapsular	50 (25.0)	4 (8.0)	46 (92.0)	
Microcalcifications				
Positive	128 (64.0)	93 (72.7)	35 (27.3)	**<0.0001**
Negative	72 (36.0)	7 (9.7)	65 (90.2)	
Orientation				
Taller-than-wide	88 (44.0)	86 (97.7)	2 (2.3)	**<0.0001**
Wider-than-tall or of other shape	112 (56.0)	14 (12.5)	98 (87.5)	
Composition				
Solid	173 (86.5)	94 (54.3)	79 (65.7)	**0.0032**
Mixed	27 (23.5)	6 (22.2)	21 (77.8)	
Echogenicity				
Hypoechogenic	106 (53.0)	84 (79.2)	22 (20.1)	**<0.0001**
Isoechogenic	94 (47.0)	16 (17.0)	78 (83.0)	
Margins				
Irregular	107 (53.5)	77 (71.9)	30 (28.1)	**<0.0001**
Well circumscribed	93 (46.5)	23 (24.7)	70 (75.3)	
Peripheral Halo				
Absent or irregular, thick	111 (55.0)	76 (68.0)	35 (32.0)	**<0.0001**
Present, thin and regular	89 (45.0)	24 (27.0)	65 (73.0)	

5. Echogenicity - understood as hypoechogenicity, defined as a reduced ("darker") echogenicity (similar to the echogenicity of muscles, surrounding the thyroid); in contrast to normal thyroid echogenicity (isoechogenicity) in benign lesions.
6. Margin - blurred and poorly defined; in contrast to well-differentiated regular margin.
7. Halo - the absence of halo, or the presence of outer shell (rim) of uneven thickness that surrounds the lesion; in contrast to the presence of thin, regular halo which speaks for a benign nature of lesion.

Statistical analysis

The statistical analysis was performed with use of the Prism 5.0 software (GraphPad, La Jolla, USA). Fisher exact test was used to analyze distribution of the obtained results between the examined benign and malignant lesions. For each tested variable – the sensitivity, specificity, positive predictive values (PPV), negative predictive values (NPV) and odds ratios were estimated. Additionally, the 95% confidence intervals of these parameters were determined. The results were regarded as significant for $p < 0.05$.

Table 2 Values of sensitivity, specificity, PPV and NPV of the analyzed US characteristics (parameters)

Parameter	Sensitivity (%)	Specificity (%)	PPV (%)	NPV (%)
Vascularity	96 (90–99)	46 (36–56)	64 (56–72)	92 (80–98)
Microcalcifications	93 (86–97)	65 (54–74)	73 (64–80)	90 (80–96)
Orientation	86 (77–92)	98 (93–99)	97 (92–99)	87 (80–93)
Composition	94 (87–97)	21 (13–30)	54 (46–61)	77 (57–91)
Echogenicity	84 (75–90)	78 (68–85)	79 (70–86)	82 (73–89)
Margins	77 (67–84)	70 (60–78)	72 (62–80)	75 (65–83)
Peripheral Halo	76 (66–84)	65 (56–74)	68 (59–77)	73 (62–82)

The 95% confidence intervals are given in the brackets.

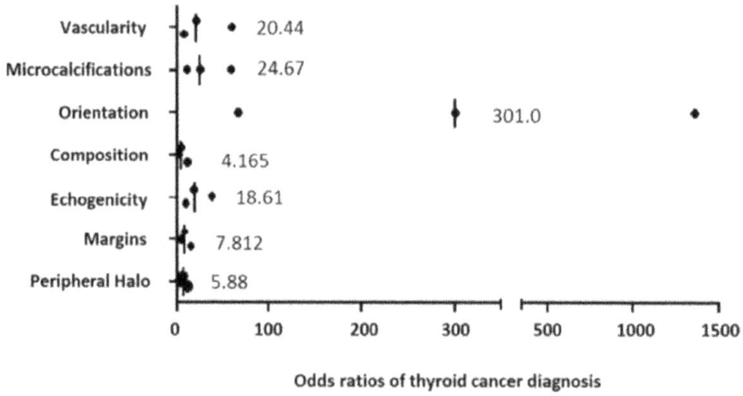

Figure 1 Odds ratios of analyzed US characteristics in diagnostics of malignant thyroid lesions. The values on the figure indicate the median odds ratio, with neighboring dots indicating the boundaries of 95% confidence intervals.

Results

The comparison of distribution of US characteristics, assessed in two (2) analyzed groups, showed the presence of significant statistical differences in the frequency of their occurrence, depending on the histopathological diagnosis (benign vs malignant lesions) (Table 1).

Table 2 presents the obtained values of sensitivity and specificity, also positive predictive values (PPV) and negative predictive values (NPV) of the analyzed parameters. Our results are comparable with data from reports of other authors [8,9,12-16].

Simultaneously, the assessment of the odds ratios of thyroid cancer diagnosis, in the presence of the particular characteristics evaluated in each case, showed the increased risk of malignancy. The highest values of odds ratios were recorded in case of lesions "taller-than-wide" in shape in transverse and/or longitudinal planes, also the presence of microcalcifications, the incorrect pattern of vascularisation (intranodular and increased or completely absent) and/or hypoechogenicity were related to the increased cancer risk. This also applied - but to a lesser extent - to the lesions such as solid composition, the absence of halo, and blurred margins (Figure 1).

In addition, data from numerous reports of other authors indicate an increased risk of malignancy, especially in the case of:

- the rapid growth of thyroid nodules/focal lesions [17] which is defined as a 20% increase in minimum two dimensions (at least - 2 mm) in the follow-up period shorter than 18 months [18];
- thyroid lesions coexisting with lymphadenopathy that may suggest nodal metastases [19,20].

It is to be recalled that cervical US is the optimal method for searching lymph node metastases [18]. This examination allows to reveal more than 90% of the current metastases [21], the presence of which is diagnosed in approximately 25% microcarcinomas and even more frequently, up to 50% in larger tumours, with significant extrathyroidal extension, *viz.* T_4 tumour stage in TNM scale [9,22]. However, it should be stressed that the simultaneous presence of the thyroid tumour and enlarged cervical lymph nodes does not necessarily constitute evidence of a direct causal relation;

Table 3 Summary of points awarded depending on the US characteristics

Most important characteristic (each feature – 3 points)	
G	Growth of nodules (resulting in rapid enlargement)
L	Pathologically altered lymph nodes
Major prognostic characteristic (each feature – 1 point)	
O	Orientation (shape)
C1	Calcifications (especially microcalcifications)
V	Vascularity (intranodular increased or absent)
E	Echogenicity (in particular hypoechogenicity)
Minor prognostic characteristic (each feature – 0.5 point)	
M	Margin (blurred and poorly defined)
H	Halo (absent or irregular and thick)
C2	Composition (solid)
D	Diameter (longer than 3.0 cm)

Table 4 The scoring system of US patterns, applied for thyroid nodules/focal lesions

Risk of malignancy, as assessed on the basis of US pattern	A total score
Low risk	0 < 4 points
Intermediate risk	≥ 4 < 7 points
High risk	≥ 7 points

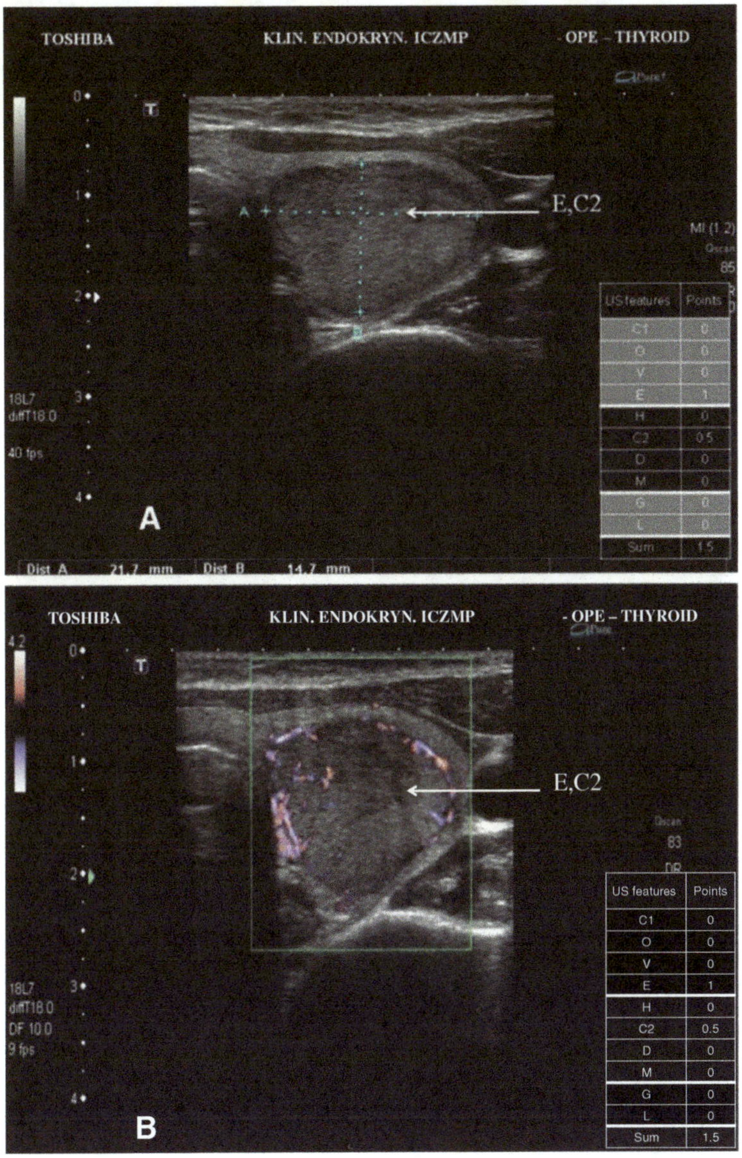

Figure 2 Low risk thyroid nodule/focal lesion US pattern. A. Ultrasound picture of the thyroid lesion (B-mode). The scoring system – 1.5 points (low risk US pattern 0 < 4 points); E – hypoechogenicity; C2 – solid composition; FNAB cytology in this case - category II TBSRTC; management - observation and repeat FNAB examination after 18 months. **B.** Ultrasound picture of the thyroid lesion (Power Doppler), peripheral blood flows.

– the presence of thyroid tumours with a diameter exceeding 3–4 cm [23]; in tumours of larger size - follicular carcinomas are diagnosed more frequently [23,24]. In these cases - FNAB, used as the sole diagnostic test, does not allow formulation of the final diagnosis and confirmation of malignant nature of tumours and its result always must be evaluated with reference to clinical and US examinations.

Three characteristics listed above (rapid growth, enlarged lymph nodes, tumour size) have not been evaluated or subjected to statistical calculations in our present study for the reasons which we would like to explain. Follow-up of changes in the size of the analyzed lesions was not possible because the majority of US examinations were performed directly prior to surgery, and the patients submitted to surgical treatment were not previously hospitalised and diagnosed in our Department.

Due to the fact that the coexistence of thyroid lesions and of abnormal lymph nodes was found exclusively in case of malignant foci, we decided to exclude that feature from the statistical evaluation.

The diameter of all lesions examined by us did not exceed 3.0 cm, thus it was not possible to use the size of

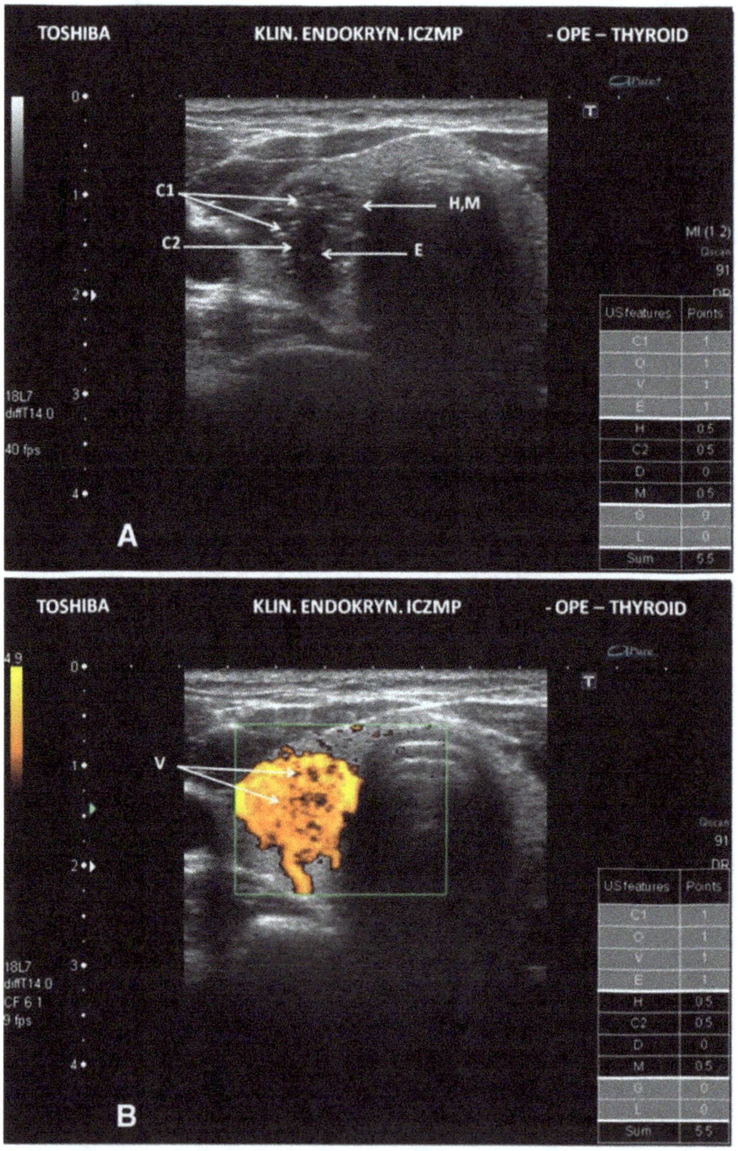

Figure 3 Intermediate risk thyroid nodule/focal lesion US pattern. A. Ultrasound picture of the thyroid lesion (B-mode). The scoring system - 5.5 points (intermediate risk US pattern ≥ 4 < 7 points); C1 – microcalcifications; O – orientation - "taller-than-wide" shape – not shown in the figure; E – hypoechogenicity; H – the absence of "halo"; C2 – solid composition; D – diameter - below 3 cm (not shown); M – irregular margin; FNAB cytology in this case - category IV TBSRTC; management - recommend surgery. **B.** Ultrasound picture of the thyroid lesion (Power Doppler). The scoring system - 5.5 points (intermediate risk US pattern ≥ 4 < 7 points); V – the increased intranodular blood flows.

lesions for differentiation of the studied groups (malignant vs benign).

Taking into account our own observations, in juxtaposition with the opinions of other authors [4,5,19,20,25-27], we propose a division of US features into 3 groups of different prognostic importance. Accordingly, microcalcifications, "taller-than-wide" orientation, the incorrect pattern of vascularisation, and hypoechogenicity constitute one group - each of the features in this group is awarded 1 point. In turn, the characteristics of minor prognostic importance, such as irregular margin, absence of halo, solid composition, and large size (a diameter longer than 3.0 cm) - are associated with the granting 0.5 points each. The most important prognostic features – a rapid growth resulting in the enlargement of nodules/focal lesions, as well as a presence of pathologically altered lymph nodes are associated with the granting 3 points for each (Table 3).

Having assigned the points for each characteristics, we created the scoring system that is applied for better assessment of thyroid US patterns in whole.

A total score constitutes the basis to assign the patients to groups of varying degree of the risk of malignancy. Accordingly, patients with a total score ranging from 0 to less than 4 points belong to the group of low risk US pattern, patients with a score from 4 to less than 7 points represent US pattern of intermediate risk of malignancy, and in patients with a score 7 points and more – US pattern of a high risk of malignancy occurs (Table 4).

We have illustrated the practical application of our scoring system of the thyroid US patterns in Figures 2A, 2B, 3A, 3B, 4A and 4B.

Discussion

It is well known that none of the individual US features allows to differentiate malignant from benign thyroid lesions. However, finding in US image of nodule/focal lesion one (1) or more than one suspicious features, correlates well with the risk of malignancy. This fact is commonly used for the qualification of patients with nodules/focal lesions for FNAB cytology.

The current system of cytological diagnoses (TBSRTC) greatly facilitates therapeutic decisions (Table 5) [6]. This

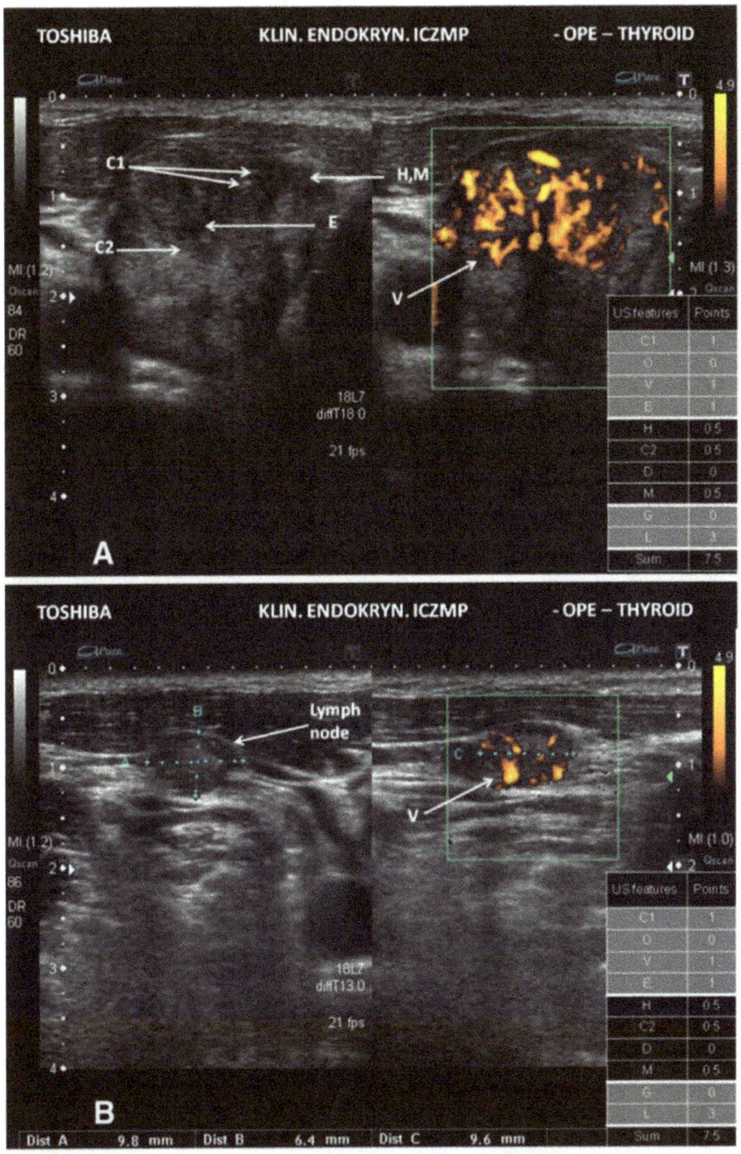

Figure 4 High risk thyroid nodule/focal lesion US pattern. A. Ultrasound picture of the thyroid lesion (B-mode, Power Doppler). The scoring system - 7.5 points (high risk US pattern ≥ 7 points); C1 – microcalcifications; O – orientation – shape other than "taller-than-wide" – not shown in the figure; V - the increased intranodular blood flows; E – hypoechogenicity; H – the absence of "halo"; C2 – solid composition; D – diameter - below 3 cm (not shown); M – irregular margin; FNAB cytology in this case - category V TBSRTC; management - recommend surgery.
B. Ultrasound picture of the metastatic lymph node in the same case (B-mode, Power Doppler). The scoring system - 7.5 points (high risk US pattern ≥ 7 points); the increased blood flows, mainly peripheral, in the metastatic lymph node.

Table 5 The Bethesda System for Reporting Thyroid Cytopathology (TBSRTC) – according to Cibas and Ali [6]

Diagnostic category	Risk of malignancy (%)
I Nondiagnostic or unsatisfactory	1-4
II Benign	0-3
III Atypia of undetermined significance or follicular lesion of undetermined significance	5-15
IV Follicular neoplasm or suspicious for a follicular neoplasm	15-30
V Suspicious for malignancy	60-75
VI Malignant	97-99

applies mainly to diagnoses of malignant lesions (category VI TBSRTC) or a suspicion of malignancy (category V TBSRTC) which both create the need for urgent referral for surgery, in order to perform a total thyroidectomy, except cases inoperable at the time of diagnosis.

Significantly more difficulties with making a therapeutic decision appear when FNAB belongs to the category IV TBSRTC - "follicular neoplasm or suspicious for a follicular neoplasm " or to category III TBSRTC - "follicular lesion of undetermined significance/atypia of undetermined significance". These diagnoses require a completely different clinical approach. Category IV TBSRTC is believed to be a final result, confirmed by the opinion of two independent pathologists. Repeating FNAB in such cases is not expected to provide additional benefits, thus, a repeated FNAB should be performed only in case of changes in the US pattern of lesions. The diagnosis of category III TBSRTC is "a category of exclusion" and should be treated as an optional diagnosis, thus, it can only ultimately be used. The main difference - when compared to category IV - is that category III requires a repeat biopsy, like in case nondiagnostic or unsatisfactory FNAB results (category I TBSRTC). One cannot forget that even in the case of benign lesions (category II TBSRTC) false-negative results are still possible and a risk of malignancy in such cases reaches up to 3% [6].

However, it should be emphasized that the thyroid US and FNAB cytology are diagnostic tests that should not always decide about the fate of our patient and about recommending him/her the surgical treatment. Many clinical parameters have long been recognized as predictors of malignancy in patients with thyroid nodules/lesions. Such factors include family medical history (genetic background), age younger than 20 and older than 60 years, irradiation of the neck and head area (particularly in the childhood) and male sex [4,18,28]. Moreover, certain clinical circumstances, e.g., if the patient complains of hoarseness (which is not a result of *stricte* laryngeal disease), or of ache in the tumour and dysphagia - usually caused by a firm thyroid tumour, may indicate a malignant character of lesion and may require an inquisitive intense diagnostics of any type, and appropriate treatment, in most cases of the radical type.

Based on the results of our observations, in combination with data of other authors, we decided to stratificate the risk of malignancy, depending on the ascertained signs and symptoms, US features, FNAB results according to TBSRTC categories, and – in consequence - we created the algorithm of diagnostic and therapeutic management, the use of which seems to be most favourable for patients with thyroid problems (nodules/focal lesions) (Figure 5).

We are aware of the fact that the assumption underlying of this study, namely comparison of distribution of US characteristics in the two groups of the same number of examined lesions, does not apply in the real epidemiological

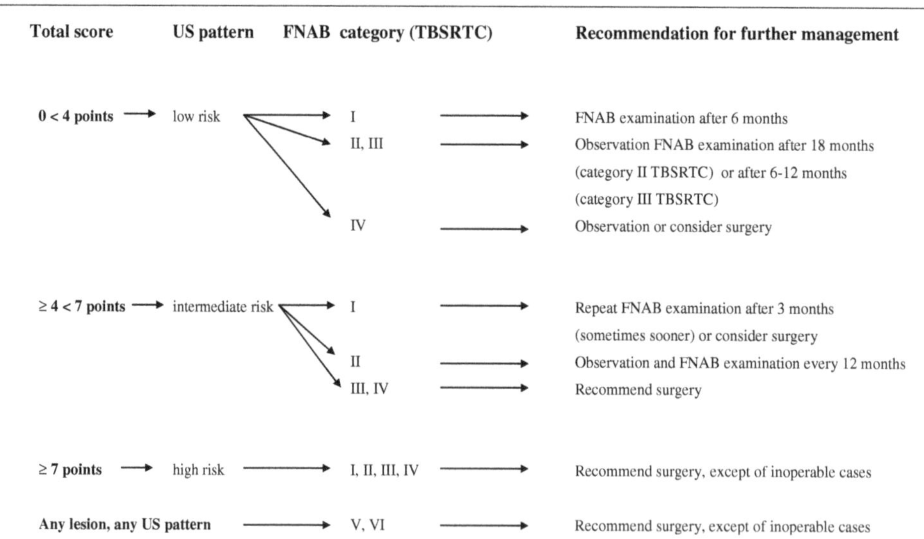

Figure 5 The algorithm of diagnostic and therapeutic management in thyroid nodules/focal lesions.

situation. However, we believe that such a design of the study highlights the most important US characteristics, the presence of which correlates - to the greatest extent - with the risk of malignancy. The presented algorithm of management in patients with thyroid problems is designed to highlight the complementarity of diagnostic procedures, such as US and FNAB. Simultaneously, we would like to stress that US is not only a tool used for selection of nodules which should be examined by FNAB but is also a diagnostic method, the outcomes of which can constitute a basis for the final therapeutic decision.

Conclusions

The presented algorithm, as many other previously developed to assess the nature of thyroid lesions, does not solve all the possible encountered clinical problems. However, by taking into consideration the important US characteristics, related to an increased risk of malignancy, in combination with cytological assessment of lesions, at the same time - by paying attention on the significance of clinical data from medical history and physical examination, it fulfils expectations in daily clinical practice and is helpful in making the proper diagnostic and therapeutic decisions.

Competing interests

The authors declare that they have no competing interests.

Authors' contributions

ZA designed the study, performed US examinations and participated in writing a manuscript. AL was involved in coordination of the study and supervised preparation of the final version of manuscript. Both authors read and approved the final manuscript.

Acknowledgments

This study was supported by statutory funds from the Medical University of Lodz, Poland (No. 503/1-107-03/503-01).

References

1. Frates MC, Benson CB, Charboneau JW, Cibas ES, Clark OH, Coleman BG, Cronan JJ, Doubilet PM, Evans DB, Goellner JR, Hay ID, Hertzberg BS, Intenzo CM, Jeffrey RB, Langer JE, Larsen PR, Mandel SJ, Middleton WD, Reading CC, Sherman SI, Tessler FN: **Management of thyroid nodules detected at US: Society of Radiologists in Ultrasound consensus conference statement.** *Ultrasound Q* 2006, **22**:231–238. discussion 239–240.
2. McCartney CR, Stukenborg GJ: **Decision analysis of discordant thyroid nodule biopsy guideline criteria.** *J Clin Endocrinol Metab* 2008, **93**:3037–3044.
3. Peli M, Capalbo E, Lovisatti M, Cosentino M, Berti E, Mattai Dal Moro R, Cariati M: **Ultrasound guided fine-needle aspiration biopsy of thyroid nodules: Guidelines and recommendations vs clinical practice; a 12-month study of 89 patients.** *J Ultrasound* 2012, **15**:102–107.
4. Horvath E, Majlis S, Rossi R, Franco C, Niedmann JP, Castro A, Dominguez M: **An ultrasonogram reporting system for thyroid nodules stratifying cancer risk for clinical management.** *J Clin Endocrinol Metab* 2009, **94**:1748–1751.
5. Kang HW, No JH, Chung JH, Min YK, Lee MS, Lee MK, Yang JH, Kim KW: **Prevalence, clinical and ultrasonographic characteristics of thyroid incidentalomas.** *Thyroid* 2004, **14**:29–33.
6. Cibas ES, Ali SZ: **The Bethesda System for Reporting Thyroid Cytopathology.** *Thyroid* 2009, **19**:1159–1165.
7. Moon WJ, Jung SL, Lee JH, Na DG, Baek JH, Lee YH, Kim J, Kim HS, Byun JS, Lee DH: **Benign and malignant thyroid nodules: US differentiation–multicenter retrospective study.** *Radiology* 2008, **247**:762–770.
8. Frates MC, Benson CB, Doubilet PM, Kunreuther E, Contreras M, Cibas ES, Orcutt J, Moore FD Jr, Larsen PR, Marqusee E, Alexander EK: **Prevalence and distribution of carcinoma in patients with solitary and multiple thyroid nodules on sonography.** *J Clin Endocrinol Metab* 2006, **91**:3411–3417.
9. Papini E, Guglielmi R, Bianchini A, Crescenzi A, Taccogna S, Nardi F, Panunzi C, Rinaldi R, Toscano V, Pacella CM: **Risk of malignancy in nonpalpable thyroid nodules: predictive value of ultrasound and color-Doppler features.** *J Clin Endocrinol Metab* 2002, **87**:1941–1946.
10. Alexander EK, Marqusee E, Orcutt J, Benson CB, Frates MC, Doubilet PM, Cibas ES, Atri A: **Thyroid nodule shape and prediction of malignancy.** *Thyroid* 2004, **14**:953–958.
11. Moon HJ, Kwak JY, Kim MJ, Son EJ, Kim EK: **Can vascularity at power Doppler US help predict thyroid malignancy?** *Radiology* 2010, **255**:260–269.
12. Bakhshaee M, Davoudi Y, Mehrabi M, Layegh P, Mirsadaee S, Rad MP, Leyegh P: **Vascular pattern and spectral parameters of power Doppler ultrasound as predictors of malignancy risk in thyroid nodules.** *Laryngoscope* 2008, **118**:2182–2186.
13. Fish SA, Langer JE, Mandel SJ: **Sonographic imaging of thyroid nodules and cervical lymph nodes.** *Endocrinol Metab Clin North Am* 2008, **37**:401–417.
14. Cappelli C, Pirola I, Cumetti D, Micheletti L, Tironi A, Gandossi E, Martino E, Cherubini L, Agosti B, Castellano M, Mattanza C, Rosei EA: **Is the anteroposterior and transverse diameter ratio of nonpalpable thyroid nodules a sonographic criteria for recommending fine-needle aspiration cytology?** *Clin Endocrinol (Oxf)* 2005, **63**:689–693.
15. Kim DL, Song KH, Kim SK: **High prevalence of carcinoma in ultrasonography-guided fine needle aspiration cytology of thyroid nodules.** *Endocr J* 2008, **55**:135–142.
16. Kim EK, Park CS, Chung WY, Oh KK, Kim DI, Lee JT, Yoo HS: **New sonographic criteria for recommending fine-needle aspiration biopsy of nonpalpable solid nodules of the thyroid.** *AJR Am J Roentgenol* 2002, **178**:687–691.
17. Hoang JK, Lee WK, Lee M, Johnson D, Farrell S: **US Features of thyroid malignancy: pearls and pitfalls.** *Radiographics* 2007, **27**:847–860. discussion 861–865.
18. Cooper DS, Doherty GM, Haugen BR, Kloos RT, Lee SL, Mandel SJ, Mazzaferri EL, McIver B, Pacini F, Schlumberger M, Sherman SI, Steward DL, Tuttle RM: **Revised American Thyroid Association management guidelines for patients with thyroid nodules and differentiated thyroid cancer.** *Thyroid* 2009, **19**:1167–1214.
19. Leboulleux S, Girard E, Rose M, Travagli JP, Sabbah N, Caillou B, Hartl DM, Lassau N, Baudin E, Schlumberger M: **Ultrasound criteria of malignancy for cervical lymph nodes in patients followed up for differentiated thyroid cancer.** *J Clin Endocrinol Metab* 2007, **92**:3590–3594.
20. Sohn YM, Kwak JY, Kim EK, Moon HJ, Kim SJ, Kim MJ: **Diagnostic approach for evaluation of lymph node metastasis from thyroid cancer using ultrasound and fine-needle aspiration biopsy.** *AJR Am J Roentgenol* 2010, **194**:38–43.
21. Krajewska J, Czarniecka A, Jarzab M, Kukulska A, Handkiewicz-Junak D, Hasse-Lazar K, Gubala E, Puch Z, Paliczka E, Roskosz J: **Relapse of differentiated thyroid carcinoma in low-risk patients.** *Pol J Endocrinol* 2006, **57**:386–391.
22. Czarniecka A, Jarzab M, Krajewska J, Chmielik E, Szcześniak-Klusek B, Stobiecka E, Kokot R, Sacher A, Poltorak S, Wloch J: **Prognostic value of lymph node metastases of differentiated thyroid cancer (DTC) according to the local advancement and range of surgical excision.** *Thyroid Res* 2010, **3**:8.
23. Mihai R, Parker AJ, Roskell D, Sadler GP: **One in four patients with follicular thyroid cytology (THY3) has a thyroid carcinoma.** *Thyroid* 2009, **19**:33–37.
24. Sillery JC, Reading CC, Charboneau JW, Henrichsen TL, Hay ID, Mandrekar JN: **Thyroid follicular carcinoma: sonographic features of 50 cases.** *AJR Am J Roentgenol* 2010, **194**:44–54.
25. Moon WJ, Baek JH, Jung SL, Kim DW, Kim EK, Kim JY, Kwak JY, Lee JH, Lee JH, Lee YH, Na DG, Park JS, Park SW: **Ultrasonography and the ultrasound-based management of thyroid nodules: consensus statement and recommendations.** *Korean J Radiol* 2011, **12**:1–14.

26. Park JY, Lee HJ, Jang HW, Kim HK, Yi JH, Lee W, Kim SH: **A proposal for a thyroid imaging reporting and data system for ultrasound features of thyroid carcinoma.** *Thyroid* 2009, **19:**1257–1264.
27. Hong YJ, Son EJ, Kim EK, Kwak JY, Hong SW, Chang HS: **Positive predictive values of sonographic features of solid thyroid nodule.** *Clin Imaging* 2010, **34:**127–133.
28. Bahn RS, Castro MR: **Approach to the patient with nontoxic multinodular goiter.** *J Clin Endocrinol Metab* 2011, **96:**1202–1212.

Protective antioxidative effects of caffeic acid phenethyl ester (CAPE) in the thyroid and the liver are similar to those caused by melatonin

Agnieszka Kokoszko-Bilska[1,3], Jan Stepniak[1], Andrzej Lewinski[2,3] and Malgorzata Karbownik-Lewinska[1,3*]

Abstract

Background: Whereas oxidative reactions occur in all tissues and organs, the thyroid constitutes such an organ, in which oxidative processes are indispensable for physiological functions. In turn, numerous metabolic reactions occurring in the liver create favourable conditions for huge oxidative stress. Melatonin is a well-known antioxidant with protective effects against oxidative damage perfectly documented in many tissues, the thyroid and the liver included. Caffeic acid phenethyl ester (CAPE), a component of honeybee propolis, has been suggested to be also an effective antioxidant.

The aim of the study was to evaluate the effects of CAPE on Fenton reaction-induced oxidative damage to membrane lipids (lipid peroxidation, LPO) in porcine thyroid and liver, and to compare the results with protective effects of melatonin.

Methods: Thyroid and liver homogenates were incubated in the presence of CAPE (500; 100; 50; 10; 5.0; 1.0 μM) or melatonin (500; 100; 50; 10; 5.0; 1.0 μM), without or with addition of $FeSO_4$ (30 μM) + H_2O_2 (0.5 mM).

The level of lipid peroxidation was measured spectrophotometrically and expressed as the amount of MDA + 4-HDA (nmol) per mg of protein.

Results: Whereas CAPE decreased the basal LPO in a concentration-dependent manner in both tissues, melatonin did not change the basal LPO level. When antioxidants were used together with Fenton reaction substrates, they prevented – in a concentration-dependent manner and to a similar extent – experimentally-induced LPO in both tissues.

Conclusions: Protective antioxidative effects of CAPE in the thyroid and the liver are similar to those caused by melatonin. CAPE constitutes a promising agent in terms of its application in experimental and, possibly, clinical studies.

Keywords: Caffeic acid phenethyl ester (CAPE), Melatonin, Oxidative stress, Lipid peroxidation (LPO), Antioxidant, Thyroid, Liver

Background

Whereas oxidative reactions occur in all tissues and organs, the thyroid gland constitutes such an organ, in which oxidative processes are indispensable for physiological functions, thyroid hormone biosynthesis included. It is estimated that huge amount of reactive oxygen species (ROS), especially of hydrogen peroxide (H_2O_2), are produced in the thyroid under physiological conditions, justifying the statement that the thyroid gland is an organ of "oxidative nature" [1,2]. However, with additional oxidative abuse caused by exogenous or endogenous prooxidants, increased oxidative damage to all major cellular components, such as lipids, proteins and DNA, may occur, leading to different thyroid diseases, cancer included [1-4].

In turn, numerous metabolic reactions occurring in the liver create favourable conditions for huge oxidative stress. ROS and reactive nitrogen species (RNS), generated during

* Correspondence: mkarbownik@hotmail.com
[1]Department of Oncological Endocrinology, Medical University of Lodz, 7/9 Zeligowski St, Lodz 90-752, Poland
[3]Polish Mother's Memorial Hospital – Research Institute, 281/289, Rzgowska St, Lodz 93-338, Poland
Full list of author information is available at the end of the article

these processes, are very important factors, not only in the physiology, but also in the pathophysiology of the hepatocyte [5,6]. The significant role of increased oxidative damage in the pathogenesis of different liver diseases, such as viral hepatitis, alcoholic hepatitis, hemochromatosis, drug-induced liver injury, hepatic insulin resistance, non-alcoholic fatty liver disease or hepatocellular cancer, has been demonstrated in many experimental and clinical studies [5-8].

Due to potential huge oxidative stress in both the thyroid and the liver, effective protective mechanisms should have been developed. In these organs, the antioxidative defence systems are very extensive and comprise both enzymatic and non-enzymatic antioxidants [2,6]. On the other hand, the use of various exogenous antioxidants in both tissues – under condition of increased oxidative stress – has been shown to be beneficial in experimental (*in vitro* or *in vivo*) studies [2,5,9,10]. Unfortunately, the applicability of different antioxidants in human thyroid or liver diseases has not been yet clearly confirmed in clinical studies and still no effective antioxidative medication is available for widespread use [6-8,10]. Moreover, some antioxidants, such as ascorbic acid (vitamin C), present a dual nature, acting in different redox environment as an antioxidant or prooxidant [11].

Melatonin (N-acetyl-5-methoxytryptamine), produced in the pineal gland, as well as in numerous other tissues and organs, is a very well-known antioxidant and free radical scavenger, with protective effects against oxidative damage perfectly documented in many tissues, the thyroid and the liver included [9,12-16].

Caffeic acid phenethyl ester (CAPE), an active component of honeybee propolis extract, is structurally related to flavonoids and has been used as a traditional medicine for many years [17-19]. It is known to possess numerous biological activities including anti-inflammatory, antiviral and immunomodulatory properties [17-19]. In experimental studies, CAPE has been shown to inhibit the growth and metastasis of different types of tumor, to protect tissues from reperfusion injury in various ischemia-reperfusion models, and to suppress inflammation in a variety of tissues [20]. It has been suggested to be also an effective antioxidant [21]. CAPE might be even used as a protective agent against chemotherapy-induced and radiotherapy-induced toxicity [17].

The aim of the study was to evaluate the effects of CAPE on experimentally-induced oxidative damage to membrane lipids (lipid peroxidation, LPO) in porcine thyroid and liver homogenates, and to compare the results with protective effects of melatonin. Substrates of Fenton reaction ($Fe^{2+} + H_2O_2 \rightarrow Fe^{3+} + {}^{\bullet}OH + OH^-$) – the most basic reaction of oxidative stress – were used to induce oxidative damage to membrane lipids.

Methods

The procedures, used in the study, were approved by the Ethics Committee of the Medical University of Lodz, Poland.

Chemicals

Caffeic acid phenethyl ester (CAPE), melatonin, ferrous sulfate ($FeSO_4$) and hydrogen peroxide (H_2O_2) were purchased from Sigma-Aldrich (St. Louis, MO). The ALDetect™ Lipid Peroxidation Assay Kit for LPO was obtained from Enzo Life Science (Farmingdale, NY). All the used chemicals were of analytical grade and came from commercial sources.

Animals

Porcine thyroids and livers were collected from twenty one (21) animals at a slaughter-house, frozen on solid CO_2 and stored at −80°C until assay. Three independent experiments were performed. Therefore, three tissue pools were prepared, with seven (7) thyroid glands used for each homogenate pool.

Incubation of thyroid and liver homogenates

Thyroid and liver tissue were homogenized in ice cold 50 mM Tris–HCl buffer (pH = 7.4) (10%, w/v), and then incubated for 30 min at 37°C in the presence of examined substances.

Tissue homogenates were incubated in the presence of:

Experiment I: CAPE (500; 100; 50; 10; 5.0; 1.0 μM) alone (to check its effect on the basal LPO) or with addition of Fenton reaction substrates [$FeSO_4$ (30 μM) + H_2O_2 (0.5 mM)].

Experiment II: melatonin (500; 100; 50; 10; 5.0; 1.0 μM) alone (to check its effect on the basal LPO) or with addition of Fenton reaction substrates [$FeSO_4$ (30 μM) + H_2O_2 (0.5 mM)].

The concentrations of $FeSO_4$ (30 μM) and H_2O_2 (0.5 mM) were selected from our previous study [12].

The reactions were stopped by cooling the samples on ice. Each experiment was run in duplicate and repeated three times.

Measurement of lipid peroxidation products

Concentrations of malondialdehyde + 4-hydroxyalkenals (MDA + 4-HDA), as an index of LPO, were measured in tissue homogenates.

The homogenates were centrifuged at 3000 x g for 10 min at 4°C. The supernatant was mixed with 650 μl of a methanol:acetonitrile (1:3, v/v) solution, containing a chromogenic reagent, N-methyl-2-phenylindole, and vortexed. After addition of 150 μl of methanesulfonic acid (15.4 M), the incubation was carried out at 45°C for 40 min. The reaction between MDA + 4-HDA and N-methyl-2-phenylindole yielded a chromophore, which was spectrophotometrically measured at the absorbance of 586 nm, using a solution of 4-hydroxynonenal (10 mM) as standard.

The level of LPO was expressed as the amount of MDA + 4-HDA (nmol) per mg of protein.

Protein measurement

Protein was measured, using Bradford's method [22], with bovine albumin as the standard.

Statistical analysis

Results are expressed as means ± SE. Data were statistically analyzed, using a one-way analysis of variance (ANOVA), followed by the Student-Neuman-Keuls' test. The level of $p < 0.05$ was accepted as statistically significant.

Statistica for Windows 10.0 software was used for the statistical analysis.

Results

In both tissue homogenates, CAPE (used in concentrations of 500, 100, 50, 10 and 5 μM) decreased the basal LPO in a concentration-dependent manner (Figures 1, 2), while melatonin (in all the used concentrations) did not change the basal LPO level (Figures 3, 4).

In all the experiments, Fenton reaction substrates ($FeSO_4$ and H_2O_2), added into the incubation medium, increased the level of LPO in both the thyroid (Figures 5, 6) and the liver (Figures 7, 8).

Antioxidants, i.e. CAPE or melatonin, prevented – in a concentration-dependent manner – experimentally-induced LPO in both the thyroid (Figures 5, 6) and the liver (Figures 7, 8), when used in the same range of concentrations (i.e. 500, 100, 50 or 10 μM).

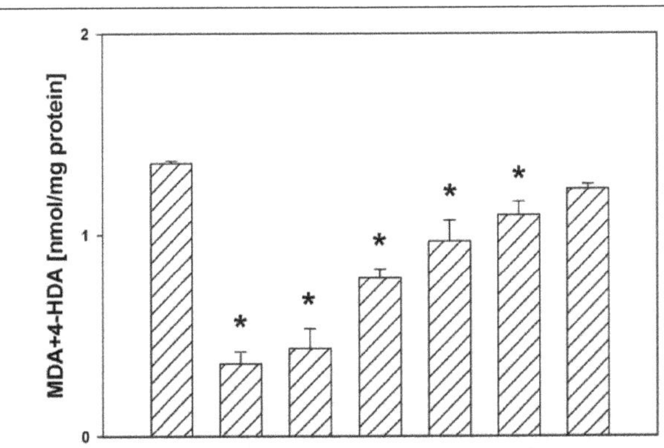

Figure 1 Concentrations of MDA + 4-HDA in porcine thyroid homogenates incubated for 30 min in presence of CAPE (500, 100, 50, 10, 5, 1 μM). Bars represent means ± SEM of three independent experiments run in duplicates. *$p < 0.05$ versus Controls.

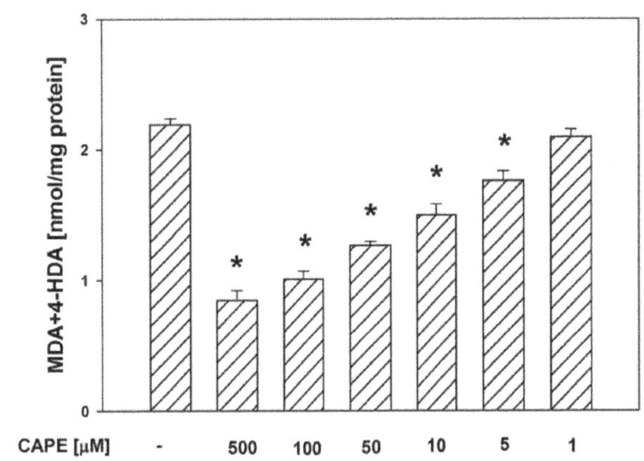

Figure 2 Concentrations of MDA + 4-HDA in porcine liver homogenates incubated for 30 min in presence of CAPE (500, 100, 50, 10, 5, 1 μM). Bars represent means ± SEM of three independent experiments run in duplicates. *$p < 0.05$ versus Controls.

Discussion

According to our knowledge, the present study has been the first attempt to evaluate the effects of CAPE on the basal and experimentally-induced LPO in the thyroid and liver homogenates under *in vitro* conditions. Also for the first time, we compared the antioxidative activities of CAPE and melatonin in the thyroid.

The selection of the thyroid and the liver for such a study is justified by several factors. The thyroid gland is an organ in which ROS are widely involved in its function and even are indispensable for physiological processes [1,2]. Hydrogen peroxide acts as an electron acceptor at each step of thyroid hormone biosynthesis and is essential for activity of thyroperoxidase (TPO) – the key enzyme in this process [1,2]. Also, the activity of antioxidative enzymes [superoxide dismutase (SOD),

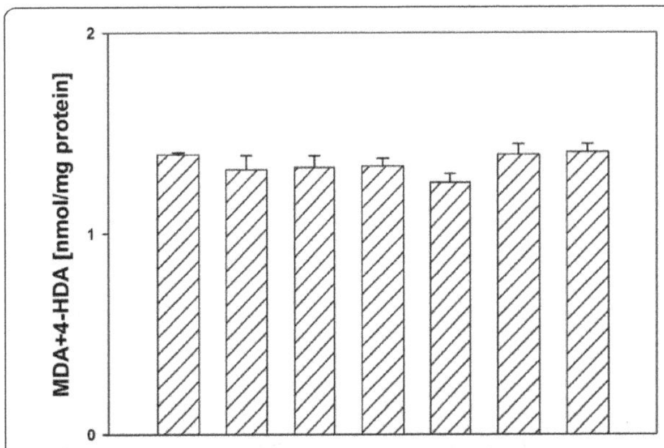

Figure 3 Concentrations of MDA + 4-HDA in porcine thyroid homogenates incubated for 30 min in presence of melatonin (500, 100, 50, 10, 5, 1 μM). Bars represent means ± SEM of three independent experiments run in duplicates.

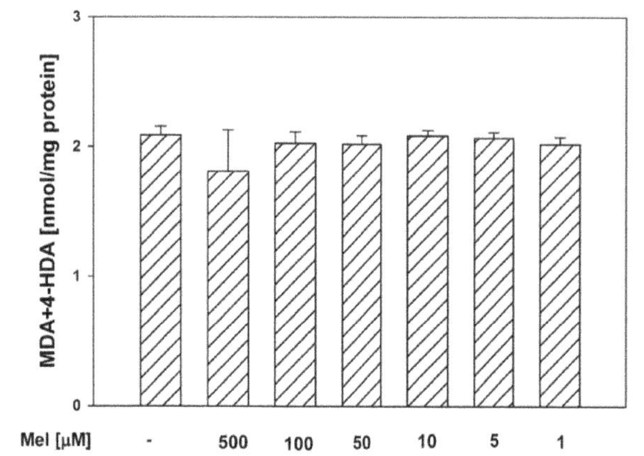

Figure 4 Concentrations of MDA + 4-HDA in porcine liver homogenates incubated for 30 min in presence of melatonin (500, 100, 50, 10, 5, 1 µM). Bars represent means ± SEM of three independent experiments run in duplicates.

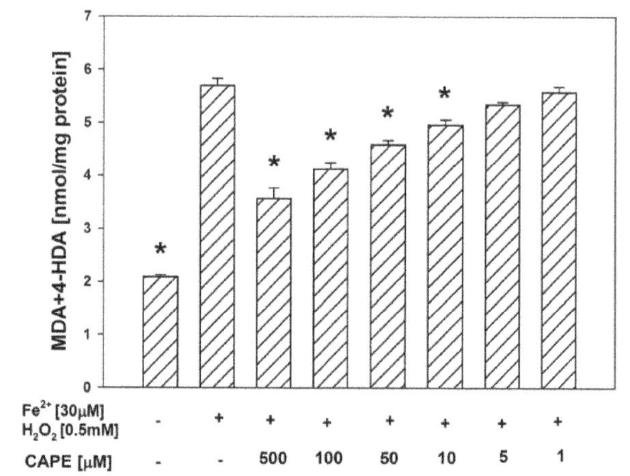

Figure 6 Concentrations of MDA + 4-HDA in porcine liver homogenates incubated for 30 min in presence of $FeSO_4$ (30 µM) + H_2O_2 (0.5 mM), or $FeSO_4$ (30 µM) + H_2O_2 (0.5 mM) + CAPE (500, 100, 50, 10, 5, 1 µM). Bars represent means ± SEM of three independent experiments run in duplicates. *$p < 0.05$ versus Fe^{2+} (30 µM) + H_2O_2 (0.5 mM).

glutathione (GSH) peroxidase (GSH-Px) and catalase (CAT)] and antioxidative proteins (such as α- and γ-tocopherols, coenzyme Q, ascorbic acid and peroxiredoxins) has been well documented in the thyroid [1,2]. The liver plays an important role in detoxifying processes. It is also one of the organs with a higher oxygen consumption rate and therefore constitutively presents a greater expression of antioxidative enzymes than those with lower oxygen consumption [5]. Hepatocytes contain a variety of antioxidant enzymatic systems (SOD, GSH-Px, CAT), so they are able to reduce the amount of oxygen free radicals generated during cellular activity [6].

Consistently with our observations, many previous studies, conducted under *in vivo* conditions, have shown that CAPE exhibits antioxidant properties in different tissues. For example, CAPE, injected intraperitoneally (*i.p.*) to 10–12 weeks old male Wistar albino rats (10 mg/kg body mass; 10-days administration), revealed protective effects on the aflatoxin B1-induced hepatoxicity by modulating free radical production: it decreased the total oxidant capacity (TOC) and glutathione S-transferase activity [23]. In another study, CAPE, given *i.p.* to 12 weeks old female Wistar albino rats (10 µmol/kg body mass; 6-days administration), prevented cisplatin-induced oxidative changes in the liver by reducing ROS production and increasing antioxidative enzyme activities (such as SOD,

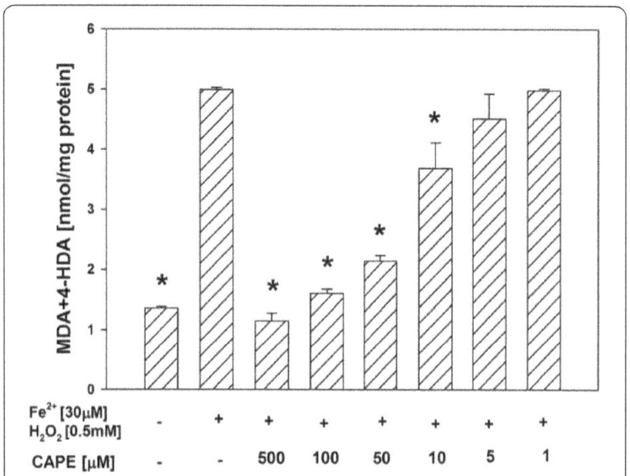

Figure 5 Concentrations of MDA + 4-HDA in porcine thyroid homogenates incubated for 30 min in presence of $FeSO_4$ (30 µM) + H_2O_2 (0.5 mM), or $FeSO_4$ (30 µM) + H_2O_2 (0.5 mM) + CAPE (500, 100, 50, 10, 5, 1 µM). Bars represent means ± SEM of three independent experiments run in duplicates. *$p < 0.05$ versus Fe^{2+} (30 µM) + H_2O_2 (0.5 mM).

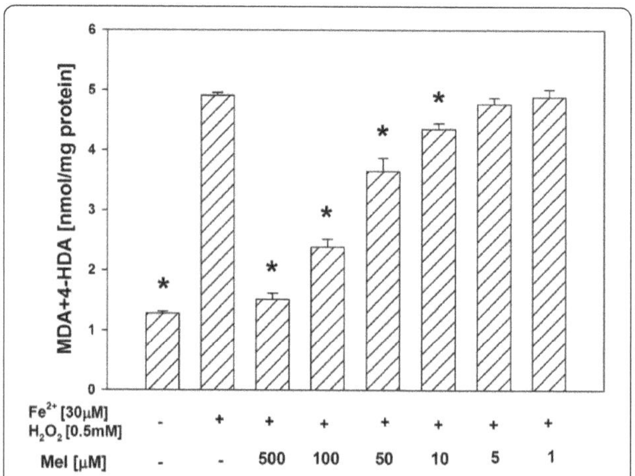

Figure 7 Concentrations of MDA + 4-HDA in porcine thyroid homogenates incubated for 30 min in presence of $FeSO_4$ (30 µM) + H_2O_2 (0.5 mM), or $FeSO_4$ (30 µM) + H_2O_2 (0.5 mM) + melatonin (500, 100, 50, 10, 5, 1 µM). Bars represent means ± SEM of three independent experiments run in duplicates. *$p < 0.05$ versus Fe^{2+} (30 µM) + H_2O_2 (0.5 mM).

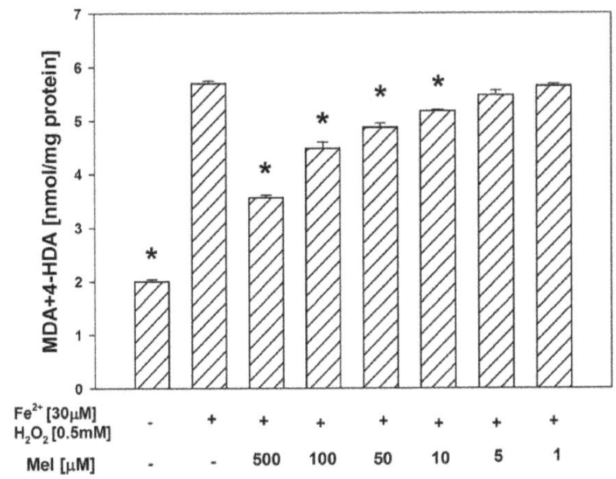

Figure 8 Concentrations of MDA + 4-HDA in porcine liver homogenates incubated for 30 min in presence of $FeSO_4$ (30 μM) + H_2O_2 (0.5 mM), or $FeSO_4$ (30 μM) + H_2O_2 (0.5 mM) + melatonin (500, 100, 50, 10, 5, 1 μM). Bars represent means ± SEM of three independent experiments run in duplicates. *$p < 0.05$ versus Fe^{2+} (30 μM) + H_2O_2 (0.5 mM).

GSH-Px and CAT) [24]. Caffeic acid phenethyl ester also revealed the protective effects against liver damage induced by cigarette smoking [25], amikacin-induced nephrotoxicity [26] and methotrexate-induced hepatorenal oxidative injury [27].

Because iron is present in TPO and H_2O_2 is indispensable for TPO activity, the thyroid gland may be exposed – under certain conditions – to excessive amounts of either Fe^{2+} or H_2O_2, or both, creating favorable conditions for additional Fenton reaction and, consequently, oxidative damage. Therefore, the observation – made by us in the present study – of the protective antioxidative effects of CAPE on Fenton reaction-induced LPO in the thyroid, seems to be of a great importance, especially that antioxidative properties of CAPE are mainly due to its free radical scavenging activity and ferrous ions chelating capacity [25]. Caffeic acid and its derivatives, such as CAPE, may chelate the ferrous ions with hydroxyl groups and then stabilizing the oxidized form of the metal ion [28].

In our study, CAPE revealed similar protective antioxidative effects to those caused by melatonin. These findings are in agreement with the results of previous studies performed under *in vivo* conditions. In 8-week old male Spraque-Dawley rats, melatonin (100 μg/kg body mass daily, for 60 days) or CAPE (10 μmol/kg body mass daily, for 60 days) preinjections reduced – to a similar extent – retinal oxidative stress caused by a long-term exposure to electromagnetic radiation (900 MHz) emitting by mobile phone [29]. In other study, melatonin and CAPE were efficient in delaying age-related cellular damage in cardiovascular system [30]. The aim of this study was to evaluate the effect of chronic melatonin (5 mg/kg body mass; injected daily for 95 days) and CAPE (15 mg/kg body mass; injected daily for 95 days) administration on the ultrastructural features, LPO levels, and enzymatic and nonenzymatic antioxidants in the heart and aorta of aged male Sprague–Dawley rats. Melatonin and CAPE administration significantly reduced the levels of MDA (as an index of LPO), increased the levels of the antioxidative enzymes and reduced age-related histological changes (such as nuclear irregularity, mitochondrial degeneration myofilament disorganization and disruption) in both heart and thoracic aorta of aged rats [30].

Of a great importance is the fact, that in the present study, in both tissue homogenates, CAPE decreased the basal LPO in a concentration-dependent manner, while melatonin (in all the used concentrations) did not change the basal LPO level. It is well known (from many *in vivo* and *in vitro* studies) that melatonin is a perfect antioxidant because of its effective protective action against damaging effects of different prooxidants and the fact that under basal conditions it does not change the level of oxidative damage to macromolecules [12,13,31,32]. The observation – made by us in the present study – of the decreasing effect of CAPE on the basal LPO level, was unexpected and also undesirable. This finding may indicate that CAPE is not as perfect antioxidant as it seemed based on the results of earlier studies. According to our knowledge, only in two studies the effect of CAPE on the basal LPO was evaluated under *in vivo* conditions [24,33]. In the quoted studies, CAPE (injected for 6 days at a dose of 10 μmol/kg body mass [24] or for 3 days at the same dose [33]) did not change the basal LPO level [24,33]. This apparent disagreement between the above quoted studies and the present results may be explained by the fact that the *in vitro* effects can not be directly extrapolated to the *in vivo* conditions.

Conclusions

In conclusion, protective antioxidative effects of CAPE in the thyroid and the liver are similar to those caused by melatonin. CAPE constitutes a promising agent in terms of its application in experimental and, possibly, clinical studies.

Abbreviations

CAPE: Caffeic acid phenethyl ester; CAT: Catalase; $FeSO_4$: Ferrous sulfate; GSH: Glutathione; GSH-Px: Glutathione peroxidase; H_2O_2: Hydrogen peroxide; LPO: Lipid peroxidation; RNS: Reactive nitrogen species; ROS: Reactive oxygen species; SOD: Superoxide dismutase; TOC: Total oxidant capacity; TPO: Thyroperoxidase.

Competing interests

The authors have declared that there is no conflict of interest.

Authors' contribution

AK-B and MK-L designed the study and prepared the final version of the manuscript. MK-L supervised the conduction of the study. AK-B and JS carried out the experiments and performed the statistical evaluation. AK-B prepared the draft of the manuscript. AL revised the final version of the manuscript. All authors read and approved the final manuscript.

Acknowledgements
The research was supported by a grant from the Medical University of Lodz [Project No. 502-03/1-107-05/502-14-014 (502-02/1-168-01/502-14-014)].

Author details
[1]Department of Oncological Endocrinology, Medical University of Lodz, 7/9 Zeligowski St, Lodz 90-752, Poland. [2]Department of Endocrinology and Metabolic Diseases, Medical University of Lodz, 281/289 Rzgowska St, Lodz 93-338, Poland. [3]Polish Mother's Memorial Hospital – Research Institute, 281/289, Rzgowska St, Lodz 93-338, Poland.

References

1. Karbownik M, Lewinski A: **The role of oxidative stress in physiological and pathological processes in the thyroid gland; possible involvement in pineal-thyroid interactions.** *Neuro Endocrinol Lett* 2003, **24**:293–303.
2. Karbownik-Lewinska M, Kokoszko-Bilska A: **Oxidative damage to macromolecules in the thyroid – experimental evidence.** *Thyroid Res* 2012, **5**:25.
3. Karbownik-Lewinska M, Stepniak J, Lewinski A: **High level of oxidized nucleosides in thyroid mitochondrial DNA; damaging effects of Fenton reaction substrates.** *Thyroid Res* 2012, **5**:24.
4. Stepniak J, Lewinski A, Karbownik-Lewinska M: **Membrane lipids and nuclear DNA are differently susceptive to Fenton reaction substrates in porcine thyroid.** *Toxicol In Vitro* 2013, **27**:71–78.
5. Tell G, Vascotto C, Tiribelli C: **Alterations in the redox state and liver damage: hints from the EASL Basic School of Hepatology.** *J Hepatol* 2013, **58**:365–374.
6. Marí M, Colell A, Morales A, von Montfort C, Garcia-Ruiz C, Fernández-Checa JC: **Redox control of liver function in health and disease.** *Antioxid Redox Signal* 2010, **12**:1295–1331.
7. Ivanov AV, Bartosch B, Smirnova OA, Isaguliants MG, Kochetkov SN: **HCV and oxidative stress in the liver.** *Viruses* 2013, **5**:439–469.
8. Leung TM, Nieto N: **CYP2E1 and oxidant stress in alcoholic and non-alcoholic fatty liver disease.** *J Hepatol* 2013, **58**:395–398.
9. Gesing A, Karbownik-Lewinska M: **Protective effects of melatonin and N-acetylserotonin on aflatoxin B1-induced lipid peroxidation in rats.** *Cell Biochem Funct* 2008, **26**:314–319.
10. Milczarek M, Stepniak J, Lewinski A, Karbownik-Lewinska M: **Potassium iodide, but not potassium iodate, as a potential protective agent against oxidative damage to membrane lipids in porcine thyroid.** *Thyroid Res* 2013, **6**:10.
11. Paolini M, Pozzetti L, Pedulli GF, Marchesi E, Cantelli-Forti G: **The nature of prooxidant activity of vitamin C.** *Life Sci* 1999, **64**:273–278.
12. Karbownik M, Lewinski A: **Melatonin reduces Fenton reaction-induced lipid peroxidation in porcine thyroid tissue.** *J Cell Biochem* 2003, **90**:806–811.
13. Karbownik M, Gitto E, Lewinski A, Reiter RJ: **Relative efficacies of indole antioxidants in reducing autoxidation and iron-induced lipid peroxidation in hamster testes.** *J Cell Biochem* 2001, **81**:693_699.
14. Karbownik M, Lewinski A, Reiter RJ: **Anticarcinogenic actions of melatonin which involve antioxidative processes: comparison with other antioxidants.** *Int J Biochem Cell Biol* 2001, **33**:735–753.
15. Altintas R, Polat A, Parlakpinar H, Vardi N, Beytur A, Oguz F, Sagir M, Yildiz A, Duran Z: **The effect of melatonin on acetylsalicylic acid-induced kidney and testis damage.** *Hum Exp Toxicol* 2014, **33**:383–395.
16. Chabra A, Shokrzadeh M, Naghshvar F, Salehi F, Ahmadi A: **Melatonin ameliorates oxidative stress and reproductive toxicity induced by cyclophosphamide in male mice.** *Hum Exp Toxicol* 2014, **33**:185–195.
17. Akyol S, Ginis Z, Armutcu F, Ozturk G, Yigitoglu MR, Akyol O: **The potential usage of caffeic acid phenethyl ester (CAPE) against chemotherapy-induced and radiotherapy-induced toxicity.** *Cell Biochem Funct* 2012, **30**:438–443.
18. Esrefoglu M, Iraz M, Ates B, Gul M: **Melatonin and CAPE are able to prevent the liver from oxidative damage in rats: an ultrastructural and biochemical study.** *Ultrastruct Pathol* 2012, **36**:171–178.
19. Gong P, Chen F, Liu X, Gong X, Wang J, Ma Y: **Protective effect of caffeic acid phenethyl ester against cadmium-induced renal damage in mice.** *J Toxicol Sci* 2012, **37**:415–425.
20. Kim H, Kim W, Yum S, Hong S, Oh JE, Lee JW, Kwak MK, Park EJ, Na DH, Jung Y: **Caffeic acid phenethyl ester activation of Nrf2 pathway is enhanced under oxidative state: Structural analysis and potential as a pathologically targeted therapeutic agent in treatment of colonic inflammation.** *Free Radic Biol Med* 2013, **65C**:552–562.
21. Abdallah FB, Fetoui H, Fakhfakh F, Keskes L: **Caffeic acid and quercetin protect erythrocytes against the oxidative stress and the genotoxic effects of lambda-cyhalothrin in vitro.** *Hum Exp Toxicol* 2012, **31**:92–100.
22. Bradford MM: **A rapid and sensitive method for the quantitation of microgram quantities of protein utilizing the principle of protein-dye binding.** *Anal Biochem* 1976, **72**:248–254.
23. Akçam M, Artan R, Yilmaz A, Ozdem S, Gelen T, Nazıroğlu M: **Caffeic acid phenethyl ester modulates aflatoxin B1-induced hepatotoxicity in rats.** *Cell Biochem Funct* 2013, **31**:692–697.
24. Iraz M, Ozerol E, Gulec M, Tasdemir S, Idiz N, Fadillioglu E, Naziroglu M, Akyol O: **Protective effect of caffeic acid phenethyl ester (CAPE) administration on cisplatin-induced oxidative damage to liver in rat.** *Cell Biochem Funct* 2006, **24**:357–361.
25. Pekmez H, Kus I, Colakoglu N, Ogeturk M, Ozyurt H, Turkoglu AO, Sarsilmaz M: **The protective effects of caffeic acid phenethyl ester (CAPE) against liver damage induced by cigarette smoke inhalation in rats.** *Cell Biochem Funct* 2007, **25**:395–400.
26. Parlakpinar H, Ozer MK, Ucar M, Gaffaroglu M, Vardi N, Koc M, Acet A: **Protective effects of caffeic acid phenethyl ester (CAPE) on amikacin-induced nephrotoxicity in rats.** *Cell Biochem Funct* 2006, **24**:363–367.
27. Çakır T, Özkan E, Dulundu E, Topaloğlu Ü, Şehirli AÖ, Ercan F, Şener E, Şener G: **Caffeic acid phenethyl ester (CAPE) prevents methotrexate-induced hepatorenal oxidative injury in rats.** *J Pharm Pharmacol* 2011, **63**:1566–1571.
28. Gülçin I: **Antioxidant activity of caffeic acid (3,4-dihydroxycinnamic acid).** *Toxicology* 2006, **217**:213–220.
29. Ozguner F, Bardak Y, Comlekci S: **Protective effects of melatonin and caffeic acid phenethyl ester against retinal oxidative stress in long-term use of mobile phone: a comparative study.** *Mol Cell Biochem* 2006, **282**:83–88.
30. Eşrefoğlu M, Gül M, Ateş B, Erdoğan A: **The effects of caffeic acid phenethyl ester and melatonin on age-related vascular remodeling and cardiac damage.** *Fundam Clin Pharmacol* 2011, **25**:580–590.
31. Karbownik M, Stasiak M, Zasada K, Zygmunt A, Lewinski A: **Comparison of potential protective effects of melatonin, indole-3-propionic acid, and propylthiouracil against lipid peroxidation caused by potassium bromate in the thyroid gland.** *J Cell Biochem* 2005, **95**:131–138.
32. Karbownik M, Stasiak M, Zygmunt A, Zasada K, Lewinski A: **Protective effects of melatonin and indole-3-propionic acid against lipid peroxidation, caused by potassium bromate in the rat kidney.** *Cell Biochem Funct* 2006, **24**:483–489.
33. Sırmalı M, Solak O, Tezel C, Sırmalı R, Ginis Z, Atik D, Agackıran Y, Koylu H, Delibas N: **Comparative analysis of the protective effects of caffeic acid phenethyl ester (CAPE) on pulmonary contusion lung oxidative stress and serum copper and zinc levels in experimental rat model.** *Biol Trace Elem Res* 2013, **151**:50–58.

Elevated thyroid stimulating hormone is associated with elevated cortisol in healthy young men and women

Kimberly N Walter[1], Elizabeth J Corwin[2], Jan Ulbrecht[1], Laurence M Demers[1,3], Jeanette M Bennett[1], Courtney A Whetzel[1] and Laura Cousino Klein[1*]

Abstract

Background: Recent attention has been given to subclinical hypothyroidism, defined as an elevation of TSH (4.5-10 uIU/L) with T4 and T3 levels still within the normal range. Controversy exists about the proper lower limit of TSH that defines patients in the subclinical hypothyroidism range and about if/when subclinical hypothyroidism should be treated. Additional data are needed to examine the relationship between markers of thyroid function in the subclinical hypothyroidism range, biomarkers of health and ultimately health outcomes.

Objective: We aimed to assess the relationship between serum TSH levels in the 0.5-10 uIU/L range and serum cortisol in a cohort of healthy young men and women without clinical evidence of hypothyroidism. Based on data in frank hypothyroidism, we hypothesized that serum TSH levels would be positively correlated with serum cortisol levels, suggesting derangement of the cortisol axis even in subclinical hypothyroidism.

Methods: We conducted a cross sectional study in 54 healthy, young (mean 20.98 +/− 0.37 yrs) men (19) and women (35). Lab sessions took place at 1300 hrs where blood was drawn via indwelling catheter for later assessment of basal serum TSH, free T3, free T4, and cortisol levels.

Results: All but 1 participant had free T3 levels within the normal reference intervals; free T4 levels for all participants were within the normal reference intervals. Linear regression modeling revealed that TSH levels in the 0.5-10 uIU/L were significantly and positively correlated with cortisol levels. This positive TSH-cortisol relationship was maintained below the accepted 4.5 uIU/L subclinical hypothyroid cutoff. Separate regression analyses conducted by systematically dropping the TSH cutoff by 0.50 uIU/L revealed that the TSH-cortisol relationship was maintained for TSH levels (uIU/L) ≤4.0, ≤3.5, ≤3.0, and ≤2.5 but not ≤2.0. Linear regression modeling did not reveal a relationship between free T3 or free T4 levels and cortisol levels.

Conclusions: Results suggest a positive relationship between TSH and cortisol in apparently healthy young individuals. In as much as this relationship may herald a pathologic disorder, these preliminary results suggest that TSH levels > 2.0 uIU/L may be abnormal. Future research should address this hypothesis further, for instance through an intervention study.

Keywords: TSH, Free T3, Free T4, Cortisol, Subclinical hypothyroidism

* Correspondence: lcklein@psu.edu
[1]Department of Biobehavioral Health, 219 Biobehavioral Health Bldg, The Pennsylvania State University, University Park, PA 16802, USA
Full list of author information is available at the end of the article

Background

Thyroxine (T4) and triiodothyronine (T3), together referred to as thyroid hormones, play an important role in basal metabolism and the functioning of almost all tissues and systems in the body [1]. In addition to T4 and T3, thyroid stimulating hormone (TSH) secretion typically is maintained within relatively narrow limits via a sensitive negative feedback loop in which TSH stimulates the synthesis and release of thyroid hormones, that in turn negatively feed back to the hypothalamus and anterior pituitary to limit further TSH release. Reduced thyroid hormone levels existing together with elevated TSH are an indication that the response of the thyroid gland to TSH is impaired, i.e. primary hypothyroidism.

Recent attention has been given to subclinical hypothyroidism, defined as a TSH elevation with T4 and T3 levels still within the normal range. Subclinical hypothyroidism is a common disorder; two large population-based studies revealed that 4% to 8.5% of individuals without known thyroid disease actually have subclinical hypothyroidism as evidenced by a mildly elevated TSH (i.e., 4.5-10 uIU/L) [2,3]. Complicating matters is the current controversy about the proper lower limit of TSH that defines patients in the subclinical hypothyroidism range (in other words, the upper limit of the normal reference range for TSH) [4-8]. In apparently healthy populations, the TSH distribution is skewed towards the lower end of the reference range, with the mean value typically being around 1.5 uIU/L, but with the range extending from 0.5–4.5 uIU/L [8]. Therefore it is possible that seemingly healthy individuals with TSH levels in the upper end of this range may in fact have elevated TSH in response to early thyroid gland failure and also should be considered to have subclinical hypothyroidism. This possibility is further supported by the fact that many patients with TSH levels in the 3.0–4.5 uIU/L range are positive for antithyroid antibodies [6,8].

Untreated hypothyroidism can lead to increased body weight, cognitive dysfunction, fatigue, abnormal serum lipids, coronary heart disease, and for women recurrent miscarriage, infertility, and possibly delayed cognitive development in their children [1,9,10]. Much controversy still exists regarding the extent to which clinically meaningful consequences result from untreated subclinical hypothyroidism or are due to TSH values in the upper range of "normal" [4-8]. Indeed, by definition the only abnormality found with subclinical hypothyroidism is a mild to modest TSH elevation that is more sensitive than either free T3 or free T4 in reflecting this condition [4]. Most clinical guidelines recommend either close observation or a therapeutic trial of levothyroxine in patients with TSH values in the 4.5-10 uIU/L range and simply observation when the TSH result is in the range of 2.5-4.5 uIU/L [5,10]. These recommendations are based on lack of conclusive evidence in either range of definitive disease. Intervention studies that examine neurocognitive symptoms in patients identified with suggestive symptoms at baseline, as well as intervention studies that focus on long-term outcomes such as atherosclerosis, have not been carried out.

More research is therefore clearly needed in this area. This preliminary study assessed the relationship between serum TSH levels in the 2.5-10 uIU/L range and serum cortisol in a cohort of healthy young men and women with no clinical history of thyroid disease or other underlying health conditions. It has long been known that frank hypothyroidism causes elevated cortisol levels, presumably due to both decreased clearance and blunted negative feedback of cortisol on the hypothalamic-pituitary-adrenal axis [11]. In the present study we hypothesized that serum TSH levels would be positively associated with serum cortisol levels even in the subclinical hypothyroidism range.

Materials and methods

Study participants

Participants were recruited through advertisements in the local newspaper and flyers posted in the local community. Research staff through telephone-screening interviews determined eligibility. Exclusion criteria included a history of smoking (<1 year ago); diagnosed heart disease, diabetes, stroke or other neurological disorders or depression; significant medication use (blood pressure, beta-blockers, inhaled beta agonists, hormonal contraceptives, corticosteroid use within prior three months, psychotropic medication use within prior eight weeks; psychiatric hospitalization within past year; and body mass index (BMI; kg/m^2) > 32. BMI was confirmed at the beginning of the study session. Women with a partial or complete hysterectomy, tubal ligations, history of menstrual irregularities, and who were pregnant or lactating within the past 12 months were also excluded from the study.

Thirty-five healthy women and 19 men, 18–30 years of age (mean age 20.98 +/– 0.37 years), were eligible. Women were randomly assigned to participate during the late luteal (N=18) or follicular (N=17) phase of their menstrual cycle because of menstrual phase effects on cortisol levels [12]. Sex steroid assays confirmed cycle phase with mean estradiol and progesterone levels for the late luteal phase at 123.94 ± 22.72 pg/mL and 18.12 ± 3.41 ng/mL, respectively, and follicular phase levels at 49.31 ± 6.13 pg/mL and 4.40 ± 0.82 ng/mL, respectively. Thirty-eight (70.4%) of the participants identified themselves as Caucasian, 4 (7.4%) African American, 4 (7.4%) Asian, 2 (3.7%) Hispanic, and 6 (10.7%) self-described as "other." The Pennsylvania

State University's Institutional Review Board reviewed and approved all study procedures.

Procedure

Lab sessions took place at 1300 hrs at The Pennsylvania State University General Clinical Research Center. Following informed consent and the measurements of body weight and height, a nurse practitioner confirmed health status and study eligibility. An indwelling catheter was then inserted and, and after a 10-minute acclimation period a 20cc blood sample was drawn and allowed to sit at room temperature for 15 minutes. Samples were centrifuged at 1500 X g at 4 degrees C for 15 minutes. Serum was stored at −80 C until hormone analysis was performed. Participants were compensated for their time.

Hormonal analyses

Cortisol, TSH, estradiol, and progesterone levels were determined at The Pennsylvania State University's GCRC using commercially available enzyme immunoassay kits (Diagnostic Systems Laboratories, Inc., Webster, Texas). Low-end assay sensitivity for cortisol, TSH, estradiol and progesterone were as follows: 0.1 ug/dL (cortisol), 0.01 uIU/L (TSH), 7 pg/mL (estradiol), and 0.13 ng/mL (progesterone). Intra-assay and inter-assay imprecision for all analytes averaged less than 10%; all samples were tested in duplicate in a single assay batch. Duplicate test values that varied by more than 5% were subject to repeat testing. The average of the duplicate test results is reported below. Serum free T3 (FT3) and free T4 (FT4) levels were determined by radioimmunoassay with reagents obtained from Siemens Medical Solutions (Hollidaysburg, PA).

Statistical analyses

Statistical analyses were performed using SPSS, version 17.0 (Chicago, IL, US). Means are reported plus or minus standard error of the mean. Statistical significance levels were set at $\alpha=0.05$ and two-tailed tests were used.

Results

Serum free T4 levels for all participants were within the normal reference interval (i.e., 0.7-1.8 ng/dl see Table 1). Serum free T3 levels fell within the normal reference interval (i.e., 2.0-5.0 pg/mL) for all but 1 participant whose level was elevated (11.5 pg/mL). We included this participant in our analyses because FT3 results are less reliable than FT4 results due to the low concentration found in the circulation and TSH and FT4 were within the normal range for this participant (TSH=3.61 uIU/L; FT4=1.6 ng/dl). It is important to note that the following results do not change as a result of removing this participant from the analyses. Overall, these FT3 and FT4 data confirm the absence of overt clinical hypothyroidism in our participants.

Table 1 Mean serum TSH (uIU/L), free T3 (pg/mL), free T4 (ng/dL), and cortisol (ug/dL), and BMI (kg/m^2) in men (N=19) and in women during the luteal (N=18) and follicular (N=14) phases of the menstrual cycle (± standard error of the mean)

	Men (N=19)	Women luteal (N=18)	Women follicular (N=14)
TSH (uIU/L)	3.25 ± 0.44	2.34 ± 0.32	2.21 ± 0.26
Free T3 (pg/mL)	3.04 ± 0.11	2.89 ± 0.11	3.29 ± 0.52
Free T4 (ng/dL)	1.28 ± 0.04	1.25 ± 0.05	1.28 ± 0.04
Cortisol (ug/dL)	14.77 ± 1.21	9.35 ± 0.87	10.94 ± 1.17
BMI (kg/m^2)	23.37 ± 0.72	23.73 ± 0.80	23.23 ± 0.82

Cortisol and TSH results were not normally distributed (i.e., were skewed). Therefore, a natural logarithmic transformation was applied to the cortisol and TSH values e.g., [13,14], which resulted in a normal distribution of the data. Thus, the transformed data were used for analyses, but the raw data are reported in Table 1 for clarity. Two serum TSH level ranges were tested in the analyses: [1] levels below the cutoff for overt hypothyroidism (<10 uIU/L) and [2] levels below the cutoff for subclinical hypothyroidism (<4.5 uIU/L). Overall, serum TSH levels varied widely among participants who otherwise presented to the study as healthy. Consistent with U.S. prevalence rates [2,3], approximately 9% of the sample population (N=5) demonstrated mildly elevated TSH levels (4.5-10 uIU/L); these participants typically would be categorized as having subclinical hypothyroid disease in a medical setting [10]. Three additional participants (all women in the follicular phase) had serum TSH levels indicative of overt clinical hypothyroidism (TSH ≥10 uIU/L) and were excluded from analyses because we were interested in the relationship between TSH and cortisol among healthy individuals. It is important to note that the following results interpretation did not change as a result of this exclusion. Serum TSH levels from the final cohort (N=51) ranged from 0.86-9.57 uIU/L (mean 2.64 ± 0.22 uIU/L). Table 1 lists the average TSH and cortisol results by hormone status group (± standard error of the mean) for the final group. Cortisol levels were in the normal range for early afternoon.

Separate one-way analyses of variance (ANOVAs) confirmed that TSH, FT3, FT4 levels, as well as body mass index (BMI), across the 3 hormone status groups were similar (see Table 1); data were therefore collapsed across hormone status groups for the subsequent analyses. Body mass index was included as a covariate in the analyses but it did not affect the statistical significance of the models. Thus, BMI was not included in the final models.

Simple linear regression modeling revealed that serum TSH levels ≤ 10 uIU/L significantly predicted serum cortisol levels [β=0.33, $t(50)$=2.80, p<0.05.]. This TSH-cortisol relationship also held for subjects who were nominally euthyroid (i.e., below the subclinical hypothyroid cutoff, i.e., TSH ≤ 4.5 uIU/L) [β=0.49, $t(46)$ =3.35, p<0.05]. To further explore the TSH-cortisol relationship, we ran separate regression analyses by systematically dropping the TSH cutoff by 0.50 uIU/L. The positive TSH-cortisol relationship was maintained for TSH levels: [1] ≤ 4.0 uIU/L [β=0.53, $t(45)$=3.51, p<0.05], [2] ≤ 3.5 uIU/L [β=0.23, $t(40)$=2.38, p<0.05], [3] ≤ 3.0 uIU/L [β=0.34, $t(37)$=3.19, p<0.05], and [4] ≤ 2.5 uIU/L [β=0.68, $t(30)$=2.89, p<0.05]. Serum TSH levels below 2.0 uIU/L were not significantly associated with serum cortisol levels [β=0.33, $t(18)$= 6.53, *ns*]. In other words, serum cortisol levels among individuals with TSH levels >2.0 uIU/L (N=31) were significantly higher than among those individuals with TSH levels ≤ 2.0 uIU/L (N=20) [13.83 ± 0.93 ug/dL vs. 8.66 ± 0.59 ug/dL, respectively, F (1,48)=14.24, p<0.0001]. There was no relationship observed between either FT3 or FT4 and cortisol levels.

Discussion

We examined the relationship between TSH levels and cortisol in a preliminary study of young, healthy adults without known thyroid disease or other underlying health conditions. The positive relationship between serum TSH and cortisol levels in a healthy population is a compelling new finding that is consistent with and extends the observation that frankly hypothyroid patients have frankly elevated cortisol levels [11].

These preliminary results raise important questions – such as whether this relationship is pathologic or physiologic and what the mechanism(s) involved in this relationship may be. While in frank hypothyroidism, it is hypothyroidism that causes elevation of cortisol by reducing peripheral disposal and blunting feedback of cortisol on the hypothalamic-pituitary-adrenal axis [11], our cross sectional data do not elucidate whether the same mechanisms hold true for TSH levels in the high normal and low elevated range. Thus more definitive population-based and intervention studies are now needed to confirm this finding and answer these questions.

Another potential explanation for the positive TSH-cortisol relationship is that hypothyroidism - subclinical or clinical - is associated with subtle metabolic stress. Metabolic stress could be imposing an effect on the adrenocorticotropin hormone-adrenal axis leading to an increase in stress hormone (i.e., cortisol) release and production. This hypothesis should be confirmed through the measurement of other stress hormones including the catecholamines, norepinephrine/epinephrine, and/or prolactin.

Although limited in sample size, our findings demonstrate that a positive relationship exists between TSH and cortisol that is maintained down to a TSH level of 2.5 uIU/L (but not below). This observation raises the possibility that negative health effects of mild, subclinical hypothyroidism with mild to modest elevations in TSH may begin at levels much lower than those currently considered abnormal based on assigned normal reference range values with an upper reference level of 4.5 uIU/L.

Chronic elevations in serum cortisol and hypothyroidism (including subclinical hypothyroidism) have been separately linked with increased rates of depression, anxiety, and poor cognitive functioning e.g., [15-17]. Thus, the association between TSH levels and cortisol suggests at least the possibility of a novel pathway through which hypothyroidism (both clinical and subclinical) may promote poor mental health; or hypothyroidism and an elevated cortisol level could be synergistic on mental health.

It is possible that the relationship described in this paper is physiologic rather than representative of pathology. Indeed, a failure to observe a relationship between TSH and cortisol for TSH < 2.5uIU/L may be a matter of methodology (assay accuracy at the lower levels, statistical power) rather than an indication that a relationship does not exist at those lower levels. Additional, larger clinical studies are needed that also include repeat TSH, FT3, FT4, cortisol, and catecholamine measurements to validate the reliability of the TSH-cortisol relationship.

A strength of this preliminary study is that we also measured FT3 and FT4 levels in this cohort of young, healthy individuals. Interestingly, while our results demonstrate that subtle elevations in TSH are associated with higher basal cortisol levels, this relationship is not apparent for FT3 or FT4 levels. One plausible explanation for the lack of an association between FT3 or FT4 and cortisol is that changes in FT3 and FT4 are slow to reflect subclinical hypothyroidism in the circulation because of adjustments made at the end organ level in both synthesis and metabolism of thyroid hormones [4]. In addition, changes in TSH are 10 times more sensitive in reflecting an abnormality in thyroid hormone homeostasis compared to FT3 or FT4 [4]. Similar to our finding, other studies of subclinical hypothyroidism typically report a relationship between the biomarker of interest (e.g., cholesterol) and TSH, but not FT3 or FT4 [18]. However, it is still possible that mechanistically the relationship that we are here reporting is indeed between T3 and/or T4 and cortisol, but that measurement of FT4 and FT3 in blood is not sensitive enough to represent effects at the tissue level.

Our results and those of Iranmanesh et al. [11] for frank hypothyroidism suggest effects of the thyroid axis on the adrenal axis where hypothyroidism causes hypercortisolemia. It is of interest to consider these observations together with the well-established opposite effects, i.e. effects of the adrenal axis on thyroid function. Thus when cortisol levels are manipulated through pathologic as well as physiologic ranges, a negative relationship is found between cortisol and TSH. Both exogenous and endogenous (i.e. Cushing's Syndrome, stress) corticosteroids suppress TSH [19-22] while low cortisol levels elevate TSH [23,24]. These studies all taken together suggest a physiologic feedback loop where lower thyroid function increases cortisol, but cortisol feeds back to reduce TSH; this hypothesis is consistent with the observations that in the case of primary hypothyroidism (elevated TSH) cortisol is elevated, but in the setting of primarily elevated cortisol TSH is suppressed. Clearly further clinical studies, for instance studies that incrementally administer TSH and evaluate cortisol levels, are needed in order to better understand the mechanisms involved in the TSH-cortisol relationship.

In summary these initial data, that add to what is already known about frank hypothyroidism and cortisol, demonstrate a potentially important relationship between TSH and cortisol in apparently healthy young individuals. The finding that this relationship appears to hold in the controversial TSH range of 2.5-10 uIU/L, but not below, is compelling and requires further scientific and clinical investigation.

Abbreviations

TSH: Thyroid stimulating hormone; T4: Thyroxine; T3: Triiodothyronine; FT4: Free T4; FT3: Free T3; BMI: Body mass index.

Competing interests

The authors have no competing interests to declare.

Authors' contributions

KNW developed the hypotheses and data analytic strategy, analyzed the data and drafted the manuscript. LCK and EJC designed the experiment and obtained funding. JU and LMD provided crucial clinical and scientific endocrine and thyroid functioning expertise. JU and LCK assisted with data analytic strategies. LMD provided funding and conducted FT4 and FT3 assays. JMB and CAW assisted with running the experiment, as well as TSH and cortisol assays. All authors made intellectual revisions to the entire manuscript, edited all sections of the manuscript and approved this version of the submitted manuscript.

Acknowledgements

This work was supported by a grant from the National Science Foundation (SBR 9905157), a seed grant from the College of Health and Human Development at Penn State (223 15 3605), and Penn State's General Clinical Research Center (NIH grant M01-RR-10732). Jeanette M. Bennett is now located at The University of North Carolina at Charlotte. We thank Michele M. Stine, our research assistants in the Biobehavioral Health Studies Lab, and the GCRC nursing staff for assistance with data collection, and Rick Ball for guidance on the biological assays. We also thank the Core Endocrine Laboratory at the Penn State Hershey Medical Center for performing the free T3 and free T4 measurements.

Author details

[1]Department of Biobehavioral Health, 219 Biobehavioral Health Bldg, The Pennsylvania State University, University Park, PA 16802, USA. [2]Nell Hodgson Woodruff School of Nursing, Emory University, Atlanta, GA 30322, USA. [3]Department of Pathology, H158 Pathology, The M.S. Hershey Medical Center, Hershey, PA 17033, USA.

References

1. Boelaert K, Franklyn JA: **Thyroid hormone in health and disease.** *J Endocrinol* 2005, **187**:1–15.
2. Canaris GJ, Manowitz NR, Mayor G, Ridgway EC: **The Colorado thyroid disease prevalence study.** *Arch Intern Med* 2000, **160**:526–534.
3. Hollowell JG, Staehling NW, Flanders WD, Hannon WH, Gunter EW, Spencer CA, Braverman LE: **Serum TSH, T-4, and thyroid antibodies in the United States population (1988 to 1994): National Health and Nutrition Examination Survey (NHANES III).** *J Clin Endocrinol Metabol* 2002, **87**:489–499.
4. Demers LM, Spencer CA (Eds): *Laboratory Medicine Practice Guidelines: Laboratory Support for the Diagnosis and Monitoring of Thyroid Disease.* Washington, DC: National Academy of Clinical Biochemistry; 2002. www.nacb.org.
5. Fatourechi V: **Subclinical Hypothyroidism: An Update for Primary Care Physicians.** *Mayo Clin Proc* 2009, **84**:65–71.
6. Spencer CA, Hollowell JG, Kazarosyan M, Braverman LE: **National health and nutrition examination survey III thyroid-stimulating hormone (TSH)-thyroperoxidase antibody relationships demonstrate that TSH upper reference limits may be skewed by occult thyroid dysfunction.** *J Clin Endocrinol Metabol* 2007, **92**:4236–4240.
7. Surks MI, Goswami G, Daniels GH: **The thyrotropin reference range should remain unchanged.** *J Clin Endocrinol Metabol* 2005, **90**:5489–5496.
8. Wartofsky L, Dickey RA: **The evidence for a narrower thyrotropin reference range is compelling.** *J Clin Endocrinol Metabol* 2005, **90**:5483–5488.
9. Roberts CGP, Ladenson PW: **Hypothyroidism.** *Lancet* 2004, **363**:793–803.
10. Surks MI, Ortiz E, Daniels GH, Sawin CT, Col NF, Cobin RH, Franklyn JA, Hershman JM, Burman KD, Denke MA, Gorman C, Cooper RS, Weissman NJ: **Subclinical thyroid disease - Scientific review and guidelines for diagnosis and management.** *J Am Med Assoc* 2004, **291**:228–238.
11. Iranmanesh A, Lizarralde G, Johnson ML, *et al*: **Dynamics of 24-hour endogenous cortisol secretion and clearance in primary hypothyroidism assessed before and after partial thyroid hormone replacement.** *J Clin Endocrinol Metabol* 1990, **70**:155–161.
12. Kirschbaum C, Kudielka BM, Gaab J, Schommer NC, Hellhammer DH: **Impact of gender, menstrual cycle phase, and oral contraceptives on the activity of the hypothalamus-pituitary-adrenal axis.** *Psychosom Med* 1999, **61**:154–162.
13. McHale SM, Blocklin MK, Walter KN, Davis KD, Almeida DM, Klein LC: **The role of daily activities in youth's stress physiology.** *J Adol Health* 2012, [published online ahead of print May 16 2012]. http://dx.doi.org/10.1016/j.jadohealth.2012.03.016.
14. Whetzel CA, Corwin EJ, Klein LC: **Disruption in Th1/Th2 immune response in young adult smokers.** *Addict Behav* 2007, **32**:1–8.
15. Almeida C, Brasil MA, Costa AJL, Reis FAA, Reuters V, Teixeira P, Ferreira M, Marques AM, Melo BA, Teixeira L, Buescu A, Vaisman M: **Subclinical hypothyroidism: psychiatric disorders and symptoms.** *Revista Brasileira De Psiquiatria.* 2007, **29**:157–159.
16. Heffelfinger AK, Newcomer JW: **Glucocorticoid effects on memory function over the human life span.** *Dev Psychopathol* 2001, **13**:491–513.
17. Sapolsky RM: **Why stress is bad for your brain.** *Science* 1996, **273**:749–750.
18. Bell RJ, Rivera-Woll L, Davison SL, Topliss DJ, Donath S, Davis SR: **Well-being, health-related quality of life and cardiovascular disease risk profile in women with subclinical thyroid disease - a community-based study.** *Clin Endocrinol* 2007, **66**:548–556.
19. Bartalena L, Martino E, Petrini L, Velluzzi F, Loviselli A, Grasso L, Mammoli C, Pinchera A: **The nocturnal serum thyrotropin surge is abolished in**

patients with adrenocorticotropin (ACTH)-dependent or ACTH-independent Cushing's syndrome. *J Clin Endocrinol Metabol* 1991, **72**:1195–1199.
20. Brabant G, Brabant A, Ranft U, Ocran K, Köhrle J, Hesch RD, von zur Mühlen A: **Circadian and pulsatile thyrotropin secretion in euthyroid man under the influence of thyroid hormone and glucocorticoid administration.** *J Clin Endocrinol Metabol* 1987, **65**:83–88.
21. Samuels MH, Luther M, Henry P, Ridgway EC: **Effects of hydrocortisone on pulsatile pituitary glycoprotein secretion.** *J Clin Endocrinol Metabol* 1994, **78**:211–215.
22. Samuels MH, McDaniel PA: **Thyrotropin levels during hydrocortisone infusions that mimic fasting-induced cortisol elevations—a clinical research center study.** *J Clin Endocrinol Metabol* 1997, **82**:3700–3704.
23. Samuels MH: **Effects of variations in physiological cortisol levels on thyrotropin secretion in subjects with adrenal insufficiency: a clinical research center study.** *J Clin Endocrinol Metabol* 2000, **85**:1388–1393.
24. Samuels MH: **Effects of metyrapone administration on thyrotropin secretion in healthy subjects—a clinical research center study.** *J Clin Endocrinal Metabol* 2000, **85**:3049–3052.

11

Phylogenetic analysis of the human thyroglobulin regions

Abdelaziz Belkadi[1,2,3*], Caroline Jacques[1,2], Frédérique Savagner[1,2] and Yves Malthièry[1,2]

Abstract

Thyroglobulin is a large protein present in all vertebrates. It is synthesized in the thyrocytes and exported to lumen of the thyroid follicle, where its tyrosine residues are iodinated . The iodinated thyroglobulin is reintegrated into the cell and processed (cleaved to free its two extremities) for thyroid hormone synthesis. Thyroglobulin sequence analysis has identified four regions of the molecule: Tg1, Tg2, Tg3 and ChEL. Structural abnormalities and mutations result in different pathological consequences, depending on the thyroglobulin region affected. We carried out a bioinformatic analysis of thyroglobulin, determining the origin and the function of each region. Our results suggest that the Tg1 region acts as a binding protein on the apical membrane, the Tg2 region is involved in protein adhesion and the Tg3 region is involved in determining the three-dimensional structure of the protein. The ChEL domain is involved in thyroglobulin transport, dimerization and adhesion. The presence of repetitive domains in the Tg1, Tg2 and Tg3 regions suggests that these domains may have arisen through duplication.

Introduction

Thyroglobulin is the precursor of the thyroid hormones triiodothyronine (T3) and thyroxine (T4). In humans, thyroglobulin is synthesized by thyroid follicle cells, which are also known as thyrocytes [1]. Thyroglobulin molecules form dimers, which are exported to the lumen of the thyroid follicles [2]. There, the thyroglobulin is immobilized on the apical membrane. The thyroid hormones process starts by the iodination of tyrosine residues. Thyroperoxidaseis activated by H_2O_2, leading to the oxidation of iodide, followed by the iodination and conjugation of some of the tyrosine residues present in the thyroglobulin molecule. The iodinated and conjugated thyroglobulin is then returned to the cell via an endocytosis process that may involve histone H1 [3], megalin (gp330) [4] and/or the N-acetylglucosamine receptor [5]. Only a very small number of iodinated tyrosine residues are involved in thyroid hormone synthesis. T4 is formed by the conjugation of two residues of diiodotyrosine followed by cleavage. T3 is formed in a similar manner, but through the conjugation of diiodotyrosine with monoiodotyrosine [6,7]. T3 is the functional form; it is generated principally by T4 deiodinases in the peripheral organs, with only 13% being formed in the thyroid gland [8]. Thyroid hormones reach their target organs via the bloodstream. Thyroglobulin has been reported to regulate some thyroid genes and the growth of epithelial cells [9,10]. It acts as both a hormone and an iodine reservoir [11].

In humans, mice and fish, thyroid hormone levels determine the basal rate of metabolism and overall energy expenditure [12-14]. In other species, such as Senegalese sole [15], amphibians [16], urochordatas [17], amphioxus [18] and lamprey [19], thyroid hormones play a critical role in the metamorphosis from larvae to juveniles. Thyroglobulin protein structure has been studied in detail [20-22]. This protein is present in all vertebrates and always has the same structure, consisting of four regions: the Tg1 (~ 10 repetitive domains), Tg2 (3 repetitive domains), Tg3 (5 repetitive domains) and ChEL regions (Figure 1-a and 1-b). The Tg1, Tg2 and Tg3 regions (moving along the molecule from its N-terminal end) consist of repetitive domains. All three regions are rich in cysteine residues, allowing them to form disulfide bonds [23]. The presence of these repetitive domains suggests their possible evolution through the duplication of source domains. The C-terminus of the molecule includes a 581-amino acid sequence displaying a high degree of similarity to the sequence of acetylcholinesterase (28% identity) [24,25]. One previous study identified the ChEL domain as the

* Correspondence: abdelaziz.belkadi@etud.univ-angers.fr
[1]INSERM U694, Institut Biologie Santé (IBS), rue des Capucins, F-49100 Angers, France
[2]University of Angers, rue de Rennes, F-49045 Angers, France
Full list of author information is available at the end of the article

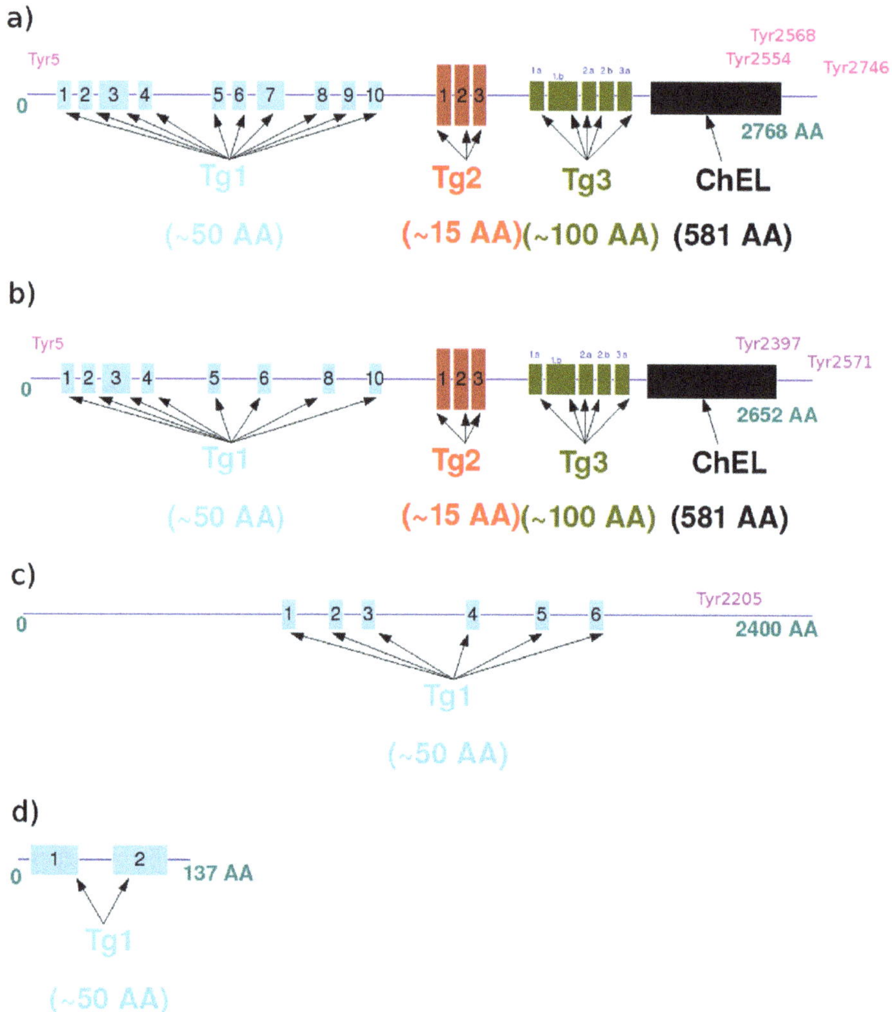

Figure 1 The structure of the thyroglobulin protein. a) Structure of the human thyroglobulin protein. **b)** Structure of the zebrafish thyroglobulin protein. **c)** Structure of the amphioxus thyroglobulin-like protein. **d)** Structure of the sea urchin thyroglobulin-like protein. Blue: Tg1 domains, red: Tg2 domains, green: Tg3 domains, black: the ChEL domain. Magenta: the location of the thyroid hormone synthesis sites on the proteins (tyrosine residues).

origininal source of thyroglobulin [26]. Thyroglobulin contains about 140 tyrosine residues, but only about 30 of these residues are iodinated and a very small number of these iodinated tyrosines undergo conjugation to form T3 and T4 [27]. Only four major thyroid hormone synthesis sites have been clearly identified in the human thyroglobulin molecule and these sites are located at either end of the protein: Tyr5, Tyr2554, Tyr2568 and Tyr2747 [21].

Thyroglobulin may thus be seen as a huge precursor of two very small products. Additional studies of its other, as yet unexplored functions in the cell may be useful. For example, this protein could potentially be involved in the trafficking of iodinefrom the thyrocyte to the follicle lumen and its storage. Many studies have made use of bioinformatics tools to analyze the evolution of proteins and genes, and such tools may be useful in this context [28,29].

We performed a phylogenetic analysis of the thyroglobulin molecule with the sequenced genomes of species corresponding to key steps in animal evolution. Our results provide clues to the evolution of thyroglobulin and potential functional roles for theTg1, Tg2, Tg3 and the ChEL regions.

Materials and methods

Sequence extraction

We extracted the available DNA and protein sequences for thyroglobulin (Tg) from the NCBI databank www.ncbi.nlm.nih.gov for four species: human [GenBank:CAA29104],rat [GenBank:AAF34909], mouse [GenBank:AAB53204], pig [GenBank:ACY66900]. We also extracted six predicted sequences: cattle [GenBank:NP_ 776308] horse [GenBank: XP 001916622] marmoset [GenBank:XP 002759270], panda [Gen-Bank:XP 002917659], zebrafish [GenBank:XP 694292] and zebra finch [GenBank:XP 002188056]. For other species, for which the amino-acid sequence of is unknown, such as opossum, and fugu, we used the human thyroglobulin genomic sequence in Blast searches of the UCSC website genome.ucsc.edu; We first translated the DNA sequence to obtain a putative amino-acid sequence. We then used Blast to check whether the predicted sequence was present in the database (chr3:411,623,333-412,004,486 and chrUn:270,007,531-270,025,053 for opossum and fugu, respectively). Homologous sequences from amphioxus [GenBank:XP 002607132] and sea urchin [Gen-Bank:XP 001202473] were also identified by BLAT analysis (chrUn:353,044,426-353,083,914 and Scaffold82420:233-1, 088 in the amphioxus and sea urchin genomes, respectively).

Sequence similarity

We searched for regions presenting sequence similarities to the constituent domains of thyroglobulin - Tgl Tg2, Tg3 and ChEL - with the Blastall command ftp://ftp.ncbi.nlm.nih.gov/blast/db/, version 2.2.19. Pairs of sequences were compared on the basis of their global alignment with the Myers & Millers algorithm manpages.ubuntu.com/manpages/karmic/man1. Results were generated in a separate text file containing alignment diagrams, scores, degrees of identity, similarity and gaps. We used ClustalX software ftp://ftpigbmc.u-strasbg.fr/pub/ClustalX/. for analysis of multiple alignments of three or more sequences. The results were output to a separate text file, but without information about score, because it was not possible to use more than two sequences for score calculation with Compositional Matrix Adjust.

Phylogeny

We used the neighbor-joining (NJ) method in PHYLIP [30] and mega 5 [31] for phylogenetic analysis. A range of analyses, from simple p distance to multiparameter models with gamma correction, were used. The significance of the phylogenetic tree was assessed by bootstrapping, with 10,000 iterations. The Jones-Taylor- Thornton (JTT) model of amino-acid sequence evolution, with gamma correction, was used for distance estimation [32]. In each case, the distance was validated with 10,000 bootstrap replications.

Results

The N-terminal Tg1 region

In humans, the first region of thyroglobulin consists of 10 Tgl repeat domains, each containing 50 amino acids and displaying 14% identity. However, Molina, et al. identified an 11th domain located after the Tg2 region [33]. A comparison of this region in all the thyroglobulin protein sequences extracted (13 species) indicated that the fish thyroglobulins (zebrafish and fugu) lacked Tgl-7 and Tgl-9 (Additional file 1: Figure S1). We used mega 5 software to calculate the distance of the whole thyroglobulin protein sequences and of each of the component regions (Additional file 2: Tables S2, Additional file 3: Table S3, Additional file 4: Table S4 and Additional file 5:Table S5). We performed a phylogenetic analysis on the thyroglobulin Tgl domains of four vertebrate species - (human (10 Tgl domains), mouse (10 Tgl domains), zebra finch (10 Tgl domains) and zebrafish (8 Tgl domains)) - six Tgl domains from amphioxus (a cephalochordate) and two Tgl domains from sea urchin (an echinoderm) (Figure 2). The sixth amphioxus Tgl domain clusteredwith the second sea urchin domain in the phylogenetic tree. With a lower bootstrap percentage, we observed two big major branches of the phylogenetic tree, the first corresponding to the sea urchin and amphioxus Tgl domains, which clustered with the thyroglobulin Tgl-8, Tgl-2, Tgl-1 and Tgl-10 domains, and the second corresponding to the Tgl-3, Tgl-4, Tgl-7, Tgl-5, Tgl-9 and Tgl-6 domains. For confirmation of these results, we performed a phylogenetic analysis on the thyroglobulin Tgl domains of 13 vertebrate species (human (10 Tgl domains), marmoset (10 Tgl domains), pig (10 Tgl domains), horse (10 Tgl domains), dog (10 Tgl domains), panda (10 Tgl domains), rat (10 Tgl domains), mouse (10 Tgl domains), cow (10 Tgl domains), opossum (10 Tgl domains), zebra finch (10 Tgl domains), zebrafish (8 Tgl domains) and fugu (8 Tgl domains)) together with six Tgl domains from amphioxus and two from sea urchin. This new tree also had two major branches (Additional file 6: Figure S2). The fish Tgl-10 domains did not cluster with the other Tgl-10 domains in either of the trees. We also investigated the genome of the urochordate Ciona intestinalis. The protein with the largest number of Tgl motifs was a predicted protein (rather than one for which the amino-acid sequence was actually known similar to entractin/nidogen (XP_ 002125504.1) and containing three Tgl motifs. We generated two phylogenetic trees, one based on 13 vertebrate Tgl regions (human, marmoset, pig, horse, dog, panda, rat, mouse, cow, opossum, zebra finch, zebrafish and fugu) (Figure 3) and the second based on 13 vertebrate thyroglobulin proteins (human, marmoset, pig, horse, dog, panda, rat, mouse, cow, opossum, zebra finch, zebrafish and fugu) together with the sequences of Thyroglobulin homologs from Ciona intestinalis, amphioxus and sea urchin (Figure 4).

We investigated the function of the Tgl region of thyroglobulin, by investigating proteins containing domains similar to the Tgl domain with cutoff e-value = 0.15 as recommended by the software. For the Tgl-1 domain, 107 proteins were selected (15 thyroglobulins, 15 nidogens, 18 testicans, 16 secreted proteins, acidic, cysteine-rich (SPARC) proteins, 13 invariant chains and 30 unnamed or hypothetical proteins). For the Tgl-2 domain, 49 proteins were

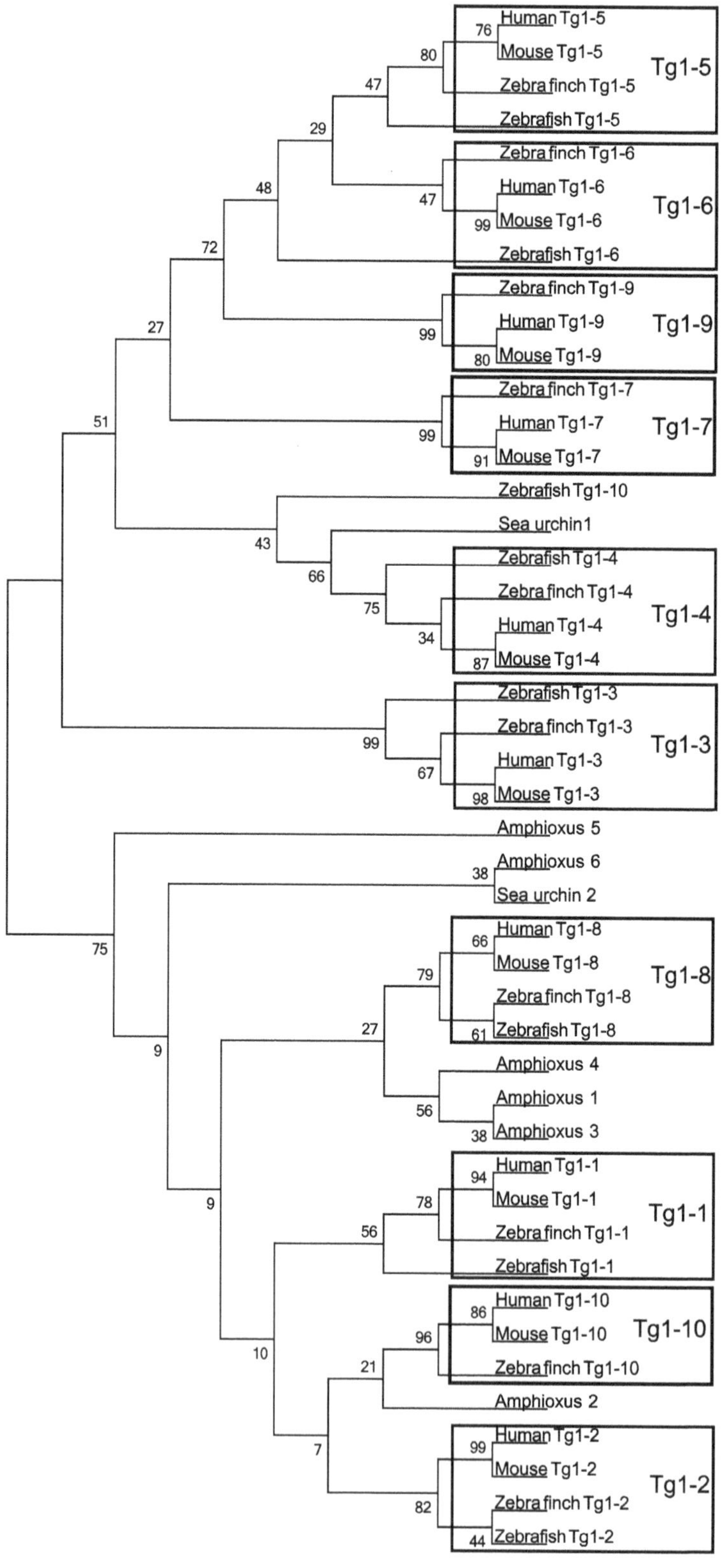

Figure 2 Phylogenetic analysis of thyroid hormone precursor Tg1 domains for six species. Phylogenetic analysis of thyroglobulin Tg1 domains from 4 species (human, mouse, zebra finch and zebrafish) and the amphioxus and sea urhin thyroglobulin-like Tg1 domains. Evolutionary history was inferred by the neighbor-joining method. The bootstrap consensus tree inferred from 1000 replicates is taken to represent the evolutionary history of the taxa analyzed. The numbers at nodes representing bootstrap support scores.

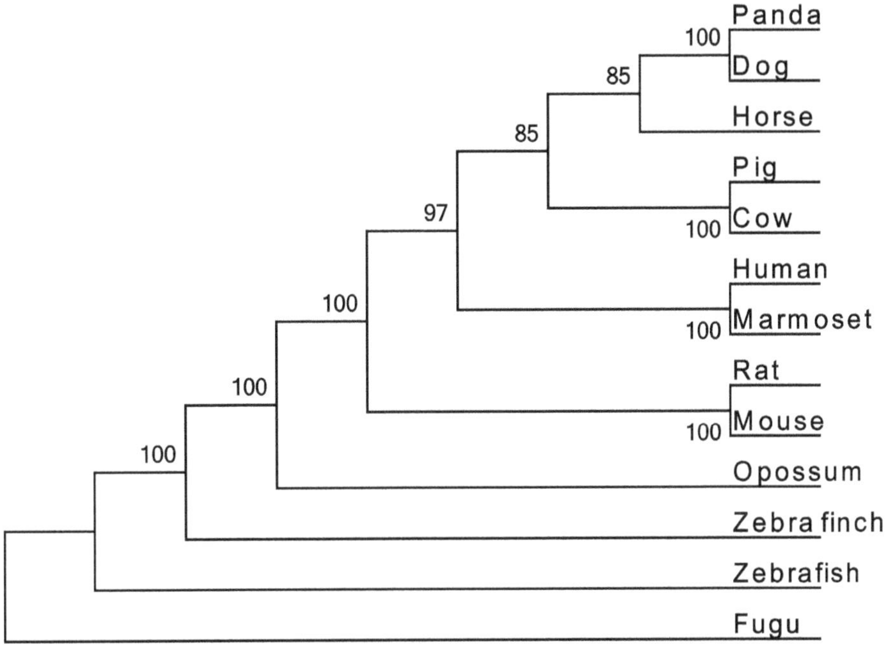

Figure 3 Phylogenetic analysis of thyroglobulin Tg1 regions from 13 species. Phylogenetic analysis of thyroglobulin Tg1 regions from 13 species (human, marmoset, rat, mouse, panda, dog, horse, pig, cow, opossum, zebra finch, zebrafish and fugu). Evolutionary history was inferred by the neighbor-joining method. The bootstrap consensus tree inferred from 1000 replicates is taken to represent the evolutionary history of the taxa analyzed. The numbers at nodes representing bootstrap support scores.

retained (15 thyroglobulins, 13 nidogens, 3 testicans, 2SPARC proteins, 3 invariant chains and 13 unnamed or hypothetical proteins). For the Tg1-3 domain, 16 proteins were found (thyroglobulins only). For the Tg1-4 domain, we retained 97 proteins (16 thyroglobulins, 13 nidogens, 10 testicans, 13 SPARC proteins, 4 invariant chains, 1 insulin-like growth factor binding protein (IGFBP) and 40 unnamed or hypothetical proteins). For the Tg1-5 domain, 103 proteins were retained (18 thyroglobulins, 6 nidogens, 11 testicans, 19 SPARC proteins, 3 invariant chains,2 IGFBPs and 44 unnamed or hypothetical proteins). For the Tg1-6 domains, 49 proteins were identified (17 thyroglobulins, 14 nidogens, 3 invariant chains and 15 unnamed or hypothetical proteins). For the Tg1-7 domain, 30 proteins were retained (10 thyroglobulins, 11 nidogens and 9 unnamed or hypothetical proteins). For the Tg1-8 domain, 105 proteins were retained (17 thyroglobulins, 13 nidogens, 9 testicans, 17 SPARC proteins, 5 invariant chains and 44 unnamed or hypothetical proteins). For the Tg1-9 domain, 11 proteins were found (thyroglobulins only). For the Tg1-10 domain, 100 proteins were retained (17 thyroglobulins, 13 nidogens, 7 testicans, 15 SPARC proteins, 3 invariant chains and 45 unnamed or hypothetical proteins). The number of thyroglobulin proteins displaying sequence similarity to the human Tg1 domains varied from 15 to 17, essentially due to the presence of incomplete thyroglobulin protein sequences in the databases we used, particularly for bears. The abovementioned proteinsdisplayed sequence similarities to the Tg1 regions of proteins from five families [34]: testicans, SPARC-related modular calcium binding (SMOC) proteins, nidogens, IGFBPs and invariant chains. Testican proteins are involved in the regulation of cell attachment, cysteine protease and metalloprotease activities [35-38]. SMOC proteins are glycoproteins present principally at the basement membrane and involved in the regulation of calcium binding [39,40]. SMOC and testican proteins are present in metazoans. Proteins of the nidogen family are known to control the three-dimensional structure of the basal membrane [41]. Nidogen proteins arealso involved in cell attachment, neutrophil chemotaxis and nervous system development [42,43]. IGFBP belongs to a family of seven proteins with high affinity for IGF with different functions in several tissues [44]. Nidogen and IGFBP are present in both tunicates and craniates. The invariant chain is involved in MHC-II cell formation [45]. This protein, like the thyroglobulin protein, is present only in vertebrates.

The Tg2 region

The second region consists of three Tg2 repetitive domains of 15 amino acids each, presenting 24% identity. The phylogenetic analysis of this region was less robust than that of the Tg1 region, due to the small size of these domains. However, we identified 33 proteins displaying sequence similarity to the Tg2 region. Nine were thyroglobulins: Bos taurus, Mus musculus, Rattus norvegicus,

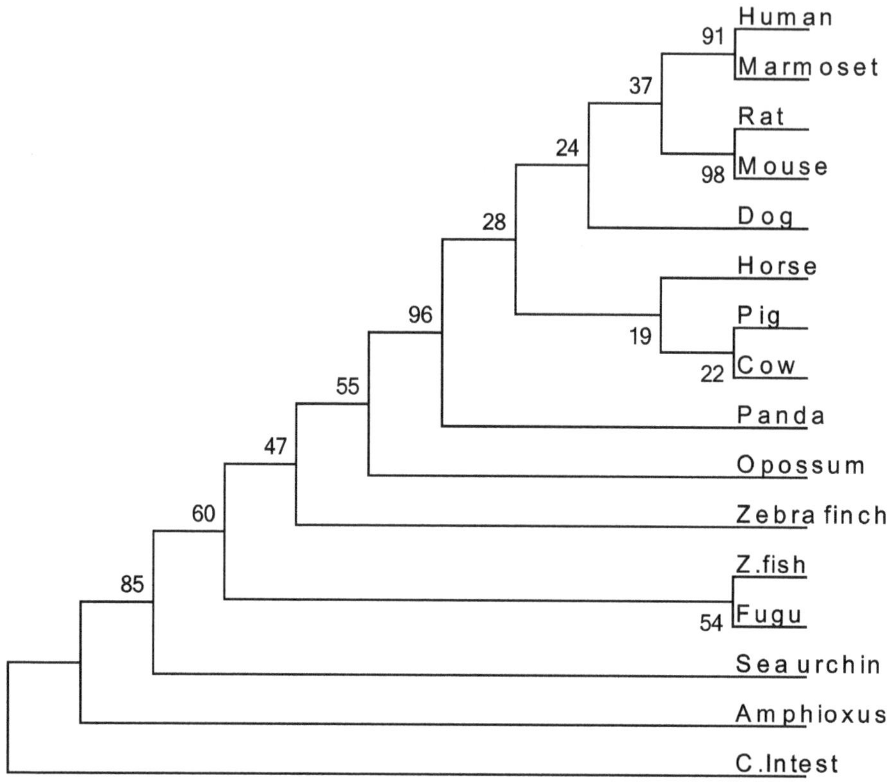

Figure 4 The phylogenetic analysis of thyroglobulins from 13 species. Phylogenetic analysis of thyroglobulins from 13 species (human, marmoset, rat, mouse, panda, dog, horse, pig, cow, opossum, zebra finch, zebrafish and fugu) and of thyroglobulin-like proteins from Ciona intestinalis, amphioxus and sea urchin. Evolutionary history was inferred by the neighbor-joining method. The bootstrap consensus tree inferred from 1000 replicates is taken to represent the evolutionary history of the taxa analyzed. The numbers at nodes representing bootstrap support scores.

Macaca mulatta, Canis lupus familiaris, Equus caballus, Sus scrofa, Taeniopygia guttata and Danio rerio. Eleven were signal peptide - CUB domain - EGF-like (SCUBE) proteins (SCUBE3: Canis familiaris, Mus musculus, Homo sapiens, Macaca mulatta, Sus scrofa and Danio rerio and/ or SCUBE1: Homo sapiens, Canis familiaris, Rattus norvegicus, Bos taurus and Danio rerio). The other 13 proteins were unnamed or hypothetical proteins. SCUBE proteins are known to involved in adhesion. Queries of the PFAM databas http://pfam.sanger.ac.uk identified a GCC2-GCC3 domain conserved in the Tg2 region of mouse and human thyroglobulins. The GCC2-GCC3 domain is also present in the human SVEP1 and mouse SCUB2 proteins.

The Tg3 region

In humans, the Tg3 region consists of five repetitive domains that can be classified into two subgroups: three domains in subgroup a (Tg3-a1: 111 AA, Tg3-a2: 98 AA, Tg3-a3: 58 AA) and two domains in subgroup b (Tg3-b1: 163 AA, Tg3-b2: 130 AA). TheseTg3 domains are 9% identical (Figure 5-a and 5-b). A search for proteins displaying sequence similarity to Tg3 domains identified only thyroglobulin proteins. Interestingly, the best conservation of cysteine residues between domains was observed in humans, with perfect conservation (100%) for Tg3-a domains and very high levels of conservation (87%) for Tg3-b domains. Furthermore, the five amino acids perfectly conserved in all Tg3 domains were cysteine residues (Figure 5-c). Cysteine residues account for 6% of all the amino acids present in the human Tg3 region and these residues were remarkably conserved in the thyroglobulin Tg3 regions of all the species studied; 100% of the 34 cysteine residues were perfectly conserved between the Tg3 regions of 12 species (human, rat, panda, marmoset, mouse, horse, dog, cow, zebra finch, zebrafish and fugu). In the opossum, two of the 34 cysteine residues in the Tg3 region were displaced (Additional file 1: Figure S1).

Tg3 domains were found only in vertebrate thyroglobulins. We investigated the origin of the Tg3 region domains, by comparing the sequences of the zebrafish Tg3 domains with the amphioxus protein. We found a similar sequence in region 413–441 of the amphioxus protein. Phylogenetic analysis including this region with the human and zebrafish thyroglobulin Tg3 domains clustered the 413–441 region of the amphioxus protein with the Tg3-2b domain of the human and the zebrafish

a)

```
Tg3-a2    CLSRCVQEHSFCQLAEITESASLYFTCTLYP---EAQVCD------DIMESN------AQ 45
Tg3-a3    CLSECS-QHEACLITTLQTQPG-AVRCMFYA---DTQSCT------HSLQG--------Q 41
Tg3-a1    CLTDCT-EDEACSFFTVSTTEP-EISCDFYAWTSDNVACMTSDQKRDALGNSKATSFGSL 58
          **: *  :.. * :  :        . * :*.    :   *         . : .

Tg3-a2    GCRLILP---QMPKALFRKKVI-LEDKVKNFYTRLPFQKLMGISIRNKVPMSEKSIS 98
Tg3-a3    NCRLLLR---EEATHIYRKP------------------------------------- 58
Tg3-a1    RCQVKVRSHGQDSPAVYLKKGQGSTTTLQKRFEPTGFQNMLSG-LYNPIVFSAS--- 111
           *..  .       .     .. *
```

b)

```
Tg3-b1    CLLACDRDLCCDGF---VLTQVQGGAIICGLLSSPSVLLCNVKDWMDPSEAWANATCPGV 57
Tg3-b2    CERRCDADPCCTGFGFLNVSQLKGGEVTCLTLNSLGIQMCSE----ENGGAWR------- 49
          *   ** * ** **     ::*::** : *   *.* .: :*.       : . **

Tg3-b1    TYDQESHQVILRLGDQEFIKSLTPLEGTQDTFTNFQQVYLWKDSDMGSRPESMGCRKDTV 117
Tg3-b2    ---------ILDCGSPDIEVHTYPFG-------------WYQKPIAQNNAPSFCPLVVL 86
                   **  *. ::     *:                * :. :...  .  *   .:

Tg3-b1    PRPASPTEAGLTTELFSPVDLNQVIVNGNQSLSSQKHW--LFKHLFSA 163
Tg3-b2    P---SLTEK-VSLDSWQSLALSSVVVDPSIRHFDVAHVSTAATSNFSA 130
          *   * **  :: : :..: *..*:*: .     .  *     .  ***
```

c)

```
Tg3-a2    CLSRCVQEHSFCQLA---EITESASLYFTCTLYP---EAQVCD--------DIMESN--- 43
Tg3-a3    CLSECS-QHEACLIT---TLQTQPG-AVRCMFYA---DTQSCT--------HSLQG---- 40
Tg3-a1    CLTDCT-EDEACSFF---TVSTTEP-EISCDFYAWTSDNVACMTSDQKR--DALGNSKAT 53
Tg3-b1    CLLACD-RDLCCDGF---VLTQVQGGAIICGLLS-SPSVLLCNVKDWMDPSEAWANATCP 55
Tg3-b2    CERRCD-ADPCCTGFGFLNVSQLKGGEVTCLTLN-SLGIQMCSEENGG----------- 46
          *   *   . *           :        . *         *

Tg3-a2    -----AQGCRLILP------------QMPKALFR--------------KKVI-LEDKV 69
Tg3-a3    ------QNCRLLLR------------EEATHIYR--------------KP-------- 58
Tg3-a1    --SFGSLRCQVKVRSHG---------QDSPAVYL--------------KKGQGSTTTL 86
Tg3-b1    GVTYDQESHQVILRLGDQEFIKSLTPLEGTQDTFTNFQQVYLWKDSDMGSRPESMGCRKD 115
Tg3-b2    -------AWRILDCGSP---------DIEVHTYPFG---------WYQKPIAQNNAPS 79
                 ::                :       :                :

Tg3-a2    KNFYTRLP-FQKLMGISIRNKVPMSEKSIS-------------------- 98
Tg3-a3    --------------------------------------------------
Tg3-a1    QKRFEPTG-FQNMLSG-LYNPIVFSAS----------------------- 111
Tg3-b1    TVPRPASP-TEAGLTTELFSPVDLNQVIVNGNQSLSSQKHW--LFKHLFSA 163
Tg3-b2    FCPLVVLPSLTEKVSLDSWQSLALSSVVVDPSIRHFDVAHVSTAATSNFSA 130
```

Figure 5 Alignment of the Tg3 domains in human thyroglobulin. a) The alignment of Tg3-a domains in human thyroglobulin: 83% of the cysteine residues are conserved in Tg3-a1, Tg3-a2 and Tg3-a3; 100% of the cysteine residues are conserved between Tg3-a1 and Tg3-a2. 55% of the conserved amino acids in Tg3-a domains are cysteine residues. **b)** The alignment of Tg3-b domains in human thyroglobulin: 100% of the cysteine residues are conserved in Tg3-b1 and Tg3-b2; 23% of the conserved amino acids in Tg3-b domains are cysteine residues. **c)** The alignment of all Tg3 domains in human thyroglobulin: 44% of the cysteine residues are conserved in all Tg3 domains; 100% of the conserved amino acids in Tg3 domains are cysteine residues.

thyroglobulins, albeit witha low bootstrap percentage (data not shown).

The C-terminal ChEL domain

The ChEL domain of human thyroglobulin consists of 581 amino acids. This region displays a high level of similarity to acetylcholinesterase, hence its name. Acetylcholinesterase catalyzes the degradation of acetylcholine in the regulation of neurotransmission [46]. Blastall analyses of the ChEL domain identified 992 proteins displaying sequence similarity to this domain: 30 thyroglobulin proteins, 598 esterases (either carboxylesterases (n = 205) or cholinesterases (n = 150)) and 35 neuroligins. Cholinesterase-like regions have previously been identified in both enzymes and structural proteins [25]. When present in structural proteins, this region is thought to be related to cell movement, as a first sign of cell differentiation [47]. The function of the ChEL domain in thyroglobulin was recently linked to its transport throughout the endoplasmic reticulum [48]. Furthermore, ChEL-truncated thyroglobulin has been shown to be unable to form homodimers [49].

Thyroid hormone synthesis sites

We determined the number of thyroid hormone synthesis sites in the thyroglobulin proteins studied here. The human thyroglobulin protein contains four major thyroid hormone synthesis sites [21]; An alignment of thyroglobulin sequences showed that the zebra finch, zebrafish and fugu proteins contained only three of the human thyroid hormone synthesis sites (Additional file 1: Figure S1). The first site (Tyr5) is the main site of hormone synthesis (more than 50%) [50] and was found to be present in all the thyroglobulin proteins studied. In amphioxus, the tyrosine residue in this position was replaced by a phenylalanine residue. Sequence alignment data showed that only the third site was present in amphioxus and that the Ciona intestinalis protein contained no thyroid hormone synthesis sites.

Discussion

The Tg1 region of thyroglobulin may be involved in binding

In vertebrates, iodination of the tyrosine residues of thyroglobulin requires the protein to be present in the lumen of the thyroid follicle. The iodinated thyroglobulin is then returned to the cell via a process called pinocytosis, which involves histone H1 [3], megalin (gp330) [4] and/or the N-acetylglucosamine receptor [5]. Our study of the thyroglobulin Tg1 region showed this region to be structurally related to proteins with binding functions from five families. Novinec et al [34] also described another protein with sequence similarity to the Tg1 domain, trophinin. This membrane protein has been shown to mediate the adhesion of homophilic cells [51]. We think the Tg1 region may mediate the binding of thyroglobulin to the thyrocyte apical membrane. The region of the H1 histone binding to thyroglobulin remains unidentified, whereas two regions of the N-acetylglucosamine receptor have been reported to bind thyroglobulin: RHL-1 subunit (N1-A500) [5] and (S789-M1,172) [52]. These receptors bind to the N-terminal end (Tg1 region) of the thyroglobulin protein. By contrast, megalin has been shown to interact with the carboxy-terminal domain of thyroglobulin, at R2,489-E2,503 [53], although the authors of this study were themselves critical of this work [54]. They reported that the region of interaction was poorly conserved between human and rat thyroglobulins and their finding that a rabbit antibody raised against R2,489-E2,503 reduced heparin-binding to rat Tg by only 70% led them to conclude that other heparin-binding sites must be involved in binding. These data, including the similarity of the Tg1 region to the extracellular matrix proteins nidogen and testican, provide support for our hypothesis that the Tg1 region is involved in the attachment and endocytosis of thyroglobulin.

Phylogeny of the Tg1 region

The function of thyroglobulin seems to depend strongly on the follicle structure of the thyroid. This follicular structure is observed only in vertebrates. Nonetheless, although it remains unclear whether a colloid is present in the endostyle of the invertebrates of the chordate group, such as cephalochordates and urochordates, the endostyle is widely considered to be homologous to the follicle of the vertebrate thyroid gland [55]. This is not consistent with the detection of a thyroglobulin protein in Eisenia fetida by Wilhelm [56]. In annelids, hormones are produced exclusively by the central nervous system. No sequence that could be unambiguously identified as corresponding to a thyroglobulin was found in the amphioxus genome [57], but a large protein (about 2,400 amino acids) with biochemical properties similar to those of thyroglobulin has been described in this organism [58]. Both T3 and T4 have also been described in this cephalochordate [59]. The 2,400-amino acid thyroglobulin-like protein of this species contains six domains displaying sequence similarity to the Tg1 region but not to the Tg2, Tg3 and ChEL domains (Figure 1-c).

Another smaller protein of about 137 amino acids that clusters with vertebrate thyroglobulin in phylogenetic analysis was identified in sea urchin (Figure 4). This protein contains two Tg1 domains but has no Tg2, Tg3 or ChEL domains (Figure 1-d). Phylogenetic analysis of a large number of sequences [60] classified the urochordates as more closely related to vertebrates than the cephalochordates (amphioxus) and echinoderms (sea urchin). On the basis of these data, we looked for a protein homologous to thyroglobulin in urochordates. Patricolo et al. demonstrated the presence of thyroid hormones and their involvement in metamorphosis in ascidian larvae from the Urochordata [17]. However, the genome of another urochordate, Ciona intestinalis, was found to contain no sequence homologous to thyroglobulin despite the presence of thyroid hormones. These data suggest that ascidians use other precursor proteins for iodotyrosine synthesis [61]. Together, these data suggest that the origins of the thyroglobulin protein lie in the Echinodermata.

We investigated the origin of the Tg1 region domains, by studying the phylogeny of the Tg1 domains in an analysis including the sea urchin protein (Echinodermata), the amphioxus protein (Cephalochordata), and the zebrafish (Teleostei), zebra finch (Aves) and human thyroglobulins. Our results suggest that the second Tg1 domain of the sea urchin protein is the ancestor of the sixth Tg1 domains of the amphioxus protein, while Tg1 domains 1, 2, 3, 4 and 5 of the amphioxus protein probably resulting from the duplication of domain 6. The phylogenetic analysis suggested that the Tg1-1, Tg1-2, Tg1-8 and Tg1-10 domains ofthyroglobulin were derived directly from the Tg1 domains of the amphioxus protein (Figure 2). The separation of thyroglobulin domains into two major branches may indicate two different origins of thyroglobulin Tg1 domains. The thyroglobulin Tg1 domains clustering with the amphioxus protein Tg1 domains are located at the end of the Tg1 region. We suggest that the thyroglobulin Tg1 domainsduplicated from the two ends to the center of the Tg1 region. The number of Tg1 domains presence increases with the number of evolutionary steps, suggesting that the evolution of thyroglobulin function may be dependent on number of Tg1 domains. However,the branching of the tree for Tg1 domains has only weak bootstrap support. (Figure 2 and Additional file 6: Figure S2), probably due to the length of time over which evolution has been occurring. Each Tg1 domain is free to evolve by itself, but the overall structure of the Tg1 region is conserved (Figure 3).

Involvement of the Tg2 region in cell adhesion

The presence of the Tg2 region in the SCUBE protein of many species suggests that these proteins may have a common function. SCUBE is a protein found in many embryonic tissues [62]. In zebrafish, mutations in the SCUBE2 gene are associated principally with developmental deficits [63]. A recent study showed that SCUBE1 was an adhesive molecule mediating platelet-matrix interaction and ristocetin-induced platelet agglutination [64]. On the basis of its secretory nature, SCUBE3 is thought to function locally or at distance, in a paracrine or endocrine fashion [65]. However, the exact functions of SCUBE3 remain elusive. On the basis of these and published results, we suggest the Tg2 region isinvolved in thyroglobulin-mediated cell adhesion. The conservation of the GCC2-GCC3 domain in the Tg2 region highlights the structural conservation of this region. The function of the GCC2-GCC3 domain remains unknown, but this domain is present in the human SVEP1 protein. The functional annotation of this protein indicates a role in cell adhesion. This is potentially consistent with our hypothesis that the Tg2 region is involved in cell adhesion.

The Tg3 region may have a structural function

Cysteine is important for the correct three-dimensional structure of a protein, through its role in the formation of disulfide bonds. Misfolded proteins are recognized as abnormal and disposed of by a non lysosomal proteolytic pathway. Hishinuma et al [66] showed that replacement of the cysteine residues of (C1236R) (C1995S) thyroglobulin prevent the protein from forming the disulfide bonds required for thyroglobulin monomer production. As a result, intracellular transport is blocked and both these mutated thyroglobulins are retained in the endoplasmic reticulum. The high degree of cysteine residue conservation in Tg3 domains and in Tg3 regions from the 13 species used to generate the phyogenetic tree, from Actinopterygii to humans, highlights the importance of correct disulfide bond formation to the the tertiary structure of thyroglobulin. In a recent study, Targovenik et al [67] reviewed the cysteine mutations in thyroglobulin andshowed that more than half these mutations (55%) occurred in the Tg3 region. They also reported changes to the three-dimensional structure of thyroglobulin in the presence of cysteine mutations in the Tg3 region. The presence of Tg3 regions only in thyroglobulin proteins may be explained by a structural function, the disulfide bonds being essential to the three-dimensional structure of the molecule. The region of homology highlighted here between the zebrafish Tg3 region and the amphioxus protein suggests that this best conserved region between Tg3 domains may be the origin of these domains. There are two Tg3 subgroups, a and b. We therefore suggest that the original sequence duplicated twice initially, to generate the Tg3-a and Tg3-b domains. The Tg3-a domain duplicated three times, generating Tg3-a1, Tg3-a2 and Tg3-a3, and the Tg3-b domain duplicated twice, giving rise to Tg3-b1 and Tg3-b2.

The ChEL domain is involved in protein transport

The two studies mentioned above [48,49] demonstrated that a role for the ChEL domain in the dimerization and transport of thyroglobulin. Kim et al [68] indicated that mutations affecting the ChEL domain of mouse thyroglobulin resulted in the synthesis of a full-length thyroglobulin that folded abnormally, preventing its transport to the Golgi complex. However, the ChEL domain is present in structural proteins, as described by Krejci et al [25]. We demonstrated the similarity of this domain between thyroglobulin, esterase and neuroligin proteins, neuroligins being heterophilic cell adhesion proteins [69]. We suggest that the ChEL domain is involved in thyroglobulin transport (thyrocyte to apical membrane) and dimerization, with a possible additional function in cell adhesion. Phylogenetic studies of esterase domains from less evolved species have indicated that the thyroglobulin ChEL and esterase domains have a common ancestor [26]. Additional file 2: Tables S2, Additional file 3: Table S3, Additional file 4: Table S4 and Additional file 5:Table S5 show the pairwise distances between whole thyroglobulin protein sequences and each region of thyroglobulin. The ChEL domain is the region of thyroglobulin for which distances were lowest between different species. This suggests that the thyroglobulin ChEL domain may have been less subject to rearrangement during evolution than the other domains.

Existence of other thyroid hormone synthesis sites

We show here that not all the thyroid hormone synthesis sites characterized to date are systematically present in all species with a thyroglobulin protein. The lack of some thyroid hormone synthesis sites in some more highly evolved species (3 in zebra finch, zebrafish and fugu), the presence of only one site in the amphioxus protein and the total absence of thyroid hormone synthesis sites in the sea urchin protein may be explained by the relocation of these sites. Thyroid hormone synthesisrequires tyrosine residue iodination. The sea urchin protein has five tyrosine residues (positions 3, 24, 31, 34 and 102) and at least one of these residues is a thyroid hormone synthesis site. The lack of sites in amphioxus, zebrafinch, zebrafish and fugu may be explained by an absence of need for large thyroid hormone production or the use of other tyrosine residues as thyroid hormone synthesis sites.

We explored the function of thyroglobulin by phylogeny; we compared the thyroglobulin regions of echinoderms and vertebrate species. Our results suggest that the Tgl region may have been the first to appear in the thyroglobulin protein. The Tgl regionwas also subject to the largest number of rearrangements during evolution. The Tg2, Tg3 and ChEL regions are present only in the thyroglobulin of vertebrates, suggesting a link between these regions and an adaptive function of thyroglobulin. The thyroglobulin protein seems to result from the assembly of the four regions. We found no precursor of thyroid hormones with only two or three of these regions in databases. We therefore suggest that the Tg2, Tg3 and ChEL regions appeared in thyroglobulin at the same time. These data support the hypothesis of potential additional functions of thyroglobulin in the cell, as an iodine reservoir, in cell-cell adhesion and in binding. As each thyroglobulin region may have a specific function in the protein, a mutation in one region may have consequences for the specific function of this region, resulting in a different pattern of phenotypic expression.

Note

A recent study raised the question of human DNA contamination in genomic databases [70], The first 5477 bp of chromosome 11 in zebrafish is 100% identical to human chromosome 4. We verified the zebrafish thyroglobulin located on chromosome 16 at position chr16:33,835,318-33,852,335, and the human thyroglobulin located on chromosome 8 at position chr8:133,909,894-134,147,141.

Additional files

Additional file 1: Figure S1. The phylogenetic analysis of Tg1 domains from the thyroglobulins of 13 species. The phylogenetic analysis of thyroglobulin Tg1 domains from 13 species (human, marmoset, rat, mouse, panda, dog, horse, pig, cow, opossum, zebra finch, zebrafish and fugu) and the Tg1 domains of thyroglobulin-like proteins from Ciona intestinalis, amphioxus and sea urchin. Evolutionary history was inferred by the neighbor-joining method. The bootstrap consensus tree inferred from 1000 replicates is taken to represent the evolutionary history of the taxa analyzed. The numbers at nodes representing bootstrap scores.

Additional file 2: Table S1. Estimation of evolutionary divergence between the thyroglobulin protein sequences of 13 species + the thryoglobulin-like sequences of Ciona intestinalis, amphioxus and sea urchin. The number of amino-acid substitutions per site between sequences is shown. Standard error estimates are shown above the diagonal and were obtained by a bootstrap procedure (10000 replicates). Analyses were conducted with the Jones-Taylor-Thornton matrix-based model. The rate variation between sites was modeled with a gamma distribution (shape parameter = 1).

Additional file 3: Table S2. Estimation of evolutionary divergence between the Tg1 region sequences of thyroglobulins from 13 species. The number of amino acid substitutions per site between sequences is shown. Standard error estimates are shown above the diagonal and were obtained by a bootstrap procedure (10000 replicates). Analyses were conducted with the Jones-Taylor-Thornton matrix-based model. The rate variation between sites was modeled with a gamma distribution (shape parameter = 1).

Additional file 4: Table S3. Estimation of evolutionary divergence between the Tg3 region sequences of thyroglobulins from 13 species. The number of amino acid substitutions per site between sequences is shown. Standard error estimates are shown above the diagonal and were obtained by a bootstrap procedure (10000 replicates). Analyses were conducted with the Jones-Taylor-Thornton matrix-based model. The rate variation between sites was modeled with a gamma distribution (shape parameter = 1).

Additional file 5: Table S4. Estimation of evolutionary divergence between the ChEL region sequences of thyroglobulins from 13 species. The number of amino acid substitutions per site between sequences is shown. Standard error estimates are shown above the diagonal and were obtained by a bootstrap procedure (10000 replicates). Analyses were conducted with the Jones-Taylor-Thornton matrix-based model. The rate variation between sites was modeled with a gamma distribution (shape parameter = 1).

Additional file 6: Figure S2. ClustalX sequence alignment for thyroglobulins from 13 species. The ClustalX sequence alignment of thyroglobulins from 13 species (human, marmoset, rat, mouse, panda, dog, horse, pig, cow, opossum, zebra finch, zebrafish and fugu) and the amphioxus and sea urchin thyroglobulin-like proteins. Red: the four humanthyroid hormone synthesis sites; in green, the 10 human Tg1 domains; in yellow, the human Tg2 region; in blue, the 5 human Tg3 domains.

Competing interests
The authors declare that they have no competing interests.

Authors' contributions
YM AB conceived the analysis. CJ FS contributed to discussion and edited the manuscript. AB analyzed data and wrote the manuscript. All authors read and approved the final manuscript.

Acknowledgements
This work was supported by the regional organization BioInformatique Ligérienne (BIL) directed by Rémi Houlgatte. We would like to thank Laurent Abel for his help. We would also like to thank La région Pays de Loire, the Institut National de Recherche Médical (INSERM) and the University of Angers.

Author details
[1]INSERM U694, Institut Biologie Santé (IBS), rue des Capucins, F-49100 Angers, France. [2]University of Angers, rue de Rennes, F-49045 Angers, France. [3]Laboratory of human genetics of infectious diseases. Necker Branch, INSERM, U980 Paris, France.

References
1. Kotlarz G, Wegrowski Y, Martiny L, Declerck P, Bellon G: **Enhanced expression of plasminogen activator inhibitor-1 by dedifferentiated thyrocytes.** *Biochem Biophys Res Commun* 2002, **295:**737–743.
2. Delom F, Mallet B, Carayon P, Lejeune P: **Role of extracellular molecular chaperones in the folding of oxidized proteins, Refolding of colloidal thyroglobulin by protein disulfide isomerase and immunoglobulin heavy chain-binding protein.** *J Biol Chem* 2001, **276:**21337–21342.
3. Brix K, Summa W, Lottspeich F, Herzog V: **Extracellularly occurring histone H1 mediates the binding of thyroglobulin to the cell surface of mouse macrophages.** *J Clin Invest* 1998, **102:**283–293.
4. Zheng G, Marino' M, Zhao J, McCluskey R: **Megalin (gp330): a putative endocytic receptor for thyroglobulin (Tg).** *Endocrinology* 1998, **139:**1462–1465.
5. Montuori N, Pacifico F, Mellone S, Liguoro D, Jeso BD, Formisano S, Gentile F, Consiglio E: **The rat asialoglycoprotein receptor binds the amino-terminal domain of thyroglobulin.** *Biochem Biophys Res Commun* 2000, **268:**42–46.
6. Dunn J, Anderson P, Fox J, Fassler C, Dunn A, Hite L, Moore R: **The sites of thyroid hormone formation in rabbit thyroglobulin.** *J Biol Chem* 1987, **262:**16948–16952.
7. Dunn J, Dunn A: **The importance of thyroglobulin structure for thyroid hormone biosynthesis.** *Biochimie* 1998, **81:**505–509.
8. Schimmel M, Utiger R: **Thyroidal and peripheral production of thyroid hormones, Review of recent findings and their clinical implications.** *Ann Intern Med* 1977, **87:**760–768.
9. Suzuki K, Lavaroni S, Mori A, Ohta M, Saito J, Pietrarelli M, Singer D, Kimura S, Katoh R, Kawaoi A, Kohn L: **Autoregulation of thyroid-specific gene transcription by thyroglobulin.** *Proc. Natl. Acad. Sci. USA* 1998, **95:**8251–8256.
10. Hayashi M, Shimonaka M, Matsui K, Hayashi T, Ochiai D, Emoto N: **Proliferative effects of bovine and porcine thyroglobulins on thyroid epithelial cells.** *Endocr J* 2009, **56:**509–519.
11. Monaco F, Roche J, Carducci C, Carlini F, Cataudella S, Felli P, Andreoli M, Dominici R: **Effect of change of habitat (sea and fresh water) on in vivo thyroglobulin synthesis in Atlantic glassed eels (Anguilla anguilla L.).** *C R Seances Soc Biol Fil.* 1981, **175:**452–456.
12. Kim B: **Thyroid hormone as a determinant of energy expenditure and the basal metabolic rate.** *Thyroid* 2008, **18:**141–144.
13. Flamant F, Baxter J, Forrest D, Refetoff S, Samuels H, Scanlan T, Vennström B, Samarut J: **International Union of Pharmacology, LIX. The Pharmacology and Classification of the Nuclear Receptor Superfamily: Thyroid Hormone Receptors.** *Pharmacol Rev* 2006, **58:**705–711.
14. Power D, Llewellyn L, Faustino M, Nowell M, Björnsson B, Einarsdottir I, Canario A, Sweeney G: **Thyroid hormones in growth and developement of fish.** *Comp Biochem Physiol C Toxicol Pharmacol.* 2001, **130:**447–459.
15. Manchado M, Infante C, Asensio E, Planas J, Canavate J: **Thyroid hormones down-regulate thyrotropin beta subunit and thyroglobulin during metamorphosis in the flatfish Senegalese sole (Solea senegalensis Kaup).** *Gen Comp Endocrino.* 2008, **155:**447–455.
16. Tata J: **Amphibian metamorphosis as a model for the developmental actions of thyroid hormone.** *Mol Cell Endocrinol* 2005, **246:**10–20.
17. Patricolo E, Cammarata M, D'Agati P: **Presence of thyroid hormones in ascidian larvae and their involvement in metamorphosis.** *J Exp Zool* 2001, **290:**426–430.
18. Paris M, Laudet V: **The history of developmental stages: metamorphosis in chordates.** *Genesis* 2008, **46:**657–672.
19. Manzon R, Holmes J, Youson J: **Variable effects of goitrogens in inducing precocious metamorphosis in sea lampreys (Petromyzon marinus).** *J Exp Zool* 2001, **289:**290–303.
20. Mercken L, Simons M, Swillens S, Massaer M, Vassart G: **Primary structure of bovine thyroglobulin deduced from the sequence of its 8,431-base complementary DNA.** *Nature* 1985, **316:**647–651.
21. Malthiéry Y, Lissitzky S: **Primary structure of human thyroglobulin deduced from the sequence of its 8448-base complementary DNA.** *Eur J Biochem* 1987, **165:**491–508.
22. de Graaf SV, Ris-Stalpers C, Pauws E, Mendive F, Targovnik H, Vijlder J: **Up to date with human thyroglobulin.** *Endocr J* 2001, **170:**307–321.
23. Veneziani B, Giallauria F, Gentile F: **The disulfide bond pattern between fragments obtained by the limited proteolysis of bovine thyroglobulin.** *Biochimie* 1999, **81:**517–525.
24. Schumacher M, Camp S, Maulet Y, Newton M, MacPhee-Quigley K, Taylor S, Friedmann T, Taylor P: **Primary structure of Tropedo californica acetylcholinesterase deduced form its cDNA sequence.** *Nature* 1986, **319:**407–409.
25. Krejci E, Duval N, Chatonnet A, Vincens P, Massoulié J: **Cholinesterase-like domains in enzymes and structural proteins: functional and evolutionary relationships and identification of a catalytically essential aspartic acid.** *Proc Natl Acad Sci USA* 1991, **88:**6647–6651.
26. Takagi Y, Omura T, Go M: **Evolutionary origin of thyroglobulin by duplication of esterase gene.** *FEBS Lett* 1991, **282:**17–22.
27. Izumi M, Larsen P: **Metabolic clearance of endogenous and radioiodinated thyroglobulin in rats.** *Endocrinology* 1978, **103:**96–100.
28. Rigden D, Mosolov V, Galperin M: **Sequence conservation in the chagasin family suggests a common trend in cysteine proteinase binding by unrelated protein inhibitors.** *Protein Sci* 2002, **11:**1971–1977.
29. Saverwyns H, Visser A, Durme JV, Power D, Morgado I, Kennedy M, Knox D, Schymkowitz J, Rousseau F, Gevaert K, Vercruysse J, Claerebout E, Geldhof P: **Analysis of the transthyretin-like (TTL) gene family in Ostertagia ostertagi - Comparison with other strongylid nematodes and Caenorhabditis elegans.** *Int J Parasitol* 2008, **38:**1545–1556.
30. Felsenstein J: **PHYLIP - Phylogeny Inference Package (Version 3.2).** *Cladistics.* 1989, **5:**164–166.
31. Tamura K, Peterson D, Peterson N, Stecher G, Nei M, Kumar S: MEGA5: Molecular Evolutionary Genetics Analysis using Maximum Likelihood, Evolutionary Distance, and Maximum Parsimony Methods. *Mol Biol and Evol* 2011, **28:**2731-2739.
32. Jones D, Taylor W, Thornton J: **A mutation data matrix for transmembrane proteins.** *FEBS Lett* 1994, **339:**269–275.
33. Molina F, Bouanani M, Pau B, Granier C: **Characterization of the type-1 repeat from thyroglobulin, a cysteine-rich module found in proteins from different families.** *Eur J Biochem* 1996, **240:**125–133.
34. Novinec M, Kordis D, Turk V, Lenarcic B: **Diversity and evolution of the thyroglobulin type-1 domain superfamily.** *Mol Biol Evol* 2006, **23:**744–755.
35. Marr H, Edgell C: **Testican-1 inhibits attachment of Neuro-2a cells.** *Matrix Biol* 2003, **22:**259–266.
36. Bocock J, Edgell C, Marr H, Erickson A: **Human proteoglycan testican-1 inhibits the lysosomal cysteine protease cathepsin L.** *Eur J Biochem* 2003, **270:**4008–4015.
37. Nakada M, Yamada A, Takino T, Miyamori H, Takahashi T, Yamashita J, Sato H: **Suppression of membrane-type 1 matrix metalloproteinase (MMP)-mediated MMP-2 activation and tumor invasion by testican 3 and its splicing variant gene product.** *N-Tes. Cancer Res.* 2001, **61:**8896–8902.
38. Nakada M, Miyamori H, Yamashita J, Sato H: **Testican 2 abrogates inhibition of membrane-type matrix metalloproteinases by other testican family proteins.** *Cancer Res* 2003, **63:**3364–3369.
39. Vannahme C, Smyth N, Miosge N, Gösling S, Frie C, Paulsson M, Maurer P, Hartmann U: **Characterization of SMOC-1, a novel modular calcium-**

binding protein in basement membranes. *J Biol Chem* 2002, **277**:37977–37986.

40. Vannahme C, Gösling S, Paulsson M, Maurer P, Hartmann U: **Characterization of SMOC-2, a modular extracellular calcium-binding protein.** *Biochem J* 2002, **373**:805–814.
41. Aumailley M, Battaglia C, Mayer U, Reinhardt D, Nischt R, Timpl R, Fox J: **Nidogen mediates the formation of ternary complexes of basement membrane components.** *Kidney Int* 1993, **43**:7–12.
42. Chakravarti S, Tam M, Chung A: **The basement membrane glycoprotein entactin promotes cell attachment and binds calcium ions.** *J Biol Chem* 1990, **265**:10597–10603.
43. Kim S, Wadsworth W: **Positioning of longitudinal nerves in C. elegans by nidogen.** *Science* 2000, **288**:150-154.
44. Rajaram S, Baylink D, Mohan S: **Insulin-like growth factor-binding proteins in serum and other biological fluids: regulation and functions.** *Endocr Rev* 1997, **18**:801–831.
45. Holst P, Sorensen M, Jensen CM, Orskov C, Thomsen A, Christensen J: **MHC class II-associated invariant chain linkage of antigen dramatically improves cell-mediated immunity induced by adenovirus vaccines.** *J Immunol* 2008, **180**:3339–3346.
46. Tsim K, Leung K, Mok K, Chen V, Zhu K, Zhu J, Guo A, Bi C, Zheng K, Lau D, Xie H, Choi R: **Expression and Localization of PRiMA-linked globular form acetylcholinesterase in vertebrate neuromuscular junctions.** *J Mol Neurosci* 2009, **40**:40–46.
47. Layer P, Kaulich S: **Cranial nerve growth in birds is preceded by cholinesterase expression during neural crest cell migration and the formation of an HNK-1 scaffold.** *Cell Tissue Res* 1991, **265**:393–407.
48. Lee J, Jeso BD, Arvan P: **The cholinesterase-like domain of thyroglobulin functions as an intramolecular chaperone.** *J Clin Invest* 2008, **118**:2950–2958.
49. Lee J, Wang X, Jeso BD, Arvan P: **The cholinesterase-like domain, essential in thyroglobulin trafficking for thyroid hormone synthesis, is required for protein dimerization.** *J Biol Chem* 2009, **284**:12752–12761.
50. Palumbo G, Gentile F, Condorelli G, Salvatore G: **The earliest site of iodination in thyroglobulin is residue number 5.** *J Biol Chem* 1990, **265**:8887–8892.
51. Fukuda M, Sugihara K, Nakayama J: **Trophinin: what embryo implantation teaches us about human cancer.** *Cancer Biol Ther* 2008, **7**:1165–1170.
52. Mezghrani A, Mziaut H, Courageot J, Oughideni R, Bastiani P, Miquelis R: **Identification of the membrane receptor binding domain of thyroglobulin, Insights into quality control of thyroglobulin biosynthesis.** *J Biol Chem* 1997, **272**:23340–23346.
53. Marino M, Friedlander J, McCluskey R, Andrews D: **Identification of a Heparin-binding Region of Rat Thyroglobulin Involved in Megalin Binding.** *J Biol Chem* 1999, **274**:30377–30386.
54. Lisi S, Pinchera A, McCluskey R, Chiovato L, Marino M: **Binding of heparin to human thyroglobulin (Tg) involves multiple binding sites including a region corresponding to a binding site of rat Tg.** *Eur J Endocrinol* 2002, **146**:591–602.
55. Ogasawara M, Lauro RD, Satoh N: **Ascidian homologs of mammalian thyroid peroxidase genes are expressed in the thyroid-equivalent region of the endostyle.** *J Exp Zool* 1999, **285**:158–169.
56. Wilhelm M, Koza A, Engelmann P, Németh P, Csoknya M: **Evidence for the presence of thyroid stimulating hormone, thyroglobulin and their receptors in Eisenia fetida: a multilevel hormonal interface between the nervous system and the peripheral tissues.** *Cell Tissue Res* 2006, **324**:535–546.
57. Paris M, Brunet F, Markov G, Schubert M, Laudet V: **The amphioxus genome enlightens the evolution of the thyroid hormone signaling pathway.** *Dev Genes Evol* 2008, **218**:667–680.
58. Monaco F, Dominici R, Andreoli M, Pirro RD, Roche J: **Thyroid hormone formation in thyroglobulin synthetized in the amphioxus (Branchiostoma lanceolatum Pallas.** *Comp Biochem Physiol* 1980, **70**:341–343.
59. Covelli I, Salvador G, Sena L, Roche J: **Sur la formation des hormones thyroïdiennes et de leurs précursseurs par Branchiostoma lanceolatum.** *C R Soc Biol Paris* 1960, **154**:1165–1169.
60. Delsuc F, Brinkmann H, Chourrout D, Philippe H: **Tunicates and not cephalochordates are the closest living relatives of vertebrates.** *Nature* 2006, **439**:965–968.
61. Campbell R, Satoh N, Degnan B: **Piecing together evolution of the vertebrate endocrine system.** *Trends Genet* 2004, **20**:359–366.
62. Grimmond S, Larder R, Hateren NV, Siggers P, Hulsebos T, Arkell R, Greenfield A: **Cloning, mapping, and expression analysis of a gene encoding a novel mammalian EGF-related protein (SCUBE1).** *Genomics* 2000, **70**:74–81.
63. Woods I, Talbot W: **The you gene encodes an EGF-CUB protein essential for Hedgehog signaling in zebrafish.** *PLoS Biol* 2005, **3**:e66.
64. Tu C, Su Y, Huang Y, Tsai M, Li L, Chen Y, Cheng C, Dai D, Yang R: **Localization and characterization of a novel secreted protein SCUBE1 in human platelets.** *Cardiovasc Res* 2006, **71**:486–495.
65. Wu B, Su Y, Tsai M, Wasserman S, Topper J, Yang R: **A novel secreted, cell-surface glycoprotein containing multiple epidermal growth factor-like repeats and one CUB domain is highly expressed in primary osteoblasts and bones.** *J Biol Chem* 2004, **279**:37485–37490.
66. Hishinuma A, Takamatsu J, Ohyama Y, Yokozawa T, Kanno Y, Kuma K, Yoshida S, Matsuura N, Ieiri T: **Two novel cysteine substitutions (C1263R and C1995S) of thyroglobulin cause a defect in intracellular transport of thyroglobulin in patients with congenital goiter and the variant type of adenomatous goiter.** *J Clin Endocrinol Metab* 1999, **84**:1438–1444.
67. Targovnik H, Esperante S, Rivolta C: **Genetics and phenomics of hypothyroidism and goiter due to thyroglobulin mutations.** *Mol Cell Endocrinol* 2009, **322**:44–55.
68. Kim P, Hossain S, Park Y, Lee I, Yoo S, Arvan P: **A single amino acid change in the acetylcholinesterase-like domain of thyroglobulin causes congenital goiter with hypothyroidism in the cog/cog mouse: a model of human endoplasmic reticulum storage diseases.** *Proc Natl Acad Sci USA* 1998, **95**:9909–9913.
69. Jaco AD, Dubi N, Comoletti D, Taylor P: **Folding anomalies of neuroligin3 caused by mutation in the α/β -hydrolase fold domain.** *Chem Biol Interact* 2010, **187**:56–58.
70. Longo M, O'Neil M, O'Neill R: **Abundant Human DNA Contamination Identified in Non-Primate Genome Databases.** *PLoS One* 2011, **6**:e16410.

12

Prevalence of diabetes mellitus in patients with newly evaluated papillary thyroid cancer

Yannis M Paulus[1], Elyn R Riedel[2], Mona M Sabra[1], Robert Michael Tuttle[1] and Marcia F Kalin[1*]

Abstract

Background: This study investigates whether diabetes mellitus is a risk factor for the development of papillary thyroid cancer, using an age-, gender-, and race-matched analysis.

Methods: We retrospectively reviewed the charts of 1559 patients with newly evaluated thyroid cancer over a 4-year period at our institution and identified 1313 patients (84%) with papillary thyroid carcinoma. Characteristics of patients with diabetes versus those without diabetes were compared with a chi-square test for categorical variables and the Wilcoxon Rank Sum test for numeric variables. The prevalence of diabetes among patients with papillary thyroid carcinoma at our institution was compared (using an age-, gender-, and race-matched analysis) with that expected based on data from the continuous National Health and Nutrition Examination Survey (NHANES) from the same time period.

Results: For patients with papillary thyroid carcinoma, the median age was 47 years; 74% were female; 83% were white; and the prevalence of diabetes was 8%. Among those with diabetes, 92% had type 2 diabetes, and 24% were treated with insulin. Risk factors for diabetes included age and race. The prevalence of diabetes among patients with papillary thyroid carcinoma of all ages versus that among patients from NHANES of all ages was not significantly different (RR 1.07, CI 0.88 - 1.28). The prevalence of diabetes among patients with papillary thyroid cancer who were 44 years of age or younger versus that among patients from NHANES who were 44 years of age or younger, however, was significantly increased (RR 2.32, CI 1.37 - 3.66). There was no significant difference when subgroup analysis was performed by gender or race.

Conclusions: We found an increased prevalence of diabetes in patients with papillary thyroid carcinoma who were 44 years of age or younger.

Keywords: Diabetes mellitus, Papillary thyroid cancer, NHANES, Risk factor

Background

Diabetes mellitus is a risk factor for cancer, specifically of breast, endometrium, bladder, liver, colorectum, and pancreas [1]. The pathophysiology of how diabetes contributes to cancer growth or development is an area of active investigation. The most commonly proposed mechanism is that hyperinsulinemia, which results as a compensatory response to the insulin resistance underlying type 2 diabetes, is mitogenic, through activation of the insulin receptor or the insulin-like growth factor-I receptor [2], which in turn stimulates cellular proliferation and inhibits cellular apoptosis [3]. Another possible mechanism is that hyperglycemia promotes carcinogenesis by increasing oxidative stress [1].

Several previous studies have tested for an association between diabetes and thyroid cancer, including one case control study and three large cohort studies. The case control study, which comprised 110 patients with anaplastic thyroid cancer, found a 4-fold increased prevalence of diabetes [4].

In the National Institutes of Health-AARP diet and health study, which involved a cohort of almost 500,000 adults, the prevalence of diabetes was 7.4% in women, and 10.1% in men. Over 10 years, 585 cases of thyroid cancer were identified. Women with diabetes had a 1.46 increased risk for all thyroid cancers, a 1.25 increased risk for papillary thyroid cancer, and a 1.92 increased

* Correspondence: kalinm@mskcc.org
[1]Memorial Sloan-Kettering Cancer Center, Department of Medicine, 1275 York Avenue, New York, NY 10065, USA
Full list of author information is available at the end of the article

risk for follicular thyroid cancer. There was no significant difference in the risk of thyroid cancer for men with diabetes or for the combined group of men and women with diabetes [5].

A cohort study of 4.5 million male veterans with 1053 cases of thyroid cancer found non-significant increases in risk for thyroid cancer among patients with diabetes: 1.2 for less than 5 years of diabetes, and 1.1 for at least 5 years of diabetes [6].

A population-based study of 1 million patients in Taiwan with 943 cases of thyroid cancer found no association between diabetes and thyroid cancer; less than 5 years of diabetes was associated with a decreased thyroid cancer risk [7]. In summary, the data from previous studies differ regarding a potential association between diabetes and thyroid cancer.

Our study is unique in that it is the only study to focus exclusively on patients with papillary thyroid carcinoma, the most common type of thyroid cancer. Using an age-, gender-, and race-matched analysis, we compared the prevalence of diabetes in patients with papillary thyroid carcinoma at our institution with that expected based on data from the continuous National Health and Nutrition Examination Survey (NHANES) [8] from the same time period.

Methods

Patient chart review

A retrospective chart review was performed after approval of an exemption from IRB/PB Review by the Memorial Sloan-Kettering Institutional Review Board/Privacy Board and in agreement with the principles of the Declaration of Helsinki involving research involving human subjects. A database was generated of all patients with newly evaluated thyroid cancer at one institution, Memorial Sloan-Kettering Cancer Center, for 4 years, from January 1, 2005, to December 31, 2008, totaling 1,559 patients. The database included patients with thyroid carcinoma newly diagnosed at our institution as well as patients with a prior diagnosis of thyroid carcinoma referred from the outside. All patients received a rigorous internal review of histology. Extracted data included age at diagnosis, gender, race, type of thyroid cancer, diagnosis of diabetes, and antidiabetic medication use at the time of papillary thyroid carcinoma evaluation. After a diagnosis of papillary thyroid carcinoma as proven by pathology was reached at our institution, a subsequent diagnosis or use of antidiabetic medications was not included.

Of the 1559 patients identified, 8 entries were duplicates; 17 patients had no primary thyroid cancer diagnosis; and 13 patients had unknown race. These 38 patients were excluded. We further restricted our cohort to those with papillary thyroid carcinoma and excluded 24 patients with anaplastic thyroid carcinoma, 40 patients with follicular thyroid carcinoma, 41 patients with Hurthle cell thyroid carcinoma, 49 patients with medullary thyroid carcinoma, 52 patients with poorly differentiated thyroid carcinoma, and 1 patient with minimally invasive hyalinizing trabecular carcinoma. Of the original 1559 patients, 1313 patients with papillary thyroid carcinoma remained for analysis (84%).

Statistical analysis

Characteristics were compared between patients with diabetes and those without diabetes using the chi-square test for categorical variables and the Wilcoxon Rank Sum test for numeric variables. To determine whether the rate of diabetes was higher than expected in the group of patients with newly evaluated papillary thyroid carcinoma at our institution, we compared their observed prevalence of diabetes to the prevalence of diabetes in patients in the National Health and Nutrition Examination Survey (NHANES). NHANES is a federal program that seeks to assess the health and nutritional status of adults and children in the United States and has a publicly available data set on the Centers for Disease Control and Prevention website. We used NHANES data for 2005–2008. The expected number of patients with diabetes was estimated by multiplying the NHANES rate of diabetes for each age, sex, and race subgroup by the number of thyroid cancer patients within those subgroups. The observed and expected numbers of cases of diabetes were then separately summed and the relative risk (RR) was expressed as the ratio of observed-to-expected cases. The 95% confidence interval was calculated based on the assumption that the observed number of patients with diabetes was distributed as a Poisson variable.

We analyzed patients 44 years of age or younger separately from those 45 years of age or older based on literature suggesting that age 45 years or older is a risk factor for diabetes [9]. We also analyzed separately patients 65–74 years of age and those 75 years of age or older to separate elderly patients who practice healthy behaviors that enhance their life span and could be protective against diabetes [10].

Results

Patient characteristics

The demographics of the patients with papillary thyroid cancer in our cohort are listed in Table 1. The median age at evaluation was 47 years, with a range from 3 to 91 years of age; 74% were female; 83% were white; and 8% had diabetes. Of the 110 patients with diabetes, 92% had type 2 diabetes, and 6% had type 1 diabetes (Table 2); 24% of patients with diabetes were taking insulin.

Prevalence of diabetes in patients with papillary thyroid cancer versus that from NHANES

Using an age-, gender-, and race-matched analysis as described in the methods, we compared the prevalence of

Table 1 Patient characteristics

		All patients N = 1313
Age at evaluation	Median (range)	47 (3–91)
	0 - 44	589 (45%)
	45 - 64	535 (41%)
	65 - 74	143 (11%)
	75+	46 (3%)
Sex	Male	347 (26%)
	Female	966 (74%)
Race	White	1096 (83%)
	Black	50 (4%)
	Hispanic	72 (5%)
	Asian	86 (7%)
	Other	9 (1%)
Diabetes at evaluation of thyroid cancer	No	1203 (92%)
	Yes	110 (8%)

diabetes in patients with newly evaluated papillary thyroid carcinoma at our institution versus that expected from NHANES data (Table 3). For patients of all ages with newly evaluated papillary thyroid carcinoma at our institution, there was a non-significant trend for a higher rate of diabetes (odds ratio 1.07, CI 0.88 - 1.28). For patients aged 0 – 44 years with newly evaluated papillary thyroid carcinoma at our institution, however, there was a statistically and clinically significant increase in the prevalence of diabetes, with more than twice the expected number of patients with diabetes (ratio 2.32, CI 1.37 - 3.66). There was no significant difference when subgroup analysis was performed with stratification based on gender or race.

Risk factors for diabetes

The characteristics of patients with diabetes versus those without diabetes were compared (Table 4). Age was found to be a significant risk factor for diabetes, with

Table 2 Characteristics of the diabetes diagnosis at the time of initial thyroid cancer evaluation

		Diabetes (n = 110)
Type of diabetes	Type 1	6 (6%)
	Type 2	101 (92%)
	Secondary to steroid use	2 (2%)
	Unknown	1
On insulin	No	84 (76%)
	Yes	26 (24%)

Table 3 Prevalence of diabetes in patients with newly evaluated papillary thyroid carcinoma at our institution compared to prevalence expected from NHANES

		Observed # of patients with diabetes	Expected # of patients with diabetes	Ratio	95% Confidence interval
All patients		110	103	1.07	0.88-1.28
By age	0-44	18	8	**2.32**	**1.37-3.66***
	45-64	61	59	1.03	0.79-1.32
	65-74	23	29	0.81	0.51-1.21
	75+	8	8	1.04	0.45-2.05
By sex	Male	31	31	0.99	0.67-1.41
	Female	79	72	1.10	0.87-1.37
By race	White	78	78	1.00	0.79-1.24
	Black	8	8	1.04	0.45-2.05
	Hispanic	10	9	1.10	0.53-2.02
	Other	14	8	1.74	0.95-2.91

*Indicates statistically significant difference.

patients aged 44 years or younger less likely to have diabetes, and an increasing frequency of diabetes with each subsequent age group. Gender was not a risk factor for diabetes, but race was a significant risk factor, with white race being protective for diabetes compared to other groups: 7% in whites, 16% in blacks, 14% in Hispanics.

Discussion

Diabetes is an epidemic disease with extensive ramifications on various organ systems. The long-term complications of diabetes comprise not only the classically cited ones, including retinopathy, nephropathy, neuropathy, coronary heart disease, stroke, and peripheral vascular disease, but also cancer. Patients with diabetes

Table 4 Risk factors for diagnosis of diabetes

		Prevalence of diabetes (%)	p-value*
Age at diagnosis of PTC	0-44	18 (3%)	<0.0001
	45-64	61 (11%)	
	65-74	23 (16%)	
	75+	8 (17%)	
Sex	Male	31 (9%)	0.65
	Female	79 (8%)	
Race	White	78 (7%)	0.003
	Black	8 (16%)	
	Hispanic	10 (14%)	
	Other **	14 (15%)	

*P-value calculated using age as a continuous variable.
**Asian and other race categories were combined to match how race is collected in NHANES.

have an increased risk of cancer of breast, endometrium, bladder, liver, colorectum, and pancreas [1].

Previous studies regarding the risk of thyroid cancer in patients with diabetes have yielded conflicting data. A case–control study showed a 4-fold increased prevalence of diabetes among 110 patients with anaplastic thyroid cancer [4]. One cohort study with 585 thyroid cancer cases showed an increased prevalence of thyroid cancer among women with diabetes but not among men with diabetes [5], whereas two other cohort studies, with 1053 [6] and 943 [7] thyroid cancer cases respectively, showed no significant increase in the prevalence of thyroid cancer among patients with diabetes.

Using a database of more than 1500 patients with thyroid cancer and an age-, gender-, and race-matched analysis, we compared the prevalence of diabetes in patients with newly evaluated papillary thyroid cancer with that expected based on NHANES data. For patients of all ages, we found a non-significant increase in the prevalence in diabetes. For patients 44 years of age or younger, we found a significant increase in the prevalence of diabetes that was more than twice expected.

This is the first study to focus on the prevalence of diabetes exclusively in patients with papillary thyroid carcinoma and the first study to demonstrate an age association between diabetes and thyroid cancer. Since the cancer was newly evaluated for inclusion in the study, the diagnosis of diabetes preceded the diagnosis of thyroid cancer, suggesting that diabetes was a risk factor for the papillary thyroid carcinoma in the subset of patients 44 years of age or younger. It is possible that the diagnosis of papillary thyroid carcinoma led to a diagnosis of diabetes by connecting young people to the healthcare system, thus accounting for a higher prevalence of diabetes compared with their peers. Akker et al. recently demonstrated an increase in insulin resistance in patients with differentiated thyroid cancer [11], however, consistent with the hypothesis that diabetes increases the risk of thyroid cancer through hyperinsulinemia and activation of the insulin receptor or the insulin-like growth factor-I receptor. Recent evidence suggests that activation of the mitogen-activated protein (MAP) kinase signaling pathway is important in the development of insulin resistance, type 2 diabetes, and cancer [12,13].

One limitation of our study is that it is retrospective, which exposes the study to bias, including selection bias of patients. Another limitation of our study is that our study population comprises newly evaluated thyroid cancer patients at a single, tertiary care referral institution over a four year period. Furthermore, our study population is predominantly Caucasian (83%). Finally, as there is no longitudinal follow-up of patients, there is no mechanism to determine the prevalence of diabetes after the diagnosis of thyroid cancer.

Conclusions

Our study suggests that diabetes is a risk factor for papillary thyroid carcinoma in patients 44 years of age or younger. Further investigation is needed regarding the relationship between diabetes and thyroid cancer and their possible shared pathophysiology.

Abbreviations

NHANES: National health and nutrition examination survey; RR: Relative risk; CI: Confidence interval; MAP: Mitogen-activated protein.

Competing interests

The authors declare that they have no competing interests.

Authors' contribution

YMP, MFK, and RMT designed the initial study and prepared the final version of the manuscript. MFK supervised the conduction of the study. RMT provided the patient database. YMP reviewed the patient charts, acquired the patient data, and prepared the draft of the manuscript. ERR performed the statistical analysis and MMS assisted with analysis and interpretation of the data revised the manuscript. All of the authors critically revised, read, and approved the final manuscript for submission and agree to be accountable for all aspects relating to the accuracy and integrity of the work.

Acknowledgements

The authors would like to thank the Heed Ophthalmic Foundation Fellowship Grant for providing the funding in part.

Author details

[1]Memorial Sloan-Kettering Cancer Center, Department of Medicine, 1275 York Avenue, New York, NY 10065, USA. [2]Memorial Sloan-Kettering Cancer Center, Department of Epidemiology and Biostatistics, 1275 York Avenue, Box 313, New York, NY 10065, USA.

References

1. Noto H, Tsujimoto T, Sasazuki T, Noda M: **Significantly increased risk of cancer in patients with diabetes mellitus: a systematic review and meta-analysis.** *Endocr Pract* 2011, **17**:616–28.
2. Malaguarnera R, Belfiore A: **The insulin receptor: a new target for cancer therapy.** *Front Endocrinol (Lausanne)* 2011, **2**:93.
3. Djiogue S, Nwabo Kamdje AH, Vecchio L, Kipanyula MJ, Farahna M, Aldebasi Y, Seke Etet PF: **Insulin resistance and cancer: the role of insulin and IGFs.** *Endocr Relat Cancer* 2013, **20**:R1–R17.
4. Zivaljevic V, Vlajinac H, Jankovic R, Marinkovic J, Diklic A, Paunovic I: **Case–control study of anaplastic thyroid cancer.** *Tumori* 2004, **90**:9–12.
5. Aschebrook-Kilfoy B, Sabra MM, Brenner A, Moore SC, Ron E, Schatzkin A, Hollenbeck A, Ward MH: **Diabetes and thyroid cancer risk in the National Institutes of Health-AARP Diet and Health Study.** *Thyroid* 2011, **21**:957–63.
6. Balasubramaniam S, Ron E, Gridley G, Schneider AB, Brenner AV: **Association between benign thyroid and endocrine disorders and subsequent risk of thyroid cancer among 4.5 million U.S. male veterans.** *J Clin Endocrinol Metab* 2012, **97**:2661–9.
7. Tseng CH: **Thyroid cancer risk is not increased in diabetic patients.** *PLoS One* 2012, **7**:e53096.
8. Centers for Disease Control and Prevention (CDC), National Center for Health Statistics (NCHS): *National Health and Nutrition Examination Survey Data.* Hyattsville, MD, USA: U.S. Department of Health and Human Services, Centers for Disease Control and Prevention; 2005–2008.
9. Cowie CC, Eberhardt MS: **Sociodemographic characteristics of persons with diabetes.** In *Diabetes in America.* 2nd edition. Edited by National Diabetes Data Group of the National Institute of Diabetes and Digestive and Kidney Disease. Bethesda, MD: National Institutes of Health; 1995:85–116.
10. Yates LB, Djoussé L, Kurth T, Buring JE, Gaziano JM: **Exceptional longevity in men: modifiable factors associated with survival and function to age 90 years.** *Arch Intern Med* 2008, **168**:284–90.

11. Akker M, Güldiken S, Sipahi T, Palabıyık O, Tosunoğlu A, Celik O, Tunçbilek N, Sezer A, Süt N: **Investigation of insulin resistance gene polymorphisms in patients with differentiated thyroid cancer.** *Mol Biol Rep* 2014, **41**:3541–7.
12. Carlson CJ, Koterski S, Sciotti RJ, Poccard GB, Rondinone CM: **Enhanced basal activation of mitogen-activated protein kinases in adipocytes from type 2 diabetes: potential role of p38 in the downregulation of GLUT4 expression.** *Diabetes* 2003, **52**:634–41.
13. Dhillon AS, Hagan S, Rath O, Kolch W: **MAP kinase signalling pathways in cancer.** *Oncogene* 2007, **26**:3279–90.

13

A patient with Graves' disease showing only psychiatric symptoms and negativity for both TSH receptor autoantibody and thyroid stimulating antibody

Hidetaka Hamasaki[1], Taro Yoshimi[2] and Hidekatsu Yanai[1*]

Abstract

Background: Both thyroid stimulating hormone (TSH) and thyroid stimulating antibody (TSAb) negative Graves's disease (GD) is extremely rare. Here we present such a patient.

Case presentation: The patient was a 76-year-old woman who was diagnosed as having schizophrenia forty years ago. She did not show characteristic symptoms for hyperthyroidism, such as swelling of thyroid, exophthalmos, tachycardia and tremor, however, she showed only psychomotor agitation. Serum free triiodothyronine and free thyroxine levels were elevated and TSH level was suppressed, suggesting the existence of hyperthyroidism. However, both the first generation TSH receptor autoantibody (TRAb1) and the thyroid stimulating autoantibody (TSAb) were negative. Slightly increased blood flow and swelling was detected by thyroid echography. Thyroid scintigraphy demonstrated diffuse and remarkably elevated uptake of ^{123}I uptake. Finally, we diagnosed her as having GD. She was treated by using methimazole, and hyperthyroidism and her psychiatric symptoms were promptly ameliorated.

Discussion: We experienced a patient with GD who did not show characteristic symptoms except for psychiatric symptoms, and also showed negativity for both TRAb1 and TSAb. Thyroid autoantibody-negative GD is extremely rare. Thyroid scintigraphy was useful to diagnose such a patient.

Keywords: Delusion, Hyperthyroidism, Scintigraphy, Thyroid stimulating autoantibody, TSH receptor autoantibody

Introduction

Graves' disease (GD) is induced by autoimmunity for the thyroid gland, and thyroid stimulating autoantibodies may be the main pathological cause of GD. We usually measure thyroid stimulating hormone (TSH) receptor autoantibodies for diagnosis for GD in medical practices. In fact, TSH receptor autoantibodies are detectable in over 90% of patients with GD [1].

Here we present a patient with GD showing the absence of characteristic symptoms and negativity for both the first generation TSH receptor autoantibody (TRAb1) and thyroid stimulating antibody (TSAb).

* Correspondence: dyanai@hospk.ncgm.go.jp
[1]Department of Internal Medicine, National Center for Global Health and Medicine Kohnodai Hospital, Chiba, Japan
Full list of author information is available at the end of the article

Case report

A 76–year-old woman was admitted to the Department of Psychiatry in our hospital because she denied medications and suffered from irritability and delusion. She had no complaints of somatic symptoms. Her thyroid function was normal at least four months before the admission, however, laboratory data on the admission revealed hyperthyroidism. She was pointed out to have thyroid disease thirty years ago, however, she was not diagnosed definitively at that time, and also did not take any medicine. She had also type 2 diabetes, hypertension, dyslipidemia, hyperuricemia and schizophrenia. The members of her family did not have thyroid disorders. She has been taking clonazepam (0.5 mg/day), trazodone (50 mg/day), nitrazepam (5 mg/day), 0.1% aripiprazole (6 ml/day), propranolol (30 mg/day) and telmisartan (40 mg/day), for the

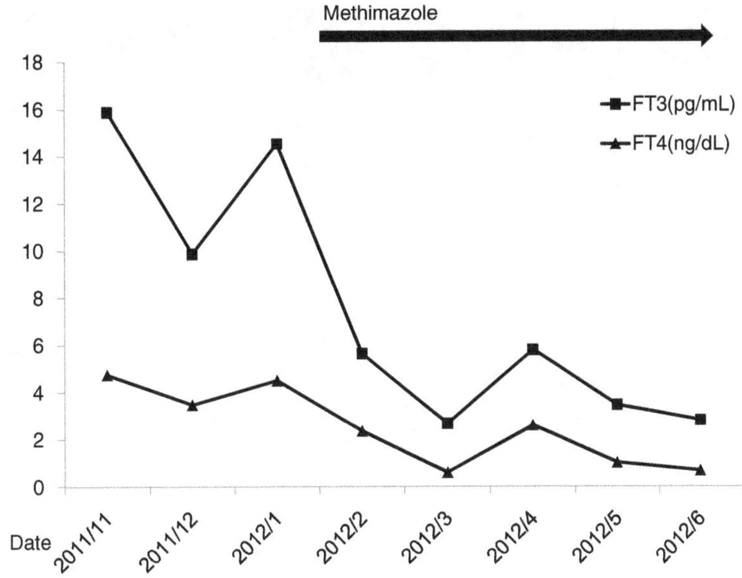

Figure 1 Changes of free triiodothyronine (FT3) and free thyroxine (FT4).

treatment for hypertension, psychiatric symptoms and schizophrenia.

Her body temperature was 35.7°C, blood pressure was 158/86 mmHg, and heart rate was 89 per minute and regular. Her thyroid was not swelled. She did not have tremor and exophthalmos. The serum TSH level was suppressed to < 0.03 μIU/mL (normal: 0.54-4.26 μIU/mL), free triiodothyronine (T3) and free thyroxine (T4) levels were elevated to 11.70 pg/mL (normal: 2.39-4.06 pg/mL) and 3.07 ng/dL (normal: 0.71-1.52 ng/dL), respectively (Figure 1). Plasma glucose level was 116 mg/dL (normal: 80–112 mg/dL), and HbA1c level was 6.6% (normal: 4.7-6.2%). Her liver and renal functions were normal, and leukocyte counts and C-reactive protein (CRP) level were not elevated.

Her serum levels of TRAb1 (7.7%; the cutoff point: 15%) and TSAb (155%; the cutoff point: 180%) were not elevated (Figure 2). Serum anti-thyroid peroxidase (TPO) antibody was elevated to 174 IU/mL (normal: < 16 IU/mL). At first, we diagnosed her as having

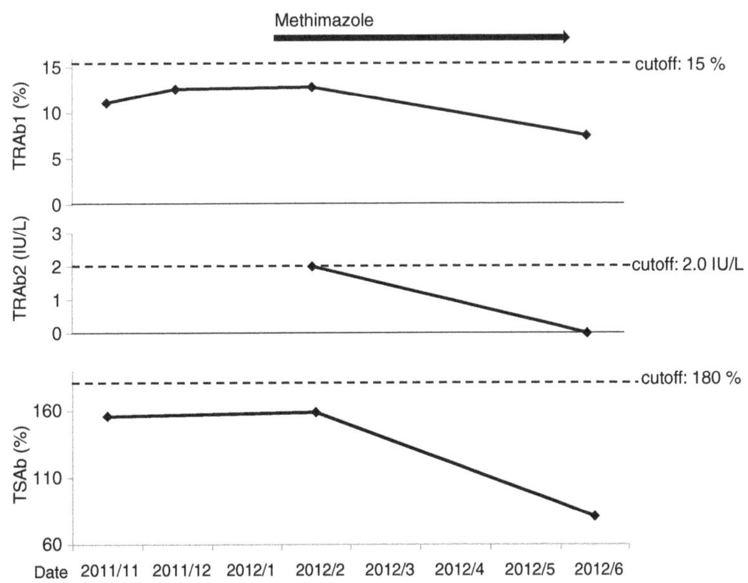

Figure 2 Changes of the first generation TSH receptor autoantibody (TRAb1), the second generation TSH receptor autoantibody (TRAb2) and thyroid stimulating antibody (TSAb). The cutoff points for TRAb1 and TSAb are values recommended by manufactures. The cutoff point for TRAb2 is value recommended by Schott M, et al. [10].

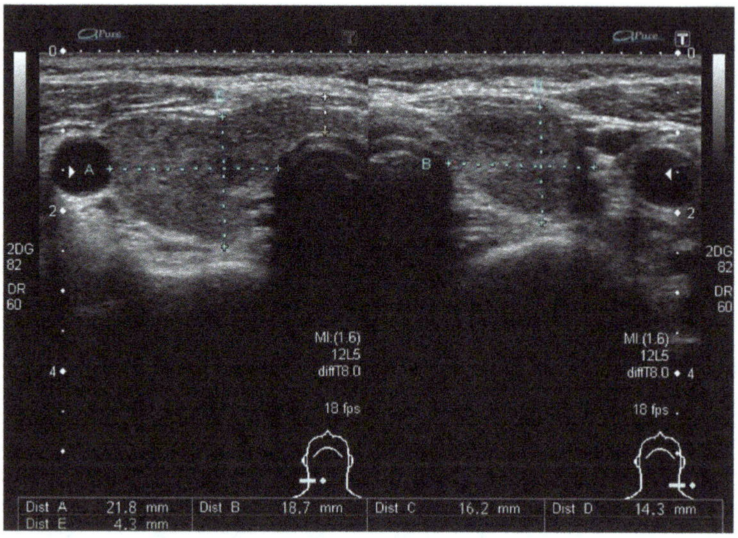

Figure 3 Echography of the thyroid glands. Bilateral thyroid glands was slightly swelled.

painless thyroiditis, and did not give her an anti-thyroid drug. Her psychiatric symptoms continued and we re-evaluated her thyroid function one month later. The serum TSH level was still suppressed to < 0.03 μIU/mL (normal: 0.54-4.26 μIU/mL), and free T3 and free T4 levels were further elevated to 15.88 pg/mL and 4.75 ng/dL, respectively (Figure 1). Thyroid echography showed slight swelling of the thyroid gland (right lobe: 52.4 mm × 21.8 mm × 16.4 mm, left lobe: 46.6 mm × 18.7 mm × 12.8 mm, isthmus size: 4.3 mm) and slightly increased blood flow (Figure 3). Thyroid scintigraphy demonstrated a diffuse and significantly elevated uptake of ^{123}I uptake in her thyroid gland (Figure 4). Uptake rate 3 and 24 hours after injection of ^{123}I was 111% and 63%, respectively Her serum levels of TRAb1 and TSAb were still not elevated (Figure 2), in spite of elevation of anti-TPO antibody (210 IU/mL; normal: < 16 IU/mL). We evaluated second generation TRAb (TRAb2), and found that her serum level of TRAb2 was very weakly positive (2.0 IU/mL; the cutoff point: 1.0 IU/mL). Because results of thyroid echography and scintigraphy strongly suggested the development of GD, we treated her by using methimazole (30 mg/day). Her thyroid function was promptly normalized one month later (Figure 1), and her psychiatric symptoms also were ameliorated. Further, the values of TRAb1, TRAb2 and TSAb were also promptly decreased under each cutoff point (Figure 2).

Discussion

Hyperthyroidism is a condition where the thyroid gland abnormally produces too much thyroid hormones. The most common cause is GD [2,3], and which is developed

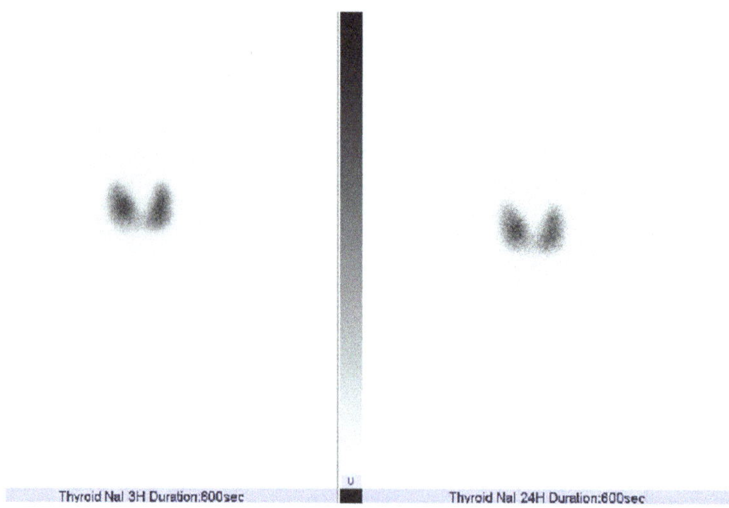

Figure 4 Scintigraphy of the thyroid glands. Uptake rate 3 and 24 hours after injection of ^{123}I was 111% and 63% respectively.

by the autoimmune stimulation of the thyroid gland [1]. Standardized diagnostic criteria for GD has not been globally established, and we usually diagnose this disease by clinical manifestations, laboratory data and imaging studies [4]. Clinical symptoms and signs include body weight loss, tremor, irritability, tachycardia, goiter, exophthalmos. Our patient had no specific somatic symptom of GD. Adrenergic hyperactivity induces psychiatric symptoms in hyperthyroidism, however. GD patients presenting only delusion like our patient are uncommon [5,6].

Paunkovic analyzed 255 patients diagnosed as having GD based on clinical manifestations and laboratory findings (free T4 and TSH). They excluded TRAb positive patients and the rest of the patients who had hyperthyroidism were re-tested with thyroid scintigraphy and serum levels of another TRAb. These results showed that TRAb were detectable in 98.7% of patients with GD. They stated TRAb negative GD was extremely rare, but there were methodological limitations in the assessment of only TRAb for the valid diagnosis of GD [7].

Our case showed no evident clinical manifestations except for psychomotor agitation which was considered to be induced by schizophrenia, and also showed negativity for both TRAb1 and TSAb. We observed a very weak positivity of TRAb2 before we started treatment. However, TRAb or TSAb have been reported to emerge in about 10% of patients with painless thyroiditis [8,9], therefore, we cannot make a definite differential diagnosis between GD and painless thyroiditis even if one of the thyroid autoantibodies is very weakly positive. The recommended cut-off value of TRAb2 used to be 2.0 IU/L and the sensitivity is 93.9% with 100% specificity [10]. It may be evident that the autoimmune stimulation of the thyroid gland is the cause of hyperthyroidism in our patient because serum levels of thyroid autoantibodies (TRAb1, TRAb2 and TSAb) were significantly decreased after starting treatment (Figure 2). We believe that present case is very rare. Our study also suggested that thyroid scintigraphy is very useful to diagnose GD patients with the absence of characteristic symptoms, TRAb and TSAb.

Thyroid autoantibody-negative GD is extremely rare. We experienced a patient with GD who did not show characteristic symptoms except for psychiatric symptoms, and also showed negativity for both TRAb1 and TSAb. Thyroid scintigraphy was useful to diagnose such a patient.

Consent

Written informed consent was obtained from the patient's relatives for publication of this case report. A copy of the written consent is available for review by the Eitor-in-Chief of this jounal.

Competing interests

The authors declare that they have no competing interests.

Authors' contributions

HH wrote the first draft. HH and TY were in a position of leadership for the patient and collected information on the patient. HY and HH did the literature searches. HY wrote the final manuscript and made appropriate revisions. All authors read through and approved the final manuscript.

Author details

[1]Department of Internal Medicine, National Center for Global Health and Medicine Kohnodai Hospital, Chiba, Japan. [2]Department of Psychiatry, National Center for Global Health and Medicine Kohnodai Hospital, Chiba, Japan.

References

1. Zöphel K, Roggenbuck D, Schott M: **Clinical review about TRAb assay's history.** *Autoimmun Rev* 2010, **9:**695–700.
2. Weetamn AP: **Graves' disease.** *N Engl J Med* 2000, **343:**1236–1248.
3. Cooper DS: **Hyperthyroidism.** *Lancet* 2003, **362:**459–468.
4. Brent GA: **Graves' Disease.** *N Engl J Med* 2008, **358:**2594–2605.
5. Bunevičius R, Prang AJ Jr: **Thyroid disease and mental disorders: cause and effect or only comorbidity?** *Curr Opin Psychiatry* 2010, **23:**363–368.
6. Ogah OS, Timeyin AO, Kayode OA, Otukoya AS, Akinyemi RO, Adeyemi FI: **Graves' disease presenting as paranoid schizophrenia in a Nigerian woman: a case report.** *Cases Journal* 2009, **2:**6708.
7. Paunkovic J, Paunkovic N: **Does autoantibody-negative Graves' disease Exist ? A second evaluation of the clinical diagnosis.** *Horm Metab Res* 2006, **38:**53–56.
8. Iitaka M, Morgenthaler NG, Momotani N, Nagata A, Ishikawa N, Ito K, Katayama S, Ito K: **Stimulation of thyroid-stimulating hormone (TSH) receptor antibody production following painless thyroiditis.** *Clin Endocrinol* 2004, **60:**49–53.
9. Takasu N, Kamijo K, Sato Y, Yoshimura H, Nagata A, Ochi Y: **Sensitive Thyroid-stimulating antibody assay with high concentrations of polyethylene glycol for the diagnosis of Graves' disease.** *Clin Exp Pharmacol Physiol* 2004, **31:**3124–3319.
10. Schott M, Feldkamp J, Bathan C, Fritzen R, Scherbaum WA, Seissler J: **Detecting TSH-receptor antibodies with the recombinant TBII assay: technical and clinical evaluation.** *Horm Metab Res* 2000, **32:**429–435.

14

Mediastinal neoplasms in patients with Graves disease: a possible link between sustained hyperthyroidism and thymic neoplasia?

Jonathan D Boyd[1] and Ridas Juskevicius[1,2*]

Abstract

Background: Anterior mediastinal masses are a rare but well documented finding in Graves disease. The vast majority of these lesions represents benign thymic hypertrophy and regress after treatment of the hyperthyroidism. A small percentage of these cases however represent neoplastic/malignant diseases which require further treatment.

Cases: 12 year old boy with one year history of refractory Graves disease was found to have an anterior mediastinal mass and underwent curative thyroidectomy for sustained hyperthyroidism. Cervical lymphadenopathy was detected during the procedure and biopsy was obtained. A 23 year old woman who presented with a one month history of hyperthyroid symptoms, was diagnosed with Graves disease and also was found to have an anterior mediastinal mass on imaging. Biopsy of the anterior mediastinal mass was obtained and subsequently the patient underwent robotic thymectomy. Histologic examination and immunophenotyping of the cervical lymph node in a 12 year old boy revealed neoplastic proliferation of T lymphoblasts diagnostic of T lymphoblastic leukemia/ lymphoma. Examination of the anterior mediastinal mass biopsy in the 23 year old woman revealed type B1 thymoma which was confirmed after examination of the subsequent robotic thymectomy specimen.

Conclusion: This is the first reported case of T cell lymphoblastic lymphoma and the third reported case of thymoma associated with sustained hyperthyroidism due to Graves disease. These cases indicate that an anterior mediastinal mass in a patient with active Graves disease may be due to a neoplastic cause, which may require definitive treatment. Caution should be exercised when dismissing a mediastinal mass as benign thymic hyperplasia in patients with active Graves disease.

Keywords: Graves disease, Hyperthyroidism, Thymoma, T Lymphoblastic leukemia/lymphoma, Thymic hyperplasia

Background

Graves disease (GD) is an autoimmune disease caused by self-reactive plasma cells which produce antibodies to the thyrotropin receptor that stimulate thyroid-stimulating hormone receptors and increase the production of thyroid hormone [1]. The relationship between Graves disease (GD) and mediastinal masses is nearly a century old having been first identified in a patient with thymic hyperplasia secondary to GD described by Halsted in 1914 [2]. With a well known benign cause of anterior mediastinal masses (AMM) in Graves disease, there is a tendency to forego tissue biopsy and re-evaluate at an unspecified time after thyroid ablation/ thyroidectomy [2-5]. Here we describe two patients with neoplastic anterior mediastinal masses associated with GD, illustrating that this may not be safe approach to all patients with anterior mediastinal masses and GD.

* Correspondence: ridas.juskevicius@vidanthealth.com
[1]Department of Pathology & Laboratory Medicine, Vidant Medical Center and Brody School of Medicine, East Carolina University, Greenville, NC, USA
[2]Department of Pathology & Laboratory Medicine, Brody School of Medicine, East Carolina University, 600 Moye Blvd, Brody Medical Sciences Building 7S18, Greenville, NC 27858-4353, USA

Case presentations

Patients

A 12 year-old African American male with a one year history of GD refractory to medical management presented with a persistent tachycardia, fever, abdominal pain, vomiting, weakness and muscle aches after discontinuing methimazole in preparation for thyroid radioablation. A 12 x 6 cm mediastinal mass had been identified radiographically which was initially thought to represent thymic hyperplasia (Figure 1A). Bilateral cervical lymphadenopathy was also detected. The decision was made to perform a curative thyroidectomy. During the procedure a cervical lymph node biopsy was performed, which demonstrated architectural effacment by a diffuse infiltrate of immature lymphoid cells (Figure 1B). The immunophenotyping by flow cytometry revealed a predominance of T lymphoblasts (CD1a+, CD2+, CD4+, CD8+, sCD3-, TdT+) consistent with T-lymphoblastic leukemia/lymphoma (T-LBL/L). Bone marrow examination identified involvement by T-LBL. The thyroidectomy specimen contained changes typical of GD. The patient was treated with induction chemotherapy for T-LBL with excellent response showing essentially complete resolution of the mediastinal mass, neck lymph nodes and no bone marrow involvement. Patient has continued to do well post thyroidectomy on levothyroxine.

The second patient is a 23-year old female without significant medical history who was transferred to our institution with increasing shortness of breath, dysphagia, cervical lymphadenopathy and a mediastinal mass identified on chest CT (Figure 1C). A TSH level was below the minimum detection limit of 0.02 uIU/m as well as a free T3 of 12.2 pg/mL (reference range: 3.4-4.8). Biopsies of the anterior mediastinal mass were obtained and showed a type B1 thymoma. Cervical lymph node biopsy revealed dermatopathic lymphadenitis. The patient underwent a robotic thymectomy and a diagnosis of type B1 thymoma was confirmed (Figure 1D). Patient had an uneventful post operative course and was discharged on post operative day 3.

Discussion

Evaluating an AMM in the setting of GD can be challenging for the clinician. There is no systematic, formal evaluation of how best to manage AMM in the setting of GD [3]. There is substantial variability in the rate of thymic involution as well as thymic size, shape and density even between individuals of the same age [6]. A retrospective study of 109 patients with AMM treated with thymectomy found that all cases with malignancy had either symptoms referable to the thymus or a discrete mass rather than a diffusely enlarged thymus gland [6]. The utility of this information is partially limited by the finding that a "discrete mass" was seen in 32% of thymic hyperplasias and 66% of histologically normal thymus glands [6]. Also, symptoms anatomically referable to enlargement of the thymus (chest discomfort, chest pain and shortness of breath) [6] can frequently also be seen in GD [7]. Prevailing wisdom from several recent case reports of thymic hyperplasia in GD is that caution should be used in evaluating AMM in the setting of GD given the known association with thymic hyperplasia [2-5]. Clinicians are urged to wait until after resolution of hyperthyroidism to follow up AMM in the absence of features concerning for malignancy (invasion, calcifications, cysts or septations) on imaging [2-5]. Reduction of thymic enlargement after achieving a euthryoid state can vary from 2 months up to 2 years [2] which could complicate following up a possibly neoplastic mediastinal mass.

These cases represent two examples of mediastinal neoplasms seen in association with GD. While the first patient represents the first documented case of T-LBL/L seen in association with GD, there are two prior case reports of thymoma occuring with GD [8,9]. On the

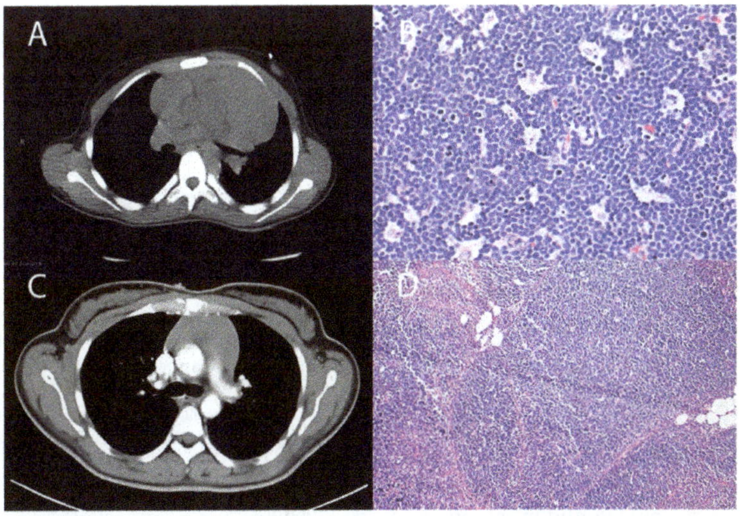

Figure 1 (A and C) Chest computed tomography images showing anterior mediastinal masses from patients with T-cell LBL/L and Type B1 thymoma. (**B** and **D**) Representative tissue sections from the same patients (Hematoxylin-Eosin, x200).

other hand, occurance of T-LBL/L with other autoimmune diseases is well documented [10-17].

Autoimmunity alters the environment of the immune system with positive selection/expansion of autoreactive T-cells in the thymus. Thymic hyperplasia is a representation of how GD, in particular, alters the microenvironment of the thymus. This is thought to be due to the hyperthyroidism associated with active GD. It is known that thyroid hormones (TH) are able to induce thymic epithelial cell (TEC) proliferation which produces cytokines (including IL-1) [18]. T3 also enhances thymic hormone thymulin secretion by TECs [18]. In turn, cytokines (e.g. IL-1) and thymulin stimulate and enhance thymocyte (immature T-cell precursor) proliferation. Thymocyte differentiation occurs as the cells migrate within thymic lobules interacting with microenvironment [18]. In active GD, thymic microenvironment may be altered due to increased proliferation of TECs driven by TH. It is unclear if thymic environment altered by the state of sustained hyperthyroidism, including increased proliferative drive on maturing thymocytes and, possibly, abnormal differentiation, may contribute to the development of genetic lesions resulting in T LBL/L in susceptible individuals. Likewise it is not unreasonable to postulate that TH driven TEC proliferation may contribute to the pathogenesis of thymoma, which is a neoplasm of thymic epithelial cells. The two patients illustrated not only raise the possibility of association between GD and mediastinal neoplasms but represent a possible reason for caution in using a watch-and-wait approach to anterior mediastinal masses in patients with GD.

Conclusions

This is the first reported case of T lymphoblastic lymphoma/leukemia and the third reported case of thymoma developing in patients with sustained poorly controlled hyperthyroidism due to Graves disease. Given the known physiologic interactions between thyroid hormones and thymic microenvironment, these cases may indicate a possible link between a sustained hyperthyroidism and the development of thymic neoplasia. In addition, our cases indicate that an anterior mediastinal mass in a patient with active Graves disease may be due to a neoplastic cause, which may require definitive treatment. Caution should be exercised when dismissing a mediastinal mass as benign thymic hyperplasia in patients with active Graves disease.

Ethical approval

This case report was based on the existing data, and the patients' identification was kept confidential in this study. This case report does not meet definition of human or animal subject research by University and Medical Center Institutional Review Board of East Carolina University, and no ethical approval was necessary for this study.

Abbreviations

GD: Graves disease; AMM: Anterior mediastinal masses; T-LBL/L: T-lymphoblastic leukemia\lymphoma.

Competing interests

The authors declare that they have no competing interests.

Authors' contributions

JB performed literature review, patient records review and drafted the manuscript. RJ conceived of the study, and participated in its design and coordination and helped to draft the manuscript. JB and RJ were directly involved in the diagnosis and care of both patients. All authors read and approved the final manuscript.

References

1. Bahn Chair RS, Burch HB, Cooper DS, Garber JR, Greenlee MC, Klein I, Laurberg P, McDougall IR, Montori VM, Rivkees SA, Ross DS, Sosa JA, Stan MN: **American Thyroid Association; American Association of Clinical Endocrinologists. Hyperthyroidism and other causes of thyrotoxicosis: management guidelines of the American Thyroid Association and American Association of Clinical Endocrinologists.** *Thyroid* 2011, **21**:593–646.
2. Popoveniuc G, Sharma M, Devdhar M, Wexler JA, Carroll NM, Wartofsky L, Burman KD: **Graves' disease and thymic hyperplasia: the relationship of thymic volume to thyroid function.** *Thyroid* 2010, **20**:1015–8.
3. Yacoub A, Gaitonde DY, Wood JC: **Thymic hyperplasia and Graves disease: management of anterior mediastinal masses in patients with Graves disease.** *Endocr Pract* 2009, **15**:534–9.
4. Budavari AI, Whitaker MD, Helmers RA: **Thymic hyperplasia presenting as anterior mediastinal mass in 2 patients with Graves disease.** *Mayo Clin Proc* 2002, **77**:495–9.
5. Yamanaka K, Nakayama H, Watanabe K, Kameda Y: **Anterior mediastinal mass in a patient with Graves' disease.** *Ann Thorac Surg* 2006, **81**:1904–6.
6. Singla S, Litzky LA, Kaiser LR, Shrager JB: **Should asymptomatic enlarged thymus glands be resected?** *J Thorac Cardiovasc Surg* 2010, **1405**:977–83.
7. Chan WB, Yeung VT, Chow CC, So WY, Cockram CS: **Gynaecomastia as a presenting feature of thyrotoxicosis.** *Postgrad Med J* 1999, **75**:229–31.
8. Levy Y, Afek A, Sherer Y, Bar-Dayan Y, Shibi R, Kopolovic J, Shoenfeld Y: **Malignant thymoma associated with autoimmune diseases: a retrospective study and review of the literature.** *Semin Arthritis Rheum* 1998, **28**:73–9.
9. Lee BW, Ihm SH, Shin HS, Yoo HJ: **Malignant thymoma associated with myasthenia gravis, Graves' disease, and SIADH.** *Intern Med* 2008, **47**:1009–12.
10. Olcay L, Koç A: **Autoimmune hemolytic anemia preceding T-ALL in a five-year-old girl.** *Pediatr Hematol Oncol* 2005, **22**:207–13.
11. Piernas S, Xicoy B, Grifols JR, Ribera JM: **Autoimmune hemolytic anemia with positive direct antiglobulin test associated with T cell acute lymphoblastic leukemia.** *Med Clin (Barc)* 2006, **126**:678–9.
12. Tsuchihashi T, Kimura N, Niho Y, Oka Y, Ikuta T, Sumita I, Otsuka M, Mitsui T, Ohara Y: **A case of cold agglutinin disease with T cell lymphoblastic lymphoma.** *Rinsho Ketsueki* 1982, **23**:743–8.
13. Uner AH, Abali H, Engin H, Akyol A, Ruacan S, Tan E, Güllü I, Altundağ K, Güler N: **Myasthenia gravis and lymphoblastic lymphoma involving the thymus: a rare association.** *Leuk Lymphoma* 2001, **42**:527–31.
14. Liu KL, Herbrecht R, Tranchant C, Gasser B, Warter JM, Wihlm JM, Oberling F: **Malignant thymic lymphoblastic lymphoma and myasthenia gravis: an exceptional association.** *Nouv Rev Fr Hematol* 1992, **34**:221–3.
15. Hansen BA, Sørensen PS, Lauritzen MJ, Iversen J, Laulund S, Petrera JE, Nielsen JB, Paulson OB: **A case of malignant lymphoma and myasthenia gravis.** *Scand J Haematol* 1983, **31**:155–60.
16. Mortimer JE, Kidd P: **Myasthenia gravis and lymphoblastic lymphoma antiacetylcholine receptor antibody as a tumor marker–a case report.** *Cancer Invest* 1989, **7**:327–31.

Increased soluble IL-2 receptor levels in serum from a patient with painless thyroiditis

Kae Hamamoto[1], Masaaki Inaba[1*], Shinsuke Yamada[1], Maki Yoda[1], Koichiro Yoda[1], Hitoshi Goto[1], Masafumi Kurajoh[2] and Hidenori Koyama[2]

Abstract

Context: Serum concentration of soluble interleukin-2 receptor (sIL-2R) has been established as a reliable marker of T-lymphocyte activation. However, there have been no reports describing the relationship between serum sIL-2R and painless thyroiditis.

Objective: We report a case of a 76-yr-old female with a significant and temporary increase of sIL-2R concomitant with painless thyroiditis.

Case illustration: The patient was diagnosed with malignant lymphoma at the age of 73. After 6 cycles of CHOP-R complete remission was induced and no recurrence was observed up to 3.5 years. At 76 years of age, she exhibited hyperthyroidism and was diagnosed with painless thyroiditis based upon US examination and ^{99m}Tc-Thyroid scintigraphy. Her AST and ALT were mildly elevated, and her serum level of sIL-2R increased up to 2230 U/mL from the approximately 540 U/mL, which had been stable for 3 years before.
These abnormal data normalized without requiring any treatment. The time-course of the reduction in sIL-2R did not correlate with FT4 or FT3, but was very similar to that of AST and ALT.

Conclusion: There was no evidence of relapse of the malignant lymphoma. We conclude that the increase of sIL-2R was associated with painless thyroiditis. Considering the similar time-course between the reduction of serum sIL-2R and those of AST and ALT, which are often accompanied by autoimmune processes in painless thyroiditis during the development of hyperthyroidism, it was suggested that the increase of serum sIL-2R in this case resulted from activation of an autoimmune process.

Keywords: Thyroiditis, sIL-2R, Autoimmune

Background

The serum concentration of soluble interleukin-2 receptor (sIL-2R), which is derived from its specific membrane receptor on activated T lymphocytes [1], has been established as a reliable marker of T-lymphocyte activation [2]. In autoimmune hyperthyroidism, such as Graves' disease, serum sIL-2R likely increases as a result of T cell activation [3]. This hypothesis is supported by the further increase of sIL-2R in patients with refractory Graves' disease [4]. However, it remains possible that hyperthyroidism alone also increases serum sIL-2R, even in the absence of autoimmune activation, based on the increase in sIL-2R that occurs with triiodothyronine replacement [5]. However, to date, there has been no report on the relationship between serum sIL-2R and painless thyroiditis, which is known as subacute variant of chronic lymphocytic thyroiditis,, which is a clinical syndrome that manifests as transient thyrotoxicosis followed by transient hypothyroidism without spontaneous pain or tenderness in thyroid gland. On histopathologic analysis, painless thyroiditis manifests as a lymphocytic infiltration of the thyroid follicles, resulting in follicular cell damage [6].

Herein, we report a case of a patient who was in remission from large cell type lymphoma with restoration of sIL-2R levels within normal range, and was being periodically monitored for any potential relapse of large cell type lymphoma. She exhibited a significant

* Correspondence: inaba-m@med.osaka-cu.ac.jp
[1]Department of Nephrology, Department of Metabolism, Endocrinology and Molecular Medicine, Osaka City University Graduate School of Medicine, 1-4-3, Asahi-machi, Abeno-ku, Osaka 545-8585, Japan
Full list of author information is available at the end of the article

and temporary increase of sIL-2R, which occurred with the same time-course as painless thyroiditis.

Case presentation

In January 2007, a 73-year-old female, developed abdominal pain with pyrexia and was diagnosed with acute appendicitis. Examination by computed tomography to further assess the appendicitis detected disseminated enlargement of the retroperitoneal lymph nodes and atrophy of the right kidney surrounded enlargement of multiple lymph nodes. Since she was suspected to be suffering from malignant lymphoma, she was then referred to the Department of Hematology, Osaka City University Hospital on February 7, 2007 for further examination.

She was diagnosed as having malignant lymphoma (follicular lymphoma Grade 3a, Stage 2), and was treated with 6 cycles of CHOP-R, which resulted in complete remission. There was no recurrence for another 3.5 years, and periodic measurements of serum sIL-2R revealed that her serum sIL-2R remained within the normal range; around 500 U/ml. In September 2010, she felt fatigue and palpitation, and subsequently developed excessive perspiration. She was identified as developing hyperthyroidism, as reflected by an increase of serum free T4 and free T3 above the normal upper limit to 3.2 ng/ml and 15.6 pg/ml respectively, with simultaneous suppression of serum TSH to <0.004 mIU/l. Of great importance was the significant increase of sIL-2R up to 2230 U/ml, which had been stable for 3 years around 540 U/ml. Once the potential relapse of malignant lymphoma had been ruled out and treatment for hyperthyroidism had been initiated, she was admitted to Osaka City University Hospital.

She was 152.0 cm in height and 51.0 kg in weight, which did not change appreciable before admission. She did not lose weight. The pulse rate was 72/min and regular, due probably to administration of atenolol at the daily dose of 50 mg, and the blood pressure was 132/68 mmHg with a body temperature of 36.0°C. She had a diffuse and elastic goiter, but she had neither spontaneous pain nor tenderness in the anterior neck area. There was no sign of a palpable cervical lymphoid node and leg edema was absent. The laboratory findings on admission are presented in Table 1. Laboratory tests confirmed primary hyperthyroidism, as indicated by the increase of serum FT4 and FT3 above the respective normal upper limits, with significant suppression of TSH to an undetectable level. She exhibited a positive test for anti-thyroglobulin antibody, but was negative for anti-TSH receptor antibody or anti-thyroid peroxidase antibody. In addition to hyperthyroidism, the abnormal findings detected on admission included a slight reduction of hemoglobin to 10.8 g/dl, mild liver dysfunction (AST 34 IU/l, ALT 36 IU/l), and slight renal dysfunction, likely due to total loss of right renal function as a result of pararenal lymph node enlargement during the onset of malignant lymphoma.

WBC, white blood cell; RBC, red blood cell; Hb, Hemoglobin; PLT, platelet; AST, asparate transaminase; ALT, alanine transaminase; ALP, alkaline phosphatase; LDH, lactate dehydrogenase; BUN, blood urea nitogen; eGFR, estimated glomerular filtration rate; CPK, creatine phosphokinase; TC, total cholesterol; TG, Triglycerides; FPG, fasting plasma glucose; CRP, C-reactive protein; ESR, erythrocyte sedimentation rate; sIL-2R, soluble interleukin-2 receptor; FT4, free thyroxine; FT3, free triiodothyronine; TSH, thyrotropin; TRAb, TSH receptor antibody; TPOAb, thyroid peroxidase antibody; TgAb, Thyroglobulin antibody.

Ultrasound examination of the thyroid gland showed destructive thyroiditis, as reflected by the apparent reduction and heterogeneity of echogenicity inside the thyroid gland. Intrathyroidal blood flow measured at the inferior thyroid artery was 24.3 cm/s, which was not as high as the mean value of 41.5 ± 26.6 m/sec, observed in untreated Graves' disease [7]. ^{99m}Tc-Thyroid scintigraphy showed essentially no uptake of 0.187% within the thyroid gland. Based on these findings, we diagnosed her etiology of primary hyperthyroidism as painless thyroiditis, and then monitored her thyroid function without any medication. Her serum FT4 and FT3 levels decreased rapidly over time without treatment, whereas her serum sIL-2R exhibited a sustained increase until the 16th Hospital day and started to decrease approximately 7 days later. (Figure 1) Therefore, the reduction of thyroid function was apparently followed by the reduction of serum sIL-2R. Of interest, the time-courses of the reductions in AST and ALT during admission were similar to that of serum sIL-2R (Figure 2). After the reduction of sIL-2R to around 500 U/ml, it was maintained at a stable range. She was discharged from our hospital after 21 Hospital days. When her serum TSH increased above the detectable lower limit to 0.013 mIu/l 35 days after admission, thyroid hormone replacement therapy was initiated at a daily dose of 50 μg L-thyroxine, and this dose was adjusted upward to 125 μg/day.

The hematologist investigated the possible recurrence of large cell type lymphoma, which had been in remission for 3 years before. However, based on her normal findings on chest and abdominal X-ray CT, with no remarkable change of LDH, an indicator of lymphoma activity, the hematologist ruled out the relapse of malignant lymphoma, which was further supported by the lack of new manifestation suggesting its recurrence for another 2 years until now.

Discussion

Herein, we report a case in which a significant and temporary increase of serum sIL-2R was detected during an episode of painless thyroiditis simultaneously with the

Table 1 Laboratory data on admission

Hematology tests			eGFR	(90<)	41 ml/min/1.7 m^2
WBC	(4300–8000)	4700 /μl	CPK	(30–140)	46 IU/l
Neut	(49.5–71.0)	56.1%	Na	(137–146)	136 mEq/l
Mono	(2.3–7.7)	10.0%	K	(3.8-5.1)	4.1 mEq/l
Eos	(0.2–6.8)	2.8%	Cl	(98–108)	105 mEq/l
Baso	(0.0–1.8)	0.4%	Ca	(7.0-10.0)	8.7 mg/dl
Lymph	(26.6–46.6)	30.7%	P	(2.9-4.3)	3.7 mg/dl
RBC	(395–465)	349 × 10^4/μl	TC	(130–220)	153 mg/dl
Hb	(11.3–14.9)	10.8 g/dl	TG	(50–150)	60 mg/dl
Hematocrit	(36–47)	32.2%	FPG	(70–109)	86 mg/dl
PLT	(18.0–34.0)	19.2 × 10^4 /μl	CRP	(0–0.4)	0.01 mg/dl
			ESR 1 h	(2–15)	5 mm
Biochemistry tests			sIL-2R	(124–466)	2230 U/ml
Total protein	(6.5–8.5)	5.8 mg/dl			
Albumin	(3.5–5.0)	3.9 g/dl	**Thyroid-related tests**		
AST	(13–33)	34 IU/l	FT4	(0.9-1.7)	3.2 ng/dl
ALT	(6–27)	36 IU/l	FT3	(2.3-4.0)	15.6 pg/ml
ALP	(115–359)	189 IU/l	TSH	(0.5-5.0)	<0.004 mIU/l
LDH	(119–229)	195 IU/l	TRAb	(<1.0)	<1.0 IU/l
BUN	(7–18)	25 mg/dl	TPOAb	(<0.3)	<0.3 IU/ml
Creatinine	(0.4–0.9)	1.0 mg/d	TgAb	(<0.3)	3.9 U/ml

Underlined data is abnormal value.

temporary increase of serum FT4 and FT3, which was supported by the periodic measurement of serum sIL-2R during ongoing follow-up for the possible relapse of her malignant lymphoma. This case showed apparent reduction of serum FT3 and FT4 by the 3rd Hospital day, although her serum sIL-2R remained at a sustained high level until the 16th Hospital day and started to decline 13 days later, after the reduction of serum FT4 and FT3 (Figure 1).

The reason for the increased sIL-2R in hyperthyroidism is mainly explained by two mechanisms. Hyperthyroidism alone could increase sIL-2R [5,8,9], in addition to the hyper-immune state with T cell auto-activation, which is often associated with hyperthyroidism [5]. Serum

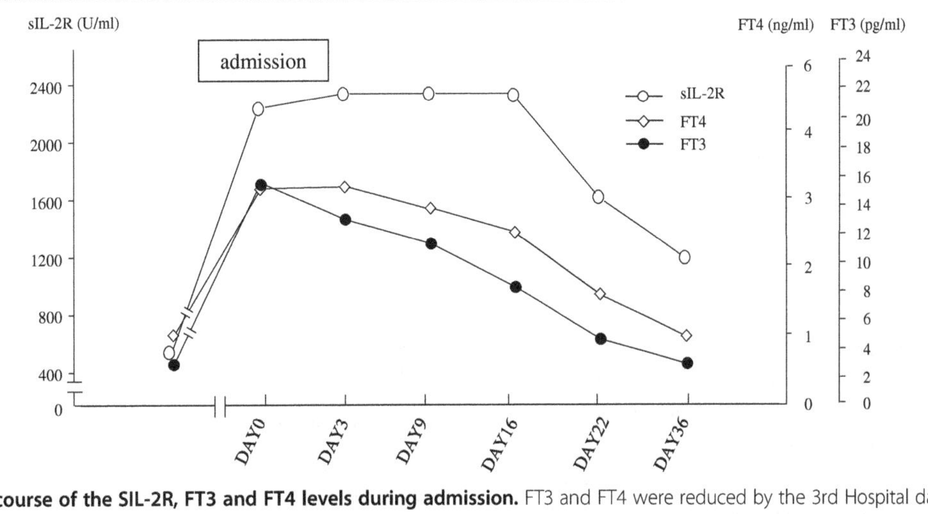

Figure 1 Time course of the SIL-2R, FT3 and FT4 levels during admission. FT3 and FT4 were reduced by the 3rd Hospital day Serum sIL-2R persisted at a high level until the 16th Hospital day and began to decline 13 days later; after reduction of serum FT4 and FT3.

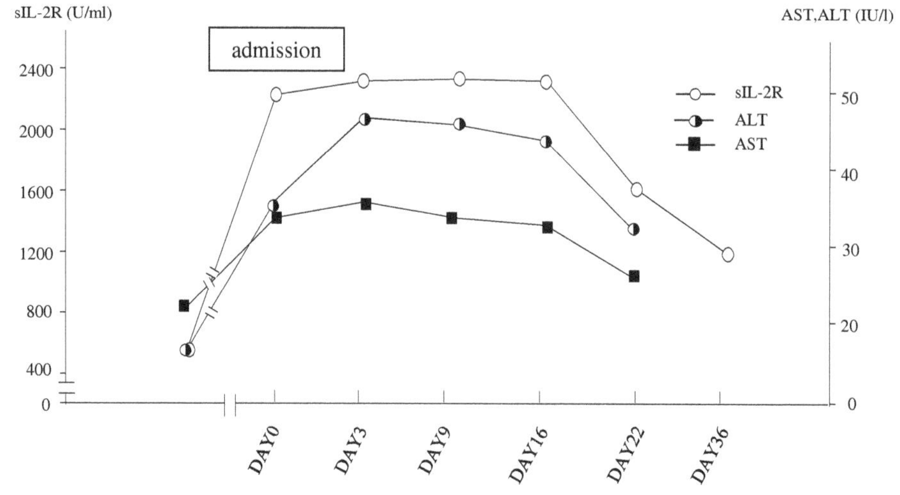

Figure 2 Time course of SIL-2R, FT3 and FT4 levels during admission. The reduction of sIL-2R was similar to that of the liver enzymes, AST and ALT.

sIL-2R has previously been demonstrated to correlate in a positive manner with serum FT3 in non-autoimmune thyroiditis, as well as in autoimmune thyroiditis [5]. Furthermore, serum sIL-2R levels have been shown to be higher in the latter group than in the former; indicating the increase of sIL-2R as a result of increased autoimmunity, in addition to hyperthyroidism [5].

Since the increase of sIL-2R persisted, despite the apparent reduction of serum FT4 and FT3 (Figure 1 above), it was suggested that hyperthyroidism alone could not be responsible for the increased sIL-2R in this patient. Further support of this hypothesis is that serum sIL-2R remained unchanged, around 800 U/ml, even after the reduction of serum FT4 and F3 below the normal lower limit, with a significant increase in serum TSH up to 17 mIu/l, although the hematologist had ruled out the possibility of recurrence of malignant lymphoma.

Another important mechanism that has been proposed to increase serum sIL-2R in hyperthyroidism is activation of the autoimmune process, since serum sIL-2R has been established as a reliable marker of T-lymphocyte activation [1]. In fact, it has previously been reported that hyperthyroid patients with refractory Graves' disease exhibited higher levels of serum sIL-2R than would be predicted from their hyperthyroid state [10]. Furthermore, it has also been reported that patients with subacute thyroiditis showed increased sIL-2R; although to date, there is no available data regarding the association of painless thyroiditis with increased sIL-2R.

Of great interest, the time course of the reduction in sIL-2R was similar to that of the liver enzymes, AST and ALT, during the episode of painless thyroiditis (Figure 2). It was previously reported that thyroid-liver interaction in autoimmune thyroid disease is partly explained by the association of intrinsic liver disease with intrinsic thyroid disease through autoimmune mechanism(s) [11-13]. Since the reductions of AST and ALT were delayed by 13 days, compared with that of serum FT3 and FT4, the increase of AST and ALT could have occurred by an autoimmune mechanism, in addition to the hepatotoxic effect of excess thyroid hormone. Considering the similar time-course of the reduction of serum sIL-2R with those of AST and ALT during the episode of hyperthyroidism, which is often accompanied by the autoimmune process in painless thyroiditis [12,13], it was suggested that the increase of serum sIL-2R in this case resulted from activation of the autoimmune process during this episode. However, since it is reported that the normalization of hypermetabolic state might be delayed for certain period even after complete normalization of serum FT4 and FT3 within their respective normal range, it could not be completely negated that the increase of sIL-2R might be explained by hyperthyroidism itself.

In conclusion, herein we report the first case of painless thyroiditis with a significant and temporary increase of serum sIL-2R.

Consent

Written informed consent was obtained from the patient for publication of this Case report and any accompanying images. A copy of the written consent is available for review by the Editor-in-Chief of this journal.

Competing interest

The authors declare that they have no competing interests.

Authors' contributions

KH wrote the first draft. MY and KY were in a position of leadership for the patients and collected information on the patients. MK, HG and HK did the literature searches. SY wrote the final manuscript and made appropriate revisions. MI supervised the writing of the manuscript. All authors read through and approved the final manuscript.

Author details
[1]Department of Nephrology, Department of Metabolism, Endocrinology and Molecular Medicine, Osaka City University Graduate School of Medicine, 1-4-3, Asahi-machi, Abeno-ku, Osaka 545-8585, Japan. [2]Department of Internal Medicine, Division of Diabetes, Endocrinology and Metabolism, Hyogo College of Medicine, Mukogawa-cho 1-1, Nishinomiya, Hyogo 663-8501, Japan.

References

1. Cantrell DA, Smith KA: **Transient expression of IL-2receptors. Conseqences for T cell growth.** *J Exp Med* 1983, **158:**1895.
2. Rubin LA, Nelson DL: **The soluble interleukin-2 receptor: biology, function and clinical application.** *Ann Intern Med* 1990, **113:**619.
3. Weryha G, Gobert B, Leclère J, Béné MC, Faure G, Hartemann P: **Dynamic changes in soluble interleukin-2 receptor levels during treatment of Graves' disease.** *Horm Res* 1991, **35:**8–12.
4. Balazs C, Farid NR: **Soluble interleukin-2 receptor in sera of patients with Graves' disease.** *J Autoimmun* 1991, **4**(4):681–688.
5. Mariotti S, Caturegli P, Barbesino G, Marinò M, Del Prete GF, Chiovato L, Tonacchera M, De Carli M, Pinchera A: **Thyroid function and thyroid autoimmunity independently modulate serum concentration of soluble interleukin 2 receptor in thyroid diseases.** *Clin Endocrinol (Oxf)* 1992, **37**(5):415–422.
6. Intenzo CM, Capuzzi DM, Jabbour S, Kim SM, dePapp AE: **Scintigraphic features of autoimmune thyroiditis.** *Radiographics* 2001, **21**(4):957–964.
7. Ueda M, Inaba M, Kumeda Y, Nagasaki T, Hiura Y, Tahara H, Onoda N, Ishikawa T, Nishizawa Y: **The significance of thyroid blood flow at the inferior thyroid artery as a predictor for early Graves' disease relapse.** *Clin Endocrinol (Oxf)* 2005, **63**(6):657–662.
8. Smallridge RC, Tsokos GC, Burman KD, Porter L, Cranston T, Sfikakis PP, Solomon BL: **Soluble interleukin-2 receptor is a thyroid hormone-dependent early-response marker in the treatment of thyrotoxicosis.** *Clin Diagn Lab Immunol* 1997, **7:**583–586.
9. Koukkou E, Panayiotidis P, Thalassinos N: **Serum soluble interleukin-2 receptors as an index of the biological activity of thyroid hormones in hyperthyroidism.** *J Endocrinol Invest* 1995, **18**(4):253–257.
10. Ohtsuka R, Abe Y, Shiratsuchi M, Suehiro Y, Karube K, Muta K, Nishimura J, Takayanagi R: **Graves' disease with splenomegaly and pancytopenia, mimicking B-cell lymphoproliferative disease.** *Rinsho Ketsueki* 2008, **49**(2):104–108.
11. Sellin JH, Vassilopoulou-Sellin R: **The gastrointestinal tract and liver in thyrotoxicosis.** In *Werner&Ingbar's The Thyroid.* 8th edition. Edited by Braverman LE, Utiger RD. Philadelphia: Lippincott Williams & Wilkins; 2000:623–624.
12. Nobili V, Liaskos C: **Autoimmune thyroiditis associated with autoimmune hepatitis.** *Thyroid* 2005, **15**(10):1193–1195.
13. Doniach D, Roitt IM, Walker JG, Sherlock S: **Tissue antibodies in primary biliary cirrhosis, active chronic (lupoid) hepatitis, cryptogenic cirrhosis and other liver disease and their clinical implications.** *Clin Exp Immunol* 1966, **1**(3):237–262.

Postoperative use of drain in thyroid lobectomy – a randomized clinical trial conducted at Civil Hospital, Karachi, Pakistan

Zahid Ali Memon[1], Gulrayz Ahmed[2*], Sarah Rafi Khan[2], Mahvesh Khalid[2] and Naheed Sultan[3]

Abstract

Background: Thyroidectomy is a common surgical procedure, after which drains are placed routinely. This study aims to assess the benefits of placing postoperative drains, its complications and affects on postoperative stay, in thyroid lobectomy.

Methodology: Randomized Clinical Trial of 60 goitre patients undergoing lobectomy was conducted at Civil Hospital Karachi, during July'11-December'11. Patients were randomly assigned into drain and non drain groups. Patient demographics, labs and complications were noted. Ultrasound of neck was performed on both groups. For drain group, the amount of fluid present in the surgical bed and redivac drain was added to calculate fluid collection while in non drain group it was calculated by ultrasound of neck on first and second post-op days. Data was entered and analyzed on SPSS v16 using Independent T tests.

Result: The mean total drain output for 2 days in non-drain group was significantly lower 10.67 (±9.072) ml while in drain group was 30.97 (±42.812) ml ($p = 0.014$). The mean postoperative stay of drain group (79.2 ±15.63 hours) was significantly higher, as compared to mean postoperative stay of non drain group (50.4 ±7.32 hours). Mean Visual Analogue Score (VAS) for pain day 1 (6.2 ±0.997) and day 2 (4.17 ±0.95) in drain group were significantly higher compared to day 1 (2.6 ±1.163) and day 2 (1.3 ±0.877) of non drain group. From drain group, 2 patients complained of stridor, dyspnea on Day 1 which subsided by Day 2 and 1 case of voice change, with no such complains in non drain group. No patients from both groups developed seroma, wound infection or hematoma.

Conclusion: In uncomplicated surgeries especially for lobectomy, use of drain can be omitted.

Keywords: Thyroidectomy, Lobectomy, Drain, Postoperative, Complications

Introduction

Thyroidectomy is one of the most commonly performed operative procedure in general surgery [1]. Indications for thyroid surgery are hyperthyroidism, thyroid swellings, and thyroid cancers. Indications for thyroid surgery are hyperthyroidism, thyroid swellings, with a prevalence of between 4.2 to 51.3% [2], and thyroid cancers.

After thyroid surgery, the chief reason for surgeons placing a drain is to detect early postoperative hemorrhage [3], and to avoid its risk of blocking the respiratory passage [4]. However, a common problem is that the drains become blocked with clotted blood and are useless in alerting the surgeon even if major bleeding occurs [1]. The probability of a postoperative hematoma forming after thyroid surgery ranges between 0 to 30% [5]. However, past studies have failed to show that placement of drains prevent the hematoma formation.

There are also very low chances of postoperative seromas forming in the absence of drains but they can be observed and allowed to resorb themselves or, if severe, aspirated [6].

Past studies conducted on the usefulness of drain placement after thyroid surgery have failed to show any benefits [7]. Instead, it was found that usage of drains increased the chances of surgical wound infections [8]. From two studies conducted in Pakistan, both reported

* Correspondence: gulrayzahmed@soch.net.pk
[2]4th Year Student, Dow Medical College, DUHS, D – 31, Block 8, Gulshan-e-Iqbal, P.O Box 75300, Karachi, Pakistan
Full list of author information is available at the end of the article

that the use of drains is not mandatory after thyroidectomy provided that strict principles of haemostasis are followed [6,9]. The study done in 2005 showed no difference in the prevalence of post thyroidectomy hematoma formation whether drains were used or not [6]. The other study reported greater fluid collection and more postoperative complications in the group of patients with drains than those without [9]. There have not been, however, many recent studies in this part of the world showing whether the use of drains is mandatory or not.

In our clinical setup, drains are commonly placed postoperatively. We have conducted this trial to see if results from other studies are relevant to ours and if disadvantages of the use of drains significantly outweigh its advantages. The use of drains after thyroid surgery is being questioned worldwide now that surgical techniques have improved for thyroid disorders. This study aims to assess the necessity of drains and to eliminate their routine use after thyroid surgery. Also, the aim for this study is to compare our findings with those of international studies and also for general awareness.

Materials and methods

A randomized clinical trial of diagnosed patients of goiter was conducted at Civil Hospital, Karachi between July 2011 and December 2011. All the patients who were to undergo sub-total lobectomy or lobectomy during the study period, were selected and randomized in to two equal groups, one with drain placed post-operatively and the other without drain. Allocation of patients to drain and non-drain group was done on the basis of computer generated random number table. Just before wound closure, the operating surgeon was informed of the group. Cases of total thyroidectomy, subtotal thyroidectomy, thyroid carcinomas or previous thyroid surgery were excluded. Cases of goiter were confirmed by all or atleast two of the following tests; ultrasound (U/S) neck, fine needle aspiration for cytology (FNAC), thyroid scan and histopathology. Indirect and direct laryngoscopy was performed preoperatively and postoperatively as a routine protocol.

The study instrument was a structured questionnaire that was filled by medical students after obtaining informed consent from the patients. The questionnaire was divided into four parts. The first part included demographics of the patient. The second part included baseline labs, including hemoglobin levels, platelet counts, total leucocytes counts, blood urea nitrogen, creatinine, serum thyroid stimulating hormone, T3 and T4 levels. The third part had details pertaining to the tests performed to confirm diagnosis of goiter. Postoperative complications were noted down in the fourth part. The patients were inquired about complications including pain, stridor, dyspnea and voice change. Pain and discomfort were evaluated by VAS (Visual Analogue Scale) with 0 being no pain and 10 being severe unbearable pain. Complications like wound infection, seroma, hemorrhage and hematoma were also noted.

Drain output was noted on post operative day 1 and day 2. In the drain group, a negative pressure drain was placed postoperatively. Ultra sound of the neck was performed in both groups, using B mode with linear frequency of 7.5 MHz. It was performed by the same radiologist with fluid volume being calculated by measuring the maximum diameter of the operative bed in three dimensions. For the drain group, the amount of fluid present in the surgical bed and Redivac drain was separately calculated and added to calculate fluid collection while in the non drain group it was calculated by ultrasound of neck. Then the calculated amount of fluid for both groups was compared. Total drain output was calculated by adding fluid collection of both groups for the two days.

Data was entered and analyzed on SPSSv16. Differences between both groups of age, postoperative hours of stay, Pain Day 1 (PD1), Pain Day 2 (PD2), Drain Output Day 1, Drain Output Day 2 and Total Drain output for two days (TD) variables was analyzed using Independent T tests with p values less than 0.05 being significant. Mean VAS scores for Pain Day 1 (PD1) and Pain Day 2 (PD2) were also analyzed using Independent T Test. Simple descriptive analysis was used to calculate frequencies, percentages and means of all variables. Results were represented in pie charts, bar charts, tables and cross tabs.

Ethical consideration

This trial was approved by the concerned Surgical Unit Ethical Committee. Written Consent was obtained from the participants after explaining the study objectives. The participants were free at all times, to withdraw from the trial without giving any reason. Strict measures for confidentiality were maintained throughout the process of data collection, entry and analysis. All efforts were made in this study to fulfill the ethical considerations in accordance with the 'Ethical principles for medical research involving human subjects' of Helsinki Declaration [10].

Result

Of the 60 patients, 6 (10%) were males and 54 (90%) were females with a ratio of 1:9. Drain group included 3 males and 27 females with mean age of 32.27 (±9.663) years, of which 16 were, diagnosed solitary thyroid nodule, 7 had nodular goitre and 7 cases of adenoma. Non drain group had 3 males and 27 females with mean age of 31.23 (±7.596) years, of which 10 were diagnosed cases of solitary thyroid nodule, 13 nodular goitre and 7

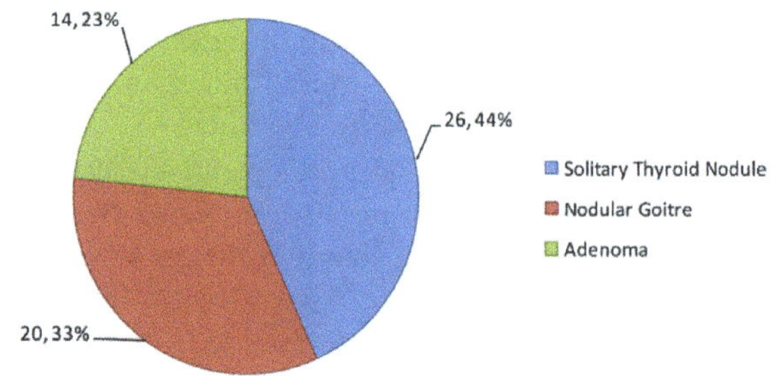

Figure 1 Total Diagnosed Cases.

adenoma. Diagnosis of all cases is represented in Figure 1.

The mean calculated TD in non drain group (10.67 ±9.072 ml) was significantly reduced as compared to drain group (30.97 ±42.812 ml, IQR = 18.25 ml, Median = 25 ml) ($p = 0.014$). The relationship between fluid collection of both groups on Day 1 and Day 2 is represented in Table 1.

The mean post-op stay of drain group was 79.2 (±15.63) hours which was significantly higher, as compared to mean post op stay of 50.4 (±7.323) hours in non drain group ($p < 0.001$). Details of post-op stay are mentioned in Table 2 and compared diagrammatically in Figure 2.

The mean VAS score also showed significance. In drain group mean VAS score for PD1 was 6.2 (±0.997) and for non drain group 2.6 (±1.163) ($p < 0.001$). For PD2 mean VAS score was also significantly higher in drain group being 4.17 (±0.95) as compared to 1.3 (±0.877) for the non drain group ($p < 0.001$).

From drain group (n = 30), 2 (6.67%) patients complained of stridor and dyspnea (respiratory complications) which subsided by Day 2, and 5 (16.7%) cases complained of voice change on Day 1, of which 1 had the same complain next day. There was no complaining of stridor, dyspnea or voice change in non drain group. Complication of hemorrhage (200 ml) was noted in a patient of drain group who was re-operated for haemostasis. None of the patients in both groups developed hematoma, wound infection or seroma. Table 3 compares the number of complications in both groups.

Table 2 Post-Op Stay

Group	Hours					Total	P value
	24	48	72	96	120		
No Drain	0	27	3	0	0	30	<0.001
%	0	90	10	0	0	100	
Drain	0	2	18	9	1	30	
%	0	6.7	60	30	3.3	100	

Discussion

Lobectomy or subtotal thyroidectomy is one of the most common surgical procedures. It is usually performed for benign thyroid disorders like multinodular goitre, nodular goiter, and adenomas.

It is common practice for surgeons to routinely insert a drain after every case of thyroid surgery [4], whether it is total thyroidectomy or lobectomy. This is mainly due to the fear of postoperative hemorrhage [3] or accumulation of excess lymphatic fluid which needs to be drained as it can compromise the airway [4]. Postoperative bleeding after thyroid surgery is reported to be as rare as 0.3 to 1% [1], while the probability of a postoperative cervical hematoma forming ranges between 0.1 to 4.7% [11]. In two studies of 250 and 400 patients no benefit of using drains after thyroid surgery has been documented [12,13]. It has been observed that if correct surgical techniques and hemostatic procedures are followed, excessive post-operative bleeding can be avoided, decreasing the incidence of hematoma formation. Precautions such as staying within the subplatysmal plane during surgery and using coagulation diathermy along with proper ligation of bleeding vessels will reduce chances of postoperative hemorrhage [6].

In real practice insertion of drain should be rationalized on the basis of the operative procedure performed and the extent of neck dissection along with patient to patient variation. Many authors recommend the use of drains only for complicated cases such as resection of substernal goiter, large dead space, raw thyroid bed [13,14] or in hypervascular diseases of thyroid (e.g. Grave's disease) or certain carcinomas [15]. In our study, only one patient with drain developed complication of hemorrhage and required reoperation in which the amount of fluid was 200 ml. Thus prevalence of this complication was 3.33% in the drain group of this

Table 1 Drain Output Day 1 and 2

	No Drain				Total	p-value	Drain				Total	p-value
	0 - 09 ml	10 - 19 ml	20 - 29 ml	> 30 ml			0 - 09 ml	10 - 19 ml	20 - 29 ml	> 30 ml		
Day 1	11	17	2	0	30`	0.228	8	11	8	3	30	0.61
%	36.67	56.67	6.67	0	100		26.67	36.67	26.67	10	100	
Day 2	22	8	0	0	30		11	12	3	4	30	
%	73.3	26.7	0	0	100		36.67	40	10	13.33	100	

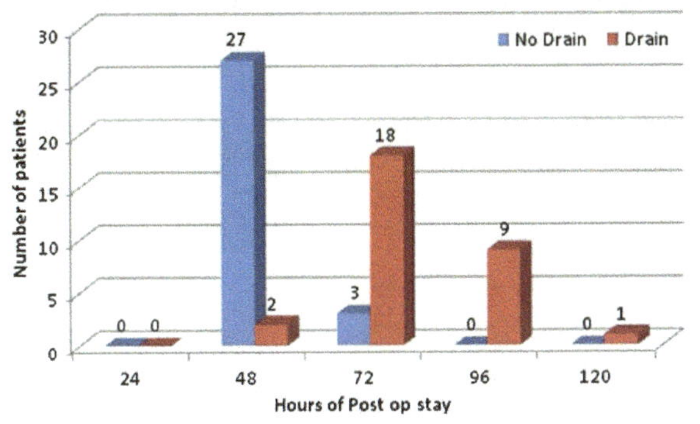

Figure 2 Post-op stay.

study which is comparable to international figures showing a variable prevalence of between 0.1 to 4.7% [11]. A study from Hyderabad, Pakistan reported 1.4% prevalence of this complication which is comparatively lower than this study [16].

In the present study, there were no cases of seroma formation in either the drain or non drain group, which coincides with the fact that seroma formation does not specifically occur when drains are not used. No patients in any group had to undergo aspirations (except for a case hemorrhage). Conversely, the placement of drains itself can lead to seroma formation since the drain is a foreign object. A study showed that there was fluid collection in the surgical field regardless of the use of a drain, the reason being, either the drain triggered inflammation and fluid formation itself or the negative pressure created by the drain sealed off the lymphatics [2]. Likewise, in this study the amount of fluid in the drain group was significantly greater [30.97 (±42.812) ml] than the non-drain group [10.67 (±9.072) ml] ($p < 0.001$). So placement of drains can initiate or even further aggravate an already developing seroma.

The insertion of drain after every thyroid surgery increases the risk of introducing infection into the patient. When compared with international literature, the incidence of wound infections after thyroid surgery in the drain group showed variable results, from no wound infections in some studies to up to 3.4% in others [1,7]. Hence, post surgical wound management and aseptic techniques used during surgery also play a major role in determining the development of infection.

Similarly, our study also suggests that insertion of drain after the thyroid surgery increases the hospital stay of the patients [79.2 (±15.63) hours] as compared to the ones that were left without the drain [50.4 (±7.323) hours]. In a study done in 2010, it was found that the

Table 3 Comparison of complications in both groups

			Drain (n = 60)		P value
			No (n = 30)	Yes (n = 30)	
Respiratory Complications Day 1	No	Count	30	28	0.150
		% within Drain No / Yes	100%	93.3%	
	Yes	Count	0	2	
		% within Drain No / Yes	0%	6.7%	
Respiratory Complications Day 2	No	Count	30	30	-
		% within Drain No / Yes	100%	100%	
	Yes	Count	0	0	
		% within Drain No / Yes	0%	0%	
Voice Change Day 1	No	Count	30	25	0.020
		% within Drain No / Yes	100%	83.3%	
	Yes	Count	0	5	
		% within Drain No / Yes	0%	16.7%	
Voice Change Day 2	No	Count	30	29	0.313
		% within Drain No / Yes	100%	96.7%	
	Yes	Count	0	1	
		% within Drain No / Yes	0%	3.3%	
Hemorrhage	No	Count	30	29	0.313
		% within Drain No / Yes	100%	96.7%	
	Yes	Count	0	1	
		% within Drain No / Yes	0%	3.3%	

No complications of Hypocalcemia, Wound Infection and Seroma reported.

length of hospital stay was increased by a day in these patients, which obviously increased overall costs [2]. Another study documents that use of drain in uncomplicated thyroid surgeries, not only increases the duration of hospital stay but also the chances of infection [17]. Hence, this also increased the cost beared by the hospital. This would not benefit a hospital setting, as in our study, which caters to an ever-growing number of patients free of cost with limited number of beds.

Patient discomfort and pain were assessed on day 1 and 2 after surgery, via the VAS (Visual Analogue Scale). It showed that the patients in the drain group felt a greater degree of pain and discomfort than those in non-drain group. The mean VAS score for PD1 and PD2 in drain group was significantly higher ($p < 0.01$) as compared to non drain group. This consequently led to a greater use of analgesics. Our results coincided with those of an African study done in 2011, which also showed the mean VAS to be significantly reduced in the non-drain group on postoperative day 0 and 1 [7]. Hematoma normally becomes clinically apparent after 4 to 6 hours of surgery [18], but no such case was recorded.

Placement of drains can also cause poor cosmetic results and create separate surgical scars. It also increases operating time by 5 minutes due to the need for an extra, irregularly shaped stab wound to be made in the lower neck or chest [6]. Other complications can include hypoparathyroidism and hypocalcemia, voice change, stridor, and dyspnea; of which there were no cases, besides one case of voice change in drain group, in our study.

The present clinical trial, in conformity with numerous international clinical trials [1,3-5,7], could not show any benefit of routinely placing drains after every case of thyroid surgery, particularly uncomplicated cases. Albeit, it did display the complications as well as life threatening conditions which can possibly occur if drains are placed routinely. This study demonstrated that prevention of postoperative hematoma did not require drain placement as much as performance of correct hemostatic techniques were needed and also that seroma formation can be triggered by drains themselves. It also showed that postoperative stay, costs, patient discomfort and pain are greater in patients which have drain placement after thyroid surgery. Major limitations of the study included patient's understanding to questions asked, unequal distribution of benign diagnosed goiter cases in both groups and chances of errors while estimating fluid volume.

Conclusion

In uncomplicated surgeries, especially in cases of lobectomy; use of drain can be omitted which will help decreasing chances of wound infection, with substantial shortening of patient stay while increasing patient comfort and satisfaction.

Abbreviations

VAS: Visual Analogue Scale; TD: Total Drain output for two days; PD1: Pain Day 1; PD2: Pain Day 2.

Competing interests

The authors declare that they have no competing interests.

Authors' contributions

ZAM and PN were involved in conceptualizing the study and final paper reviewing. GA was also involved in the conceptualization of this study, questionnaire development and wrote the initial and final paper and performed data analysis with assistance from SRK. MK supervised the data collection, entered and verified the data and helped in drafting the initial paper. All authors read and approved the final manuscript.

Acknowledgement

We would like to acknowledge our colleagues Faiq Hamirani and Sameer Hanfi who helped us in data collection.

Author details

[1]Senior Registrar, Surgical Unit 1, Civil Hospital, Karachi, Pakistan. [2]4th Year Student, Dow Medical College, DUHS, D – 31, Block 8, Gulshan-e-Iqbal, P.O Box 75300, Karachi, Pakistan. [3]Dean Surgery and Allied, Incharge Surgical Unit 1, Dow University of Health Sciences, Civil Hospital, Karachi, Pakistan.

References

1. Tahsin C, Tamer A, Ozgur T, Hakan C, Bora U, Arzu K, *et al*: **Drainage after total thyroidectomy or lobectomy for benign thyroidal disorders.** *J Zhejiang Univ Sci B* 2008, **9**(4):319–323.
2. Prichard RS, Murphy R, Lowry A, McLaughlin R, Malone C, Kerin MJ: **The routine use of post-operative drains in thyroid surgery: an outdated concept.** *Ir Med J* 2010, **103**(1):26–27.
3. Wihlborg O, Bergljung L, Martensson H: **To drain or not to drain in thyroid surgery. A controlled clinical study.** *Arch Surg* 1988, **123**(1):40–41.
4. Khanna J, Mohil RS, Chintamani D, Dinesh B, Mittal MK, Sahoo M, *et al*: **Is the routine drainage after surgery for thyroid necessary? A prospective randomized clinical study.** *BMC Surg* 2005, **19**:5–11.
5. Lee SW, Choi EC, Lee YM, Lee JY, Kim SC, Koh YW: **Is lack of placement of drains after thyroidectomy with central neck dissection safe? A prospective, randomized study.** *Laryngoscope* 2006, **116**(9):1632–1635.
6. Gooda MR, Oonwala ZG, Khan S: **Use of Drainage after Thyroid Surgery: Is it Evidence based?** *Pak J Surg* 2007, **23**(3):173–176.
7. Chalya PL, Gilyoma JM, Mchembe M: **Drain versus No Drain after Thyroidectomy: A prospective Randomized Clinical Study.** *East Cent. Afr J Surg* 2011, **16**(22)):55–61.
8. Ozlem N, Ozdogan M, Gurer A, Gomceli I, Aydin R: **Should the thyroid bed be drained after thyroidectomy?** *Langenbecks archives of surgery Deutsche Gesellschaft fur Chirurgie* 2006, **391**(3):228–230.
9. Ishaq I, Iqbal J, Ajmal R, Afzal M, Munir K: **The role of drainage after thyroid surgery. Is it mandatory?** *A.P.M.C* 2008, **2**(1):46–49.
10. World Medical Association, Inc: *WMA Declaration of Helsinki*; 2009. http://www.wma.net/en/30publications/10policies/b3/index.html.
11. Calo PG, Pisano G, Piga G, Medas F, Tatti A, Donati M, Nicolosi A: **Postoperative hematomas after thyroid surgery, Incidence and risk factors in our experience.** *Ann Ital Chir* 2010, **81**:343–347.
12. Arriyanayagam DC: **Narayan Singh V, Busby D, Sieunarine K, Raju G: Thyroid surgery without drainage; 15 years of clinical experience.** *J Roy Coll Surg Edinb.* 1993, **38**:69–70.
13. Shaha AR, Jaffe BM: **Selective use of drains in thyroid surgery.** *J Surg Oncol* 1993, **52**(4):241–3.
14. Schoretsanitis G, Melissas J, Sanidas E, *et al*: **Does draining the neck affect morbidity following thyroid surgery?** *Am Surg* 1998, **64**:778–780.
15. Hurtado-Lopez LM, Lopez-Romero S, Rizzo-Fuentes C, *et al*: **Seletive use of drains in thyroid surgery.** *Head Neck* 2001, **23**:189–193.

16. Khanzada TW, Samad A, Memon W, Kumar B: **Post thryoidectomy complications: the Hyderabad experience.** *J Ayub Med Coll Abbotabad* 2010, **22**(1):65–68.
17. Suslu N, Vural S, Oncel M: **Is the insertion of drains after uncomplicated Thyroid surgery always necessary?** *Surg Today* 2006, **36**(3):215–218.
18. Shaha AR, Jaffe BM: **Practical management of postthyroidectomy hematoma.** *J Surg Oncol* 1994, **57**:235–238.

17

The use of semi-quantitative ultrasound elastosonography in combination with conventional ultrasonography and contrast-enhanced ultrasonography in the assessment of malignancy risk of thyroid nodules with indeterminate cytology

Massimo Giusti[1,4*], Claudia Campomenosi[1], Stefano Gay[1], Barbara Massa[2], Enzo Silvestri[3], Eleonora Monti[1] and Giovanni Turtulici[3]

Abstract

Background: The pre-surgical selection of thyroid nodules with indeterminate cytology (Thy 3 according to British Thyroid Association) after fine-needle aspiration biopsy (FNAB) is currently required in order to reduce unnecessary total thyroidectomy. The objective of our study was to use a surgical series of Thy 3 nodules to evaluate the predictive role of ultrasound elastosonography (USE) and contrast-enhanced ultrasonography (CEUS) in pre-surgical diagnoses of malignancy.

Subjects and methods: We enrolled 63 patients with Thy 3 nodules in which cytological–histological correlation was available. The ELX 2/1 strain index was obtained by means of semi-quantitative USE, which was performed before surgery in addition to conventional ultrasonography (US) and contrast-enhanced US (CEUS) on the Thy 3 nodules. The ELX 2/1 strain index, a five-item US score and both peak (P) index and time to peak (TTP) index from CEUS were correlated with the histological results. After surgical diagnosis, the data were analysed by using a receiver-operating characteristic (ROC) curve.

Results: Histology was benign in 50 and malignant in 13 Thy 3 nodules. No difference in maximal diameter was noted between benign (22.8 ± 1.6 mm) and malignant (18.9 ± 2.9 mm) nodules. Significant correlations were found between histology and cumulative US findings ($p=0.005$), ELX 2/1 index ($p=0.002$), P index ($p=0.01$) and TTP index ($p=0.02$). On analysing data from US, USE and CEUS, significant ROC areas under the curve were observed ($p<0.0001$). A cut-off value was set for US (>2), ELX 2/1 (>0.95), P index (<0.99) and TTP index (>0.98) scores. The diagnostic power of the cumulative pre-surgical analysis of Thy 3 nodules with US, USE and CEUS, considering the experimental cut-off points obtained from the ROC curves was: sensitivity 64%, specificity 92%, PPV 75% and accuracy 84%.

(Continued on next page)

* Correspondence: magius@unige.it
[1]Endocrine Unit, IRCCS Azienda Ospedaliera Universitaria San Martino – IST Istituto Nazionale per la Ricerca sul Cancro, Genoa, Italy
[4]UO Clinica Endocrinologica, Viale Benedetto XV, 6, I-16100 Genoa, Italy
Full list of author information is available at the end of the article

(Continued from previous page)

Conclusion: The ELX 2/1 index in conjunction with the US score can be useful in orienting surgical strategies in Thy 3 nodules. The information added by CEUS is less sensitive than that provided by US and USE. The use of a cut-off based on histology can reduce thyroidectomy. Observation should be the first choice when not all instrumental results are suspect.

Keywords: Thyroid nodules, Indeterminate cytology, Ultrasosonography, Ultrasound elastosonography, Strain index, Contrast-enhanced ultrasonography, Cytological–histological correlation, ROC analysis

Introduction

The prevalence of diagnoses of thyroid nodules often varies according to the method of examination used [1-3]. The current thyroid nodule and thyroid cancer epidemic can be explained by the worldwide diffusion of ultrasonography (US) equipment [4,5]. When a nodule is found, the most important clinical problem is to exclude malignancy, which accounts for approximately 5%-15% of all thyroid nodules [6-8]. A combination of clinical factors (age, sex, exposure to radiation, familial traits) and US features determines whether or not the clinician should proceed with further tests or observation. The accuracy of US in predicting thyroid cancer has recently been reviewed by Brito et al. [9]. Only two US findings – spongiform and cystic thyroid nodule features – seem to provide sufficient probability to help rule out cancer and to suggest observation at first, while all other US findings, when assessed individually, might not be able to rule in or rule out malignancy, owing to their modest likelihood ratio [9]. Therefore, in order to distinguish malignant from benign thyroid nodules, cytological investigation by means of fine-needle aspiration biopsy (FNAB) must be performed under US guidance in nodules larger than 10 mm or with suspicious US findings [10-13]. Thyroid cytology is usually reported both descriptively and as suggested categories with different risks of malignancy. Both the Bethesda system and the British Thyroid Association (BTA) category (Thy 1 – Thy 5) are used. The ultimate aim of FNAB is to reassure the patient and to avoid surgery if not otherwise indicated [13]. FNAB yields useful cytological results in about 80% of cases, but has several weaknesses, including false negative (about 1-2%), non-diagnostic (3-16%) and indeterminate (follicular lesions; 6-20%) results [13-16]. The low risk of underestimating a thyroid cancer supports the recommendation for repeat thyroid nodule evaluation 2–4 years after initial benign (Thy 2) FNAB [16], while the very high probability (77-100%) [17-21] of cancer in nodules "suspicious for malignancy" (Thy 4) obliges surgery, as in the case of findings that are "diagnostic of malignancy" (Thy 5). Core-needle biopsy seems more useful than FNAB repetition in reducing non-diagnostic (Thy 1) cytology [22], but its utility in cases of indeterminate cytology after FNAB is still debated [22,23]. As indeterminate lesions (Thy 3) are associated with an approximately 25% risk of malignancy [12,17,19,24-27], histological examination is still required by the current guidelines of thyroid societies. Rago et al. [27] recently reported an overall good prognosis in Thy 3 lesions with malignant histology, which suggests the possibility that more exhaustive pre-surgical evaluation might reduce unnecessary (about 70% of cases) surgery. In this context, the role of US in distinguishing malignant from benign Thy 3 nodules is still uncertain, though in the large series of Thy 3 nodules examined in Rago's study, blurred nodule margins and spots of microcalcification were significantly associated with malignancy.

The introduction of novel diagnostic tools may provide a more reliable approach to assessing the risk of malignancy in Thy 3 nodules. Recently, the determination of somatic mutation in FNAB specimens from Thy 3 nodules has been proposed [17,28,29], and may also help in deciding the extent of surgery [30]. However, the role of molecular screening could be overestimated, as this technique increases FNAB sensitivity from 67% to only 75% in indeterminate lesions [31]. On the other hand, a search for several gene expressions conducted in 326 nodules with indeterminate cytology has demonstrated the substantial impact of this approach on clinical care recommendations, though site-to-site variation exists [32] and this evaluation is not yet universally available.

US elastography (USE) and contrast-enhanced US (CEUS) are another two innovative techniques under evaluation for the detection of malignancy in thyroid nodules, but they still need validation. USE has been likened to "electronic palpation" and provides reproducible stiffness measurements even in otherwise non-palpable thyroid lesions [33]. At present, heterogeneity among different USE technologies (difference in compression source, modality of processing, stiffness expression), equipment and applications explains why USE is not yet part of routine nodule management [19,33]. USE should primary be implemented in the pre-surgical differential diagnosis between benign and malignant nodules; however, its accuracy is debated and surgery has not always been taken as the reference in evaluating USE data [17-21,25]. In addition, a certain risk of false negative results has been reported, especially in cases of follicular [34,35] or medullary thyroid cancer [36]. CEUS is a dynamic evaluation which enables thyroid nodules to be characterized by studying vascular enhancement patterns, which it does better than conventional US. Some authors have reported that the absence of ring enhancement and the presence of heterogeneous enhancement [37-39] or a shorter time to peak of the perfusion curve [40] could characterize malignant nodules. However, these data are still controversial [19,41].

The pre-surgical diagnostic role of USE [17-19,21,25,42,43] and CEUS [19,37] in nodules with indeterminate cytology has been considered uncertain because of the low number of these nodules in the series analyzed. Two recently published studies have focused on USE in indeterminate nodules. In 169 patients in whom histology was available after qualitative USE, Rago et al. [27] reported that high elasticity is closely associated with benign histology, with a negative predictive value of 97%. In addition, in a series of 270 nodules with atypia of indeterminate significance evaluated by means of semi-quantitative USE, Cakir et al. [44] reported a higher median strain index in the malignant group than in the benign group. To our knowledge, no data are available in the literature on large series of Thy 3 nodules evaluated by CEUS in order to judge the pre-surgical role of this technique.

The aim of the present study was to retrospectively evaluate the pre-surgical role of both USE and CEUS together with US findings in our series of patients with indeterminate cytology and known histology. The construction of a validate cut-off for numerical indices could be used to avoid surgical procedures in Thy 3 patients in whom all tests (US, USE, CEUS) yield "benign" results. The cost and time consumption of these techniques could be lower than those of unnecessary thyroid surgery.

Materials and methods

Patients

This prospective study enrolled 78 consecutive patients (60 female, 18 male; age: 20–82 yrs; mean ± SD: 55.4 ± 14.7 yrs) with thyroid nodules observed at the out-patient Thyroid Cancer Unit. On FNAB, performed as previously reported [19], all patients had an indeterminate thyroid lesion (Thy 3) according to the 2009 BTA classification. These patients were considered candidates for surgery in accordance with the cytological result. In 47% of these patients, the Thy 3 nodule was found in a multinodular goitre, while 53% had a uninodular goiter. In 8 patients, laboratory data were compatible with Hashimoto's thyroiditis, while one patient had a single Thy 3 nodule in a diffuse toxic goiter. Levothyroxine was being taken by 20% of patients, either for hypothyroidism (n=3) or as a TSH-reducing therapy (n=13). Three patients were on methimazole therapy for pre-toxic goiter. All patients underwent laboratory evaluations. TSH and free-T4 (f-T4) were measured by means of ultra-sensitive chemiluminescence immunoassay (Roche Diagnostics, Mannheim, Germany). Normal ranges are: 0.3-4.2 mIU/l for TSH and 12.0-22.0 pmol/l for f-T4. Thyroperoxidase antibodies (TPOAb) were evaluated by means of the Dia Sorin assay (Saluggia, Italy); concentrations <100 mIU/l were regarded as negative. Serum calcitonin (CT) was assayed by chemiluminescence immunoassay (Dia Sorin); in our laboratory, the upper limit of the normal CT range is 10 ng/l. All patients were invited to undergo further sonographic evaluation. All patients gave their informed consent to participate in the study. The collection of patient's data and subsequent analysis was performed in compliance with the Helsinki declaration and was approved by University of Genoa Ethical Committee.

Thyroid US, USE and CEUS

All patients were examined in the supine position with the neck extended. Scans of both thyroid lobes and isthmus were obtained in both transverse and longitudinal planes. The Thy 3 nodules were examined by means of conventional high-resolution US with a colour-Doppler module (MyLab40, Esaote Biomedica, Genoa) equipped with a 7.5 MHz linear probe. In 23 subjects, a further FNAB was performed with the aid of this equipment. As previously reported [19] and in accordance with US guidelines [45], the following parameters were investigated: echogenicity *vs.* non-nodular tissue, presence or absence of halo sign, presence or absence of microcalcifications, and flow pattern of the nodule. All USE examinations were performed by the same operator (GT) by means of a MyLab 70 XvG US scanner (Esaote Biomedica) equipped with an LA-522 linear probe working in the range of 7–12 MHz and software for the quantification of the USE features of the tissue. Static and moving images were recorded, as already reported by Lyshchik et al. [34], at least 3 times in order to obtain mean values. The elasticity score (ELX 2/1) index was calculated at the same depth as the ratio between the elasticity feature of the selected region-of-interest (ROI) located on US-normal thyroid tissue and the ROI of the nodule under investigation. As previously reported [19], we considered the ELX 2/1 index directly reported on the screen of the equipment, as this is a less operator-dependent variable than the elasticity colour-scale extrapolated from breast tissue to the thyroid gland by some authors [18,25,35,46]. CEUS images were acquired by the MyLab 70 US scanner, as previously reported [19], by using a non-destructive US mode after bolus injection of SonoVue (4.8 ml; Bracco, Milan). CEUS video-clips were digitally recorded and analysed by means of Q-Contrast software V.4.0. (Bracco). Time-intensity curves within selected ROI and colour maps were acquired. Nodule and healthy thyroid tissue values of peak contrast enhancement (Peak) and time to peak (TTP) were calculated. Peak and TTP are reported as indexes (Peak index, TTP index) derived from the ratio between the values from the ROI of the nodule and the ROI of normal thyroid tissue [19].

Statistical analysis

Non-parametric tests were used to compare averages; the correlation coefficient r was calculated by means of Spearman correlation (Sr) (GraphPad 6.0 Software, San Diego, CA, USA). Data are reported as mean ± standard error of mean (SEM) if not otherwise reported. Significance was set at $p \leq 0.05$. A US score (from 0 to 5) was arbitrarily calculated for the nodule under evaluation, with one point being assigned for the presence of each of the following radiological findings: solid, hypo-echoic, microcalcification, internal vascularisation, and irregular shape [19]. All cytological and histology diagnoses were made by a pathologist (BM) with 10 years' experience in the pathologic analysis of thyroid cancer. After surgery, Thy 3 lesions were classified as malignant or benign. The diagnostic value of the ELX 2/1 index from USE or the P index and TTP index from CEUS in distinguishing between benign and malignant nodules was analysed by means of the receiver-operating characteristic (ROC) curve and calculated area under the curve. After using this curve to establish a cut-off point, we established sensitivity and specificity values and likelihood ratios. The cumulative results from US, USE and CEUS were evaluated for sensitivity, specificity, positive predictive value and accuracy. Thy 3 nodules that fitted all experimental cut-off points obtained from ROC curves were considered true positive if they proved malignant and false positive if they proved benign on histological examination. In addition Thy 3 nodules that did not fit all experimental cut-off points obtained from ROC curves were considered true negative if they proved benign and false negative if they proved malignant on histology.

Results

At the time of FNAB evaluations, all patients had normal f-T4 (15.1 ± 0.3 pmol/l) and TSH (2.0 ± 0.2 mIU/l) levels. CT was in the normal range in all but two patients; in these two patients, CT levels above the upper limit of the normal range (20 ng/l and 27 ng/l) were recorded. Surgery was performed in 63 of the 78 patients (81%). Surgery was not performed in 19% of Thy 3 nodules for the following reasons: down-grading of BTA classification from Thy 3 to Thy 2 (benign lesion) after the second FNAB (n=6), patient lost (n=4), patient request for further follow-up (n=2), patient refusal (n=2) and severe comorbidity (n=1). After surgery, a benign histological diagnosis of the cytological Thy 3 nodule was found in 50 cases (25 hyperplastic nodules; 18 follicular adenomas; 6 Hürthle cell adenomas; 1 intra-thyroid parathyroid adenoma). In 9 of these 50 cases (18%) an extra-nodular focal lymphocytic thyroiditis pattern was found, and in 6 (12%) a micro-papillary carcinoma of the isthmus (n=1) or in the contralateral lobe (n=5) was incidentally found. In one patient, C-cell hyperplasia was described. A final diagnosis of malignancy in the cytological Thy 3 nodules was reported in 13 cases (21%) (5 papillary thyroid carcinomas; 5 follicular variants of papillary thyroid carcinomas; 2 follicular carcinomas; 1 medullary thyroid carcinoma). Table 1 reports the clinical details of patients with thyroid

Table 1 Clinical and instrumental data on Thy 3 nodules with proven malignancy on histology

#	Age (yrs)	Sex	Nodule size (mm)	US (score)	USE (ELX 2/1)	CEUS P index	TTP index	Histology (°)	Tumour stage (*)
1	23	m	25	3	1.10	0.75	0.90	FTC	1
2	34	m	9	3	1.90	0.86	1.10	MTC	1
3	36	f	20	3	1.53	0.69	1.07	FvPTC	1
4	40	f	15	1	1.50	1.00	1.00	FTC	1
5	45	f	30	4	3.00	0.69	1.25	FvPTC	3
6	45	f	44	4	ne	0.82	1.62	FvPTC	3
7	46	f	7	4	1.00	0.60	0.63	PTC	1
8	46	f	9	3	1.30	0.95	1.20	FvPTC	1
9	50	m	13	3	1.80	0.33	1.00	PTC	3
10	54	m	20	3	1.70	0.90	2.40	PTC	1
11	66	m	23	5	1.50	0.80	1.01	PTC	1
12	71	f	7	3	1.90	0.77	1.00	PTC	1
13	74	f	22	3	2.00	0.90	1.00	PTC	1

(°) FTC = follicular thyroid carcinoma; MTC = medullary thyroid carcinoma; FvPTC = follicular variant of papillary thyroid carcinoma; PTC = papillary thyroid carcinoma.
(*) Tumour stage on diagnosis according to AJCC/UICC 2010 Seventh Edition criteria.
ne = not evaluable owing to coarse calcification (case #6).

malignancy. No difference in maximal diameter was noted between Thy 3 nodules with benign (22.8 ± 1.6 mm) or malignant (18.9 ± 2.9 mm) histology.

A significant correlation was seen between cumulative US findings and histology (n=63, Sr 0.35; p=0.005). A ROC curve was obtained (Figure 1) with an area under the curve (AUC) of 0.97 ± 0.01 (p<0.0001). By establishing a cut-off level that classified Thy 3 nodules with a US score greater than 2 as malignant, we were able to achieve a sensitivity of 79.0% and a specificity of 100%, with a 5.0 likelihood ratio.

USE was available in 61 Thy 3 nodules before surgery. In the remaining 2 cases, the ELX 2/1 index was unobtainable owing to coarse calcification of a 44 mm malignant nodule and the loss of data in a 23 mm benign nodule. A significant correlation was seen between the ELX 2/1 index and histology (Sr 0.39; p=0.002). A ROC curve was obtained (Figure 2) with an AUC of 0.95 ± 0.02 (p<0.0001). By establishing a cut-off level that classified Thy 3 nodules with an ELX 2/1 index greater than 0.95 as malignant, we were able to achieve a sensitivity of 83.6% and a specificity of 80.3%, with a 4.2 likelihood ratio. No significant correlation was found between the ELX 2/1 index and nodule (maximal) size or cumulative US findings (score).

CEUS was performed on 53 Thy 3 nodules; no side effects were recorded during or immediately after injection of the contrast agent. CEUS could not be performed in 10 Thy 3 nodules owing to refusal of intravenous injection of the contrast agent (n=5), technical impossibility of recording adequate video-clips (n=3) and loss of data (n=2). All these Thy 3 nodules (size-range: 14–30 mm) had benign histology. A significant inverse correlation was observed between histology and P index (Sr −0.37; p=0.01) while a significant positive correlation was found between histology and TTP index (Sr 0.32; p=0.02). ROC curves were obtained for the P index and TTP index, with an AUC of 0.83 ± 0.04 (p<0.0001) and 0.86 ± 0.04 (p<0.0001), respectively (Figure 3). By establishing a cut-off level that classified Thy 3 nodules with a P index lower than 0.99 as malignant, we were able to achieve a sensitivity of 37.7% and a specificity of 75.5%, with a 1.5 likelihood ratio. By establishing a cut-off level that classified Thy 3 nodules with a TTP index greater than 0.98 as malignant, we were able to achieve a sensitivity of 56.6% and a specificity of 75.5%, with a 2.3 likelihood ratio. A significant inverse correlation was found between P index and US findings (score) (Sr −0.44; p=0.001). The peak index was not related to nodule size, while the TTP index was not related to either US findings (score) or nodule size.

A cohort of 51 Thy 3 cases underwent US-guided FNAB, USE and CEUS before surgery. In 9 out of 12 (75%) histologically malignant Thy 3 nodules, all indictors were positive for malignancy, while they were all positive in 5 out of 39 (13%) histologically benign Thy 3 nodules. The diagnostic power of the cumulative pre-surgical analysis of Thy 3 nodules by means of US, USE and CEUS, considering the experimental cut-off points obtained from ROC curves was: sensitivity 64%, specificity 92%, PPV 75%, and accuracy 84%.

Discussion

The number of thyroid cancer diagnoses is currently increasing. This is probably the result of a reservoir

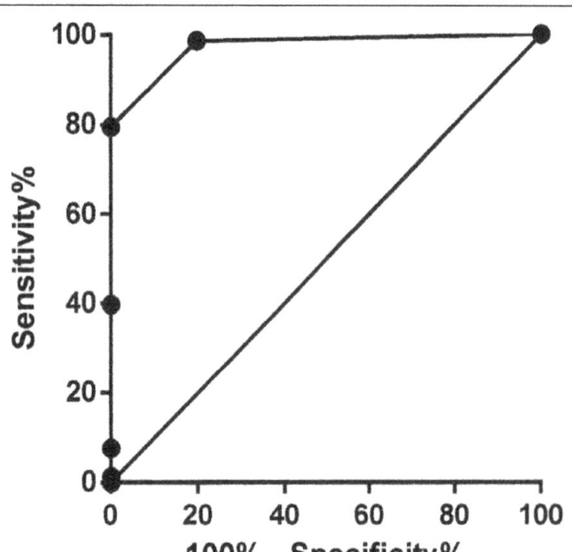

Figure 1 ROC curve created with histology as a reference for distinguishing malignant from benign Thy 3 nodules according to US score. The best cut-off was >2.

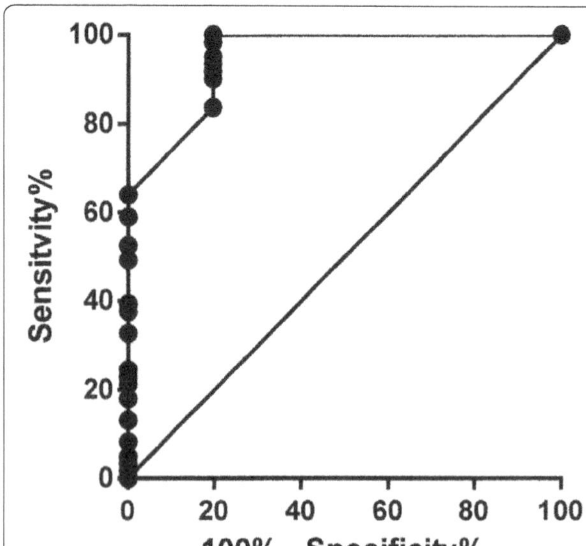

Figure 2 ROC curve created with histology as a reference for distinguishing malignant from benign Thy 3 nodules according to USE ELX 2/1 strain index. The best cut-off was >0.95.

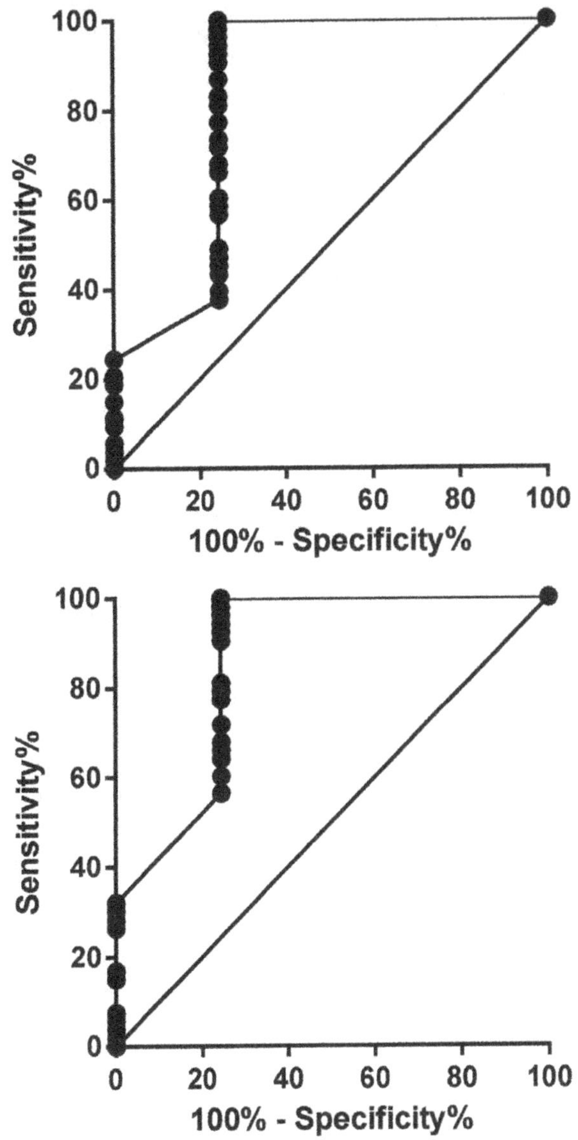

Figure 3 ROC curve created with histology as a reference for distinguishing malignant from benign Thy 3 nodules according to CEUS. The upper panel reports the P index; the best cut-off was <0.99. The lower panel reports the TTP index; the best cut-off was >0.98.

of asymptomatic (subclinical) malignant nodular thyroid disease which is disclosed in parallel with the "epidemic" of thyroid nodules due to the increase in instrumental, mainly US, diagnostics. Current clinical efforts should be aimed at defining the nature (malignant or benign) of a given nodule and identifying the relatively rare malignant nodules, in order to reduce unnecessary invasive surgical procedures.

US, which is the most sensitive means of evaluating thyroid morphology, can evaluate the size and characteristics of non-palpable nodules, reveal lymph-node metastases and guide FNAB. It is well known that no single US pattern can be used alone as a definite criterion of malignancy [45], and individual US features are not now considered accurate predictors of thyroid cancer [9].

The present study demonstrates that, in Thy 3 nodules, nodule size is not a useful means of distinguishing malignant from benign nodules, as already reported by several other authors [12,27,47]. In a previous study involving five US parameters (hypoechogenic, solid, intra-nodular vascularization, microcalcifications, and irregular margins), we found that the diagnostic power of color-Doppler US was high; indeed, 100% of nodules in which four or five these parameters were positive proved to be malignant [19]. Similarly, on using the so-called "thyroid imaging reporting and data system", Horvath et al. [48] found malignancy in 80% of nodules classified as probably malignant on US. A limitation of these studies, however, was the 5-14% of false negative results in nodules with a low number of suspicious US features [19,48]. In a very large series of Thy 3 nodules, Rago et al. [27] recently reported a significant association of three suspicious US features (blurred margins, spot microcalcifications and hypoechogeneicity) with malignancy. Moreover, in the present study, a significant correlation was found between cumulative US findings and histology, and the ROC curve analysis indicated that the presence of more than two suspicious US findings in Thy 3 nodules reached a sensitivity of 82% and a specificity of 100%, with a 5.0 likelihood ratio. In a series of 40 Thy 3 nodules with US available for review, Matthey-Gie et al. [49] reported that high nodule vascularity associated with ill-defined borders was a suspicious US finding linked to malignancy. In a series of 78 indeterminate lesions, Batawil and Alkordy [50] found that solid structure and irregular border were the most suspicious findings. Yoo et al. [26] examined a selected series of 249 nodules which met the criteria of atypia or follicular lesion of indeterminate significance and in which core-biopsy or surgery were used as references; they observed that taller-than-wide shape and marked hypoechogenicity were highly suspicious US findings. In 61 follicular neoplasms and 99 Hürthle cell neoplasms, Tutuncu et al. [51] did not report the role of cumulative US findings; however, they indicated that hypoechogenicity and microcalcification had the highest odds ratios. In sum, in Thy 3 nodules, US is helpful to the initial decision-making process, but combination with other evaluations is needed.

More recently, USE machines able to measure tissue hardness qualitatively (colour score), semi- quantitatively (strain ratio), or quantitatively (elasticity index, shear-wave velocity) have been introduced into the clinical setting in order to overcome the limitations of FNAB and US in thyroid nodules [33]. The efficacy of USE in distinguishing benign from malignant thyroid nodules varies widely among studies [17-20,25,34,35,46,47,52]). In a 2013 meta-analysis by Razavi et al. [53], in which 24 studies comprising 3531 nodules were evaluated and the results were compared with those yielded by US, USE was reported to be more sensitive (colour score 82%; strain ratio 89%) and specific (colour score and strain ratio 82%) than each individual US feature. However, in a previous study in which we evaluated a subset of 27 Thy 3 nodules with cytological-histological correlation by means of semi-quantitative USE, we were unable to distinguish these nodules from cytological benign (Thy 2) or malignant (Thy 5) nodules on the basis of the ELX 2/1 strain index [19]. The only reported finding was an increasing trend in low-range ELX 2/1 strain index values from Thy 2 to Thy 5 nodules [19]. In the present study, which involved a higher number of Thy 3 nodules, the ELX 2/1 strain index showed a significant correlation with histology, and the established cut-off level, which classified Thy 3 nodules with an ELX 2/1 index greater than 0.95 as malignant, showed better sensitivity of 83.6% and specificity of 80.3%, with a 4.2 likelihood ratio. In the study by Rago et al. [27], qualitative USE was performed in 169 Thy 3 nodules in which cytological-histological correlation was available, and low stiffness was found in nodules with benign diagnoses, the negative predictive value of 97% increasing the predictivity of US features. In several other studies on the pre-surgical utility of USE in thyroid nodules, the number of indeterminate lesions was limited, ranging from 9 to 58 [17,21,43,47,53], and separate data analysis was either not done [17] or, when done, was poorly understandable [21] or revealed low sensitivity (78%) and specificity (44%) [47]. Similarly, a very low specificity (6%) was observed in a study by Lippolis et al. [46], which evaluated 103 nodules with indeterminate cytology. On the other hand, in 270 nodules cytologically classified as atypia of undetermined significance by means of qualitative and semi-quantitative USE, Cakir et al. [44] reported favourable conclusions, suggesting the use of this technique in the pre-surgical evaluation of indeterminate nodules. The best strain index value in distinguishing between cytologically benign and cytologically malignant nodules reaches a sensitivity of 99% and a specificity of 96%.

Overall, the diagnostic utility of USE in Thy 3 nodules remains under evaluation. However, qualitative and semi-quantitative methods and definite cut-off values obtained in large numbers of subjects have yielded promising results (present study, [27,44]), thus supporting a less aggressive strategy, especially when no suspicious features are noted on US.

The latest technique involving US for the study of thyroid vascularization uses a microbubble contrast agent. It is well known that the thyroid gland has an abundant microvasculature, and that the parenchyma of normal thyroid shows rapid and uniform enhancement after intravenous injection of contrast agents. By contrast, the vascular structure of nodules differs from the normal pattern, and hence enhancement differs from that of the normal parenchyma. Argalia et al. [54] have shown that CEUS time-intensity curves can provide an indirect description of intra-nodular vascularization, which seems to be anarchic in malignant nodules. Literature data on the utility of CEUS in distinguishing malignant from benign nodules are controversial. Zhang et al. [37] reported that heterogeneous enhancement rendered a thyroid nodule suspicious for malignancy, while Friedrich-Rust et al. [41] reported that the time-intensity CEUS curve did not prove useful in distinguishing between benign and malignant nodules. Moreover, in our previous report [19], the P index and TTP index were found to be unrelated to cytological and histological results. More recently, two studies involving Chinese patients examined the role of CEUS in distinguishing between malignant and benign thyroid nodules. In 175 nodules, without histological reference in all cases, Deng J et al. [39] reported a CEUS sensitivity of 82% and a specificity of 85%. Their study was based on the impression that hypo-enhancement could be regarded as an indicator of malignancy. Ma et al. [38] studied the preoperative diagnostic role of CEUS combined with US in 172 nodules, all surgically removed. Both US and CEUS areas under the ROC curves were significant, but the best sensitivity (89%) and specificity (94%) was reached by considering five positive features (ring enhancement, homogeneity of enhancement, arrival time of the nodule at CEUS, microcalcifications, and halo sign on US) on combining US and CEUS.

To our knowledge, no studies on CEUS have focused on the subpopulation of indeterminate nodules. In our previous study on CEUS in thyroid nodules, CEUS was available in 17 indeterminate nodules with cytological-histological correlation [19]. Regarding the indicators P index and TTP index, no differences were noted among the nodules scored according to the Thy classification [19]. The present study provided more interesting data. Significant correlations were noted between histology and both P index (negative) and TTP index (positive). The areas under the ROC curves for the P index and TTP index were significant at an established cut-off level that classified Thy 3 nodules as malignant when the P index was lower than 0.99 (sensitivity 37.7%; specificity 75.5%) and the TTP index was greater than 0.98 (sensitivity 56.6%; specificity 75.5%). Our experience of Thy 3 nodules seems to indicate a greater diagnostic role of semi-quantitative USE than of CEUS. In the study by Deng et al. [39], however, quantitative USE and CEUS displayed the same value in distinguishing between benign and malignant nodules.

The simultaneous evaluation of different indicators from US, USE and CEUS and the use of validated cut-off levels for interpreting data – without or with low subjectivity – is crucial in clinical decision-making when cytological results are indeterminate and lobectomy or thyroidectomy is indicated by the guidelines. In the 51 cases that were fully evaluable, our study indicates that the diagnostic power of the cumulative pre-surgical analysis of Thy 3 nodules by means of US, USE and CEUS does not increase sensitivity (64%) but improves specificity (92%); moreover, it showed interesting levels of PPV (75%) and accuracy (84%). While false negative (25%) and false positive (13%) results are limitations, these preliminary data on the combination of US, USE and CEUS with FNAB seem to provide promising indications that unnecessary lobectomy/thyroidectomy can be reduced. To our knowledge there are no studies on Thy 3 nodules in which results obtained from conventional US, USE and CEUS have been simultaneously scored in order to make a clinical decision. In our opinion, US-guided FNAB remains the gold standard in solid nodules. However, when an indeterminate response emerges from cytology, surgery may be postponed if no suspicious findings are observed (in our hands: US score ≤ 2, ELX 2/1 <0.95, P index >0.99 and TTP index <0.98).

There are some limitations to this study. First, the number of fully evaluable Thy 3 nodules was small. As the thyroid tissue adjacent to the Thy 3 nodule may not be normal, both USE and CEUS may sometimes be impracticable. Moreover, injection of the contrast agent before CEUS is sometimes refused by the patient. Second, we did not divide FNAB results into Thy 3 atypia and Thy 3 follicular neoplasm, as suggested by the BTA in 2014 [27,43]. Larger numbers of Thy 3 nodules could necessary in order to compare USE and CEUS data in these two Thy 3 subpopulations. Third, genetic markers were not considered in the present study; however, BRAF, the most frequent mutation in thyroid cancer, seems to be less important in follicular neoplasms [31]. Fourth, this was a single-centre study. However, pooling data from different centres for qualitative and semi-quantitative USE remains impracticable, since different devices may yield various types of strain indices, such as maximum ratio or simple ratio. While we used an average ELX 2/1 index from at least 3 measures, it is unclear whether the average index is truly representative of nodular stiffness. Among our Thy 3 lesions, medullary carcinomas and follicular carcinomas were rare (25% of Thy 3 nodules with histological malignancy). According to some authors [34-36,39], however, false negative results from these tumours should be taken into consideration when USE and CEUS data are evaluated.

In conclusion, in cytologically Thy 3 nodules, conventional US must be associated, when feasible, to the combined application of USE and CEUS. The use of a cut-off based on histology can reduce the surgical approach. Observation should be the first choice when not all instrumental results are suspect.

Competing interests

The authors declare that they have no competing interests.

Authors' contributions

MG and GT designed the initial study and prepared the final version of the paper. ST and EM provided patients data and analysis. BM carried out the cytological and histological examinations. CC. GT and ES carried out radiological examinations. All authors had read and approval the final manuscript.

Author details

[1]Endocrine Unit, IRCCS Azienda Ospedaliera Universitaria San Martino – IST Istituto Nazionale per la Ricerca sul Cancro, Genoa, Italy. [2]Cytopathology and Pathology Unit, IRCCS Azienda Ospedaliera Universitaria San Martino – IST Istituto Nazionale per la Ricerca sul Cancro, Genoa, Italy. [3]Radiology Unit, Ospedale Evangelico, Genoa, Italy. [4]UO Clinica Endocrinologica, Viale Benedetto XV, 6, I-16100 Genoa, Italy.

References

1. Mortensen JD, Woolner LB, Bennett WA: **Cross and microscopic findings in clinically normal thyroid gland.** *J Clin Endocrinol Metab* 1955, **15**:1270–1280.
2. Vander JB, Gaston EA, Dawber TR: **The significance of nontoxic thyroid nodules. Final report of a 15-year study of the incidence of thyroid malignancy.** *Ann Intern Med* 1968, **69**:537–540.
3. Guth S, Theune U, Aberle J, Galach A, Bamberger CM: **Very high prevalence of thyroid nodules detected by high frequency (13 MHz) ultrasound examination.** *Eur J Clin Invest* 2009, **39**:699–706.
4. Udelsman R, Zhang Y: **The epidemic of thyroid cancer in the United States: the role of endocrinologists and ultrasounds.** *Thyroid* 2014, **24**:472–479.
5. Van der Bruel A, Francart J, Dubois C, Adam A, Vlayen J, De Schutter H, Stordeur S, Decallonne B: **Regional variation in thyroid cancer incidence in Belgium is associated with variation in thyroid imaging and thyroid disease management.** *J Clin Endocrinol Metab* 2013, **98**:4063–4071.
6. Hegedus L: **Clinical practice. The thyroid nodule.** *N Engl J Med* 2004, **351**:1764–1771.
7. Jin J, McHenry CR: **Thyroid incidentaloma.** *Best Pract Res Clin Endocrinol Metab* 2012, **26**:83–96.
8. Frates MC, Benson CB, Doubilet PM, Kunreuther E, Contreras M, Cibas ES, Orcutt J, Moore FR Jr, Larsen PR, Marqusee E, Alexander EK: **Prevalence and distribution of carcinoma in patients with solitary and multiple thyroid nodules on sonography.** *J Clin Endocrinol Metab* 2006, **91**:3411–3417.
9. Brito JP, Gionfriddo MR, Al Nofal A, Boehmer KR, Leppin AL, Reading C, Callstrom M, Elraiyah TA, Prokop LJ, Stan MN, Murad MH, Morris JC, Montori VM: **The accuracy of thyroid nodule ultrasound to predict thyroid cancer: systemic review and meta-analysis.** *J Clin Endocrinol Metab* 2014, **99**:1253–1263.
10. Lee TI, Yang HJ, Lin SY, Lee MT, Lin HD, Braverman LE, Tang KT: **The accuracy of fine-needle aspiration biopsy and frozen section in patients with thyroid cancer.** *Thyroid* 2002, **19**:619–626.
11. Nam-Goong IS, Kim HY, Gong G, Lee HK, Hong SJ, Kim WB, Shong YK: **Ultrasonography-guided fine-needle aspiration of thyroid incidentaloma: correlation with pathological findings.** *Clin Endocrinol (Oxf)* 2004, **60**:21–28.
12. Sidoti M, Marino G, Resmini E, Augeri C, Cappi C, Cavallero D, Lagasio C, Ceppa P, Minuto F, Giusti M: **The rational use of fine-needle aspiration biopsy (FNAB) in diagnosing thyroid nodules.** *Minerva Endocrinol* 2006, **31**:159–172.
13. Castro MR, Gharib H: **Thyroid fine-needle aspiration biopsy: progress, practice, and pitfalls.** *Endocr Pract* 2003, **9**:128–136.
14. Gharib H, Papini E: **Thyroid nodules: clinical importance, assessment, and treatment.** *Endocrinol Metab Clin North Am* 2007, **36**:707–735.
15. Cibas ES, Ali SZ, NCI Thyroid FNA State of the Science Conference: **The Bethesda system for reporting thyroid cytopathology.** *Am J Clin Pathol* 2009, **132**:658–655.
16. Nou E, Kwong N, Alexander LK, Cibas ES, Marqusee E, Alexander EK: **Determination of optimal time interval for repeat evaluation following a benign thyroid nodule aspiration.** *J Clin Endocrinol Metab* 2014, **99**:510–516.
17. Nacamulli D, Nico L, Barollo S, Zambonin L, Pennelli G, Girelli ME, Casal Ide E, Pelizzo MR, Vianello F, Negro I, Watutantrige-Fernando S, Mantero F, Rugge M, Mian C: **Comparison of the diagnostic accuracy of combined elastosonography**

and BRAF analysis *vs* cytology and ultrasonography for thyroid nodule suspected of malignancy. *Clin Endocrinol (Oxf)* 2012, **77**:608–614.

18. Trimboli P, Guglielmi R, Monti S, Misischi I, Graziano F, Nasrollah N, Amendola S, Morgante SN, Deiana MG, Valabrega S, Toscano V, Papini E: **Ultrasound sensitivity for thyroid malignancy is increased by real-time elastosonography: a prospective multicenter study.** *J Clin Endocrinol Metab* 2012, **97**:4524–4530.
19. Giusti M, Orlandi D, Melle G, Massa B, Silvestri E, Minuto F, Turtulici G: **Is there a real diagnostic impact of elastosonography and contrast-enhanced ultrasonography in the management of thyroid nodules?** *J Zhejiang Univ Sci B* 2013, **14**:195–206.
20. Magri F, Chytiris S, Capelli V, Gaiti M, Zerbini F, Carrara R, Malovini A, Rotondi M, Bellazzi R, Chiovato L: **Comparison of elastographic strain index and thyroid fine–needle aspiration cytology in 631 thyroid nodules.** *J Clin Endocrinol Metab* 2013, **98**:4790–4797.
21. Guazzaroni M, Spinelli A, Coco I, Del Giudice C, Girardi V, Simonetti G: **Value of strain-ratio on thyroid real-time sonoelastography.** *Radiol Med* 2014, **119**:149–155.
22. Na DG, Kim JH, Sung JY, Beak JH, Jung KC, Lee H, Yoo H: **Core-needle biopsy is more useful than repeat fine-needle aspiration in thyroid nodules read as nondiagnostic or atypia of undetermined significance by Bethesda system for reporting thyroid cytopathology.** *Thyroid* 2012, **22**:468–475.
23. Hakala T, Kholova I, Sand J, Saaristo R, Kellokumpu-Lehtinen P: **A core needle biopsy provides more malignancy-specific results than fine-needle aspiration biopsy in thyroid nodules suspicious for malignancy.** *J Clin Pathol* 2013, **66**:1046–1050.
24. Mihai R, Parker AJ, Roskell D, Sadler GP: **One in four patients with follicular thyroid cytology (THY 3) has a thyroid carcinoma.** *Thyroid* 2009, **19**:33–37.
25. Rago T, Scutari M, Santini F, Loiacono V, Piaggi P, Di Coscio G, Basolo F, Berti P, Pinchera A, Vitti P: **Real-time elastosonography: useful tool for refining the presurgical diagnosis in thyroid nodules with indeterminate or nondiagnostic cytology.** *J Clin Endocrinol Metab* 2010, **95**:5274–5280.
26. Yoo WS, Choi HS, Cho SW, Moon JH, Kim KW, Park HJ, Park SY, Choi SI, Choi SH, Lim S, Yi KH, Park Do J, Jang HC, Park YJ: **The role of ultrasound findings in the management of thyroid nodules with atypia or follicular lesions of undetermined significance.** *Clin Endocrinol (Oxf)* 2014, **80**:735–742.
27. Rago T, Scutari M, Latrofa F, Loiacono V, Piaggi P, Marchetti I, Romani R, Basolo F, Miccoli P, Tonacchera M, Vitti P: **The large majority of 1520 patients with indeterminate thyroid nodules at cytology have a favorable outcome and a clinical risk score has a high negative predictive value for a more cumbersome cancer disease.** *J Clin Endocrinol Metab* 2014, **99**:3700–3007.
28. Nikiforov YE, Steward DL, Robinson-Smith TM, Haugen BR, Klopper JP, Zhu Z, Fagin JA, Falciglia M, Weber K, Nikiforova MN: **Molecular testing for mutations in improving the fine-needle aspiration diagnosis of thyroid nodules.** *J Clin Endorinol Metab* 2009, **94**:2092–2098.
29. Ferraz C, Eszlinger M, Paschke R: **Current state and future perspective of molecular diagnosis of fine-needle aspiration biopsy of thyroid nodules.** *J Clin Endocrinol Metab* 2011, **96**:2016–2026.
30. Gomberawalla A, Elaraj DM: **How to use molecular testing to guide surgery: a surgeon's perspective.** *Curr Opin Oncol* 2014, **26**:14–21.
31. Eszlinger M, Krogdahl A, Munz S, Rehfeld C, Precht Jensen EM, Ferraz C, Bosenberg E, Drieschner N, Scholz M, Hegedus L, Paschke R: **Impact of molecular screening for point mutations and rearrangements in routine air-dried fine-needle aspiration samples of thyroid nodules.** *Thyroid* 2014, **24**:305–313.
32. Alexander EK, Schorr M, Klopper J, Kim C, Sipos J, Nabhan F, Parker C, Steward DL, Mandel SJ, Haugen BR: **Multicenter clinical experience with the Afirma gene expression classifier.** *J Clin Endocrinol Metab* 2014, **99**:119–125.
33. Andrioli M, Persani L: **Elastographic techniques of thyroid gland: current status.** *Endocrine* 2014, **46**:455–461.
34. Lyshchik A, Higashi T, Asato R, Tanaka S, Ito J, Mai JJ, Pellot-Barakat C, Insana MF, Brill AB, Saga T, Hiraoka M, Togashi K: **Thyroid gland tumor diagnosis at US elastography.** *Radiology* 2005, **237**:202–2011.
35. Vorlander C, Wolff J, Saalabian S, Lienenluke RH, Wahl RA: **Real-time ultrasound elastography – a non invasive diagnostic procedure for evaluating dominant thyroid nodules.** *Langenbecks Arch Surg* 2010, **395**:865–871.
36. Andrioli M, Trimboli P, Amendola S, Valabrega S, Fukunari N, Mirella M, Persani L: **Elastographic presentation of medullary thyroid carcinoma.** *Endocrine* 2013, **45**:153–155.
37. Zhang B, Jiang YX, Liu JB, Yang M, Dai Q, Zhu QL, Gao P: **Utility of contrast-enhanced ultrasound for evaluation of thyroid nodules.** *Thyroid* 2010, **20**:51–57.
38. Ma JJ, Ding H, Xu BH, Xu C, Song LJ, Huang BJ, Wang WP: **Diagnostic performances of various gray-scale, color Doppler, and contrast-enhanced ultrasonography findings in predicting malignant thyroid nodules.** *Thyroid* 2014, **24**:355–363.
39. Deng J, Zhou P, Tian SM, Zhang L, Li JI, Qian Y: **Comparison of diagnostic efficacy of contrast-enhanced ultrasound, acoustic radiation force impulse imaging, and their combined use in differentiating focal solid thyroid nodules.** *PLoS One* 2014, **9**:e90674.
40. Spiezia S, Farina R, Cerbone G, Assanti AP, Iovino V, Siciliani M, Lombardi G, Colao A: **Analysis of color Doppler signal intensity variation after levovist injection: a new approach to the diagnosis of thyroid nodules.** *J Ultrasound Med* 2001, **20**:223–231.
41. Friedrich-Rust M, Sperber A, Holzer K, Diener J, Grunwald F, Badenhoop K, Weber S, Kriener S, Herrmann E, Bechstein WO, Zeuzem S, Bojunga J: **Real-time elastography and contrast-enhanced ultrasound for the assessment of thyroid nodules.** *Exp Clin Endocrinol Diabetes* 2010, **118**:602–609.
42. Ragazzoni F, Deandrea M, Mormile A, Ramunni MJ, Garino F, Magliona G, Motta M, Torchio B, Garberoglio R, Limone P: **High diagnostic accuracy and interobserver reliability of real-time elastography in the evaluation of thyroid nodules.** *Ultrasound Med Biol* 2012, **38**:1154–1162.
43. Mehrotra P, McQueen A, Kolla S, Johnson SJ, Richardson DL: **Does elastography reduce the need for thyroid FNAs?** *Clin Endocrinol (Oxf)* 2013, **78**:942–949.
44. Cakir B, Ersoy R, Cuhaci FN, Aydin C, Polat B, Kilic M, Yazgan A: **Elastosonographic strain index in thyroid nodules with atypia of undetermined significance.** *J Endocrinol Invest* 2014, **37**:127–133.
45. Moon WJ, Baek JH, Jung SL, Kim DW, Kim EK, Kim JY, Kwak JY, Lee JH, Lee JH, Lee YH, Na DG, Park JS, Korean Society of Thyroid Radiology (KSThR); Korean Society of Radiology, Park SW: **Ultrasonography and the ultrasound-based management of thyroid nodules: consensus statement and recommendations.** *Korean J Radiol* 2011, **12**:1–14.
46. Lippolis PV, Tognini S, Materazzi G, Polini A, Mancini R, Ambrosini CE, Dardano A, Basolo F, Seccia M, Miccoli P, Monzani F: **Is elastography actually useful in the presurgical selection of thyroid nodules with indeterminate cytology?** *J Clin Endocrinol Metab* 2011, **96**:E1826–E1830.
47. Unluturk U, Erdogan MF, Demir O, Gullu S, Baskal N: **Ultrasound elastography is not superior to grayscale ultrasound in predicting malignancy in thyroid nodules.** *Thyroid* 2012, **22**:1031–1038.
48. Horvath E, Majlis S, Rossi R, Franco C, Niedmann JP, Castro A, Dominguez M: **An ultrasonogram reporting system for thyroid nodules stratifying cancer risk for clinical management.** *J Clin Endocrinol Metab* 2009, **94**:1748–1751.
49. Matthey-Gie ML, Walsh SM, O'Neill AC, Lowery A, Evoy D, Gibbson D, Prichard RS, Skehan S, McDermott EW: **Ultrasound predictors of malignancy in indeterminate thyroid nodules.** *Ir J Med Sci*, in press
50. Batawil N, Alkordy T: **Ultrasonographic features associated with malignancy in cytologically indeterminate thyroid nodules.** *Eur J Surg Oncol* 2014, **40**:182–186.
51. Tutuncu Y, Berker D, Isik S, Akbaba G, Ozuguz U, Kucukler FK, Gocmen E, Yalcin Y, Aydin Y, Guler S: **The frequency of malignancy and the relationship between malignancy and ultrasonographic features of thyroid nodules with indeterminate cytology.** *Endocrine* 2014, **45**:37–45.
52. Rivo-Vazquez A, Rodriguez-Lorenzo A, Rivo-Vazquez JE, Paramo-Fernandez C, Garcia-Lorenzo F, Pardellas-Rivera H, Casal-Nunez JE, Gil-Gil P: **The use of ultrasound elastography in the assessment of malignancy risk in thyroid nodules and multinodular goitres.** *Clin Endocrinol (Oxf)* 2013, **79**:887–891.
53. Razavi SA, Hadduck TA, Sadigh G, Dwamena BA: **Comparative effectiveness of elastographic and B-mode ultrasound criteria for diagnostic discrimination of thyroid nodules: a meta-analysis.** *AJR Am J Roentgenol* 2013, **200**:1317–1326.
54. Argalia G, De Bernardis S, Mariani D, Abbattista T, Taccaliti A, Ricciardelli L, Faragona S, Gusella PM, Giuseppetti GM: **Ultrasonographic contrast agent: evaluation of time-intensity curves in the characterisation of solitary thyroid nodules.** *Radiol Med* 2002, **103**:407–413.

18

A rare malignant thyroid carcinosarcoma with aggressive behavior and DICER1 gene mutation

Jing Yang, Carmen Sarita-Reyes, David Kindelberger and Qing Zhao*

Abstract

Background: Malignant biphasic tumor also known as carcinosarcoma is an uncommon neoplasm that is composed of both malignant epithelial and mesenchymal components. Most reported cases of carcinosarcoma affect the female genital tract; however, other sites including head and neck, lung, and breast have been described. Carcinosarcoma of the thyroid is an extremely rare and aggressive malignancy with an ominous clinical course similar to anaplastic carcinoma.

Case presentation: We report a case of a 45-year-old female who was found to have a biphasic thyroid carcinosarcoma. Her clinical course declined significantly shortly after she underwent a total thyroidectomy and she developed distant metastases to the lungs. Histopathological features of the primary and metastatic tumor were identical. The tumor is composed of an intimately intermixed epithelial component of poorly differentiated follicular thyroid carcinoma and a spindle cell sarcoma with rhabdomyosarcoma differentiation. Molecular analysis using a next-generation sequencing based assay revealed a *DICER1* (E1705K) point mutation in neoplastic cells.

Conclusion: To our knowledge, the E1705K point mutation within the *DICER1* gene is the first reported mutation in carcinosarcoma of the thyroid. A comprehensive review of the relevant literature is also included for discussion.

Keywords: Thyroid, Carcinosarcoma, Biphasic tumor, Lung metastasis, DICER1 mutation

Background

Thyroid carcinosarcoma is a rare and aggressive malignant thyroid tumor [1]. These tumors are usually found to infiltrate the surrounding soft tissue at the time of diagnosis. The overall survival rate for these patients is only a few months and most of the cases occur in women who are older than 50 years of age. To date, less than 30 cases of thyroid carcinosarcoma have been reported in the literature (Table 1) [1–8]. According to the latest World Health Organization (WHO 2017) classification for thyroid tumors, carcinosarcoma is considered to be a variant of anaplastic carcinoma [9]. Recently, Agrawal et al. proposed that, with the presence of both malignant epithelial and mesenchymal cells, 'thyroid carcinosarcoma' should be considered a distinct entity from anaplastic carcinoma [6].

The pathogenesis of thyroid carcinosarcoma is not fully understood. Carcinosarcoma of the thyroid has been suggested to originate from both malignant epithelial (carcinoma) and mesenchymal (sarcoma) elements of the thyroid [1, 6]. Positive immunohistochemical (IHC) staining for thyroglobulin in carcinomatous cells, and positive staining for vimentin in mesenchymal cells supports a diagnosis of carcinosarcoma [1]. In contrast, studies from anaplastic thyroid carcinoma suggested a monoclonal origin of the tumor [2]. The sarcoma-like morphology of the tumor is thought to be de-differentiated from the epithelial component during the process of carcinogenesis.

In 2013, Agrawal et al. reviewed 25 cases reported in the literature as carcinosarcoma of the thyroid. Since

* Correspondence: Grace.Zhao@bmc.org
Department of Pathology and Laboratory Medicine, Boston University Medical Center, 670 Albany St. Biosquare III, Boston, MA 02118, USA

Table 1 Summary of all reported cases of thyroid carcinosarcoma in English literature

Author; year; Ref [#]	Morphology	Metastasis	Treatment	Survival (months)
Rasheed; 2017; [8]	Follicular carcinoma with sarcoma	none	total thyroidectomy, chemotherapy	3
Ekici; 2015; [7]	Papillary carcinoma with sarcoma	none	total thyroidectomy	2
Agrawal; 2013; [6]	Papillary carcinoma with sarcoma	lymph nodes	total thyroidectomy, right neck dissection	12
Naqiyah; 2010; [5]	Follicular carcinoma with sarcoma	none	total thyroidectomy, radiation	8
Guiffrida; 2000; [1]	Follicular carcinoma with sarcoma	bilateral lung, lymph nodes	total thyroidectomy lymph node dissection and chemoradiation therapy	6
Al-Sobhi; 1997; [4]	Follicular carcinoma with sarcoma	lung	total thyroidectomy, radiation	8
Cooper; 1989; [3]	Follicular carcinoma with chondrosarcoma	N/A	subtotal thyroidectomy	5
Donnell; 1987; [2]	Follicular carcinoma with osteosarcoma and chondrosarcoma	lung	subtotal thyroidectomy	26

then, there have been two additional cases reported. Among the reported cases, most were described as fibrosarcoma or osteosarcoma with co-existing differentiated thyroid carcinoma, such as follicular or papillary carcinoma [1–8]. In most of the cases, the tumors behaved aggressively, with death from disease occurring within 2 months to 26 months following diagnosis [1–8]. No specific molecular signatures or genetic alteration have been reported. The current report presents a case of a young female patient with a biphasic thyroid carcinosarcoma. Next generation sequencing (NGS) analysis revealed a novel point mutation in the *DICER1* gene (E1705K) in neoplastic cells.

Case presentation

A 45-year-old woman presented to our hospital with multiple lung nodules. She had a history of poorly differentiated thyroid carcinoma, diagnosed 7 months prior to admission, at an outside hospital. The patient was healthy otherwise and reported no radiation exposure or any family history of thyroid cancer. The initial work-up at the time of discovery of the right thyroid nodule included fine needle aspiration and core biopsy, with findings consistent with poorly differentiated thyroid carcinoma. The patient then underwent a total thyroidectomy and central neck lymph node dissection. The pathologic diagnosis from the outside hospital reported a 2.8 × 2.4 × 1.1 cm tumor in the right thyroid without extrathyroidal extension or lymph node metastasis. However, both capsular invasion and extensive vascular space invasion were noted. Based on the tumor size, tumor extension and lymph node status, the tumor was designated as Stage II (pT2 pN0 pMx). IHC staining showed that the tumor cells were positive for thyroglobulin and thyroid transcription factor 1 (TTF1). An immunostain for p53 was also performed at the outside hospital and showed a small focus (< 1 cm) with p53 positivity, suggesting a diagnosis of anaplastic thyroid carcinoma.

At our institution, the diagnosis was revised, based on review of both the primary thyroid tumor and the current lung metastases. Both tumors were remarkable for biphasic malignant components: the carcinoma and the sarcoma. The carcinoma component showed a poorly differentiated microfollicular type thyroid carcinoma, composed of sheets and islands of tightly packed thyroid follicles with dense colloid. The tumor nuclei were small and round with vesicular chromatin, resembling those of typical poorly differentiated follicular thyroid carcinoma. Admixed with the epithelial component were malignant spindle cells with small round blue cell type morphology. Focally, rhabdomyosarcoma-like cells with eosinophilic cytoplasm were appreciated. No heterologous cartilage or bone components were identified. The IHC staining performed at the outside hospital showed that the thyroid carcinoma (epithelial) component was positive for thyroglobulin, PAX8 and TTF1 (Fig. 1). The sarcoma (spindled) component was negative for all thyroid carcinoma markers (TTF-1, thyroglobulin and PAX8), but was positive for vimentin and focally positive for myogenin (supporting skeletal muscle differentiation) consistent with mesenchymal differentiation. Interestingly, the foci of vascular space invasion contained both epithelial and mesenchymal components as well.

The patient received Taxol with Carboplatin for 7 weeks followed by radiation therapy. Her thyroglobulin level rose from 1.2 ng/mL to 25.40 ng/mL 5 months after completion of the chemo-radiation therapy, suggesting progression of the disease. A follow-up CT scan of the chest showed multiple newly developed nodules (ranging from 1 to 2 cm) in the right lung, highly suspicious for metastases. The patient underwent a right thoracotomy, right lung resection/metastasectomy. The surgery was uneventful with negative resection margins. However, the patient's general condition deteriorated and she succumbed to the disease 4 months later.

Histological examination of the lung nodules revealed similar tumor morphology and tumor differentiation

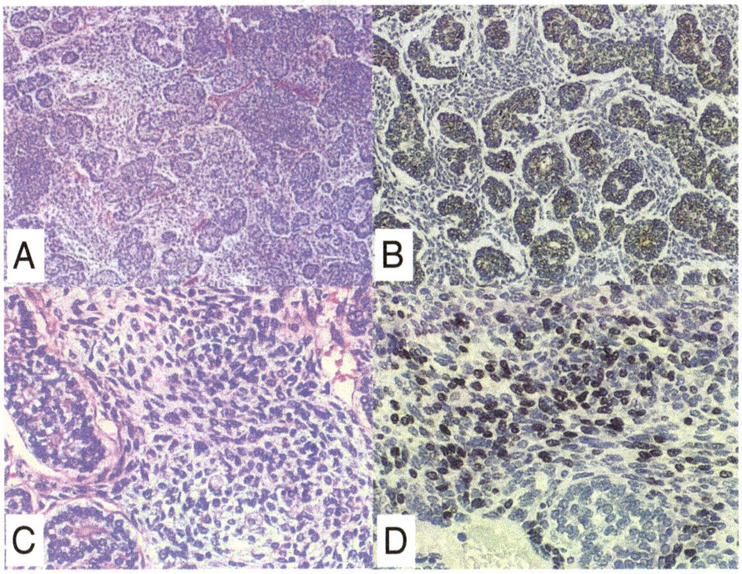

Fig. 1 Immunohistochemical stains demonstrated biphasic components. The carcinoma component (**a**) showed positivity for thyroglobulin (**b**). The sarcoma component (**c**) showed positivity for myogenin (**d**). All pictures are at 200×

when compared to the original thyroid tumor, which is somewhat unusual for a biphasic carcinosarcoma (Fig. 2). Tumor necrosis was also present. Mutational analysis using a next-generation sequencing based assay showed that the neoplastic cells from the lung metastasis were devoid of genomic alterations for known thyroid cancers, including *BRAF*, *RAS* family (*KRAS*, *NRAS* and *HRAS*), *EGFR*, *PTEN*, *TERT*, *PI3Kinase* or *RET*. *BRAF* or *RAS* family are known as the most commonly altered genes in papillary thyroid cancers. Other molecular mutations reported in the development of anaplastic thyroid carcinoma include p53, *PAX8/PPAR* gamma rearrangement [10]. None of the mentioned gene mutations were identified in our patient.

However, an interesting finding in this case is the presence of a point mutation in *DICER1* (E1705K) that has

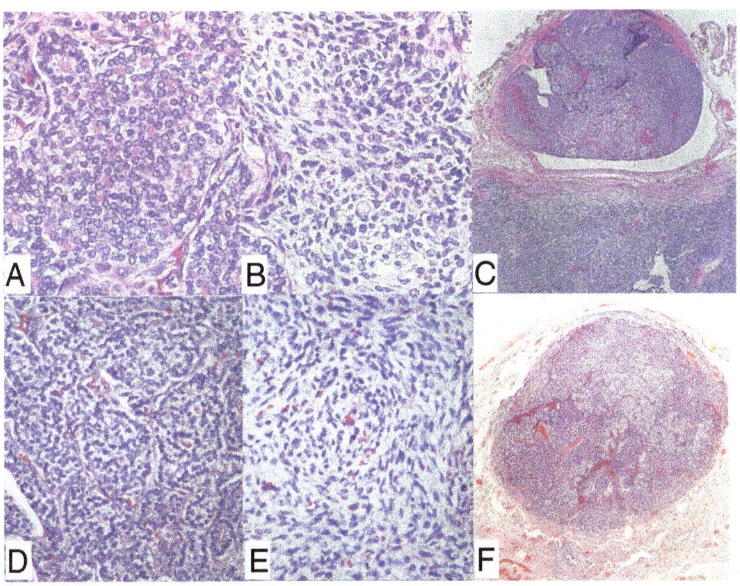

Fig. 2 Histological features of primary thyroid cancer and metastatic lung nodules. The epithelial component in the thyroid cancer (**a**) is morphologically similar to the epithelial component in the lung nodule (**d**). The sarcomatous component is composed of spindle cells both in the thyroid cancer (**b**) and in the lung nodule (**e**). There is vascular invasion in the thyroid cancer (**c**). Low power review of a small lung nodule (40×) in (**f**)

previously been associated with differentiated thyroid carcinoma [11, 12]. Whether the *DICER1* (E1705K) mutation is the underlying genetic event leading to the initiation of tumorigenesis or is downstream to other gene alterations in tumor development is largely unknown. Additional mutations of unknown significance were also detected in this tumor including *FLCN* (R239H), *POLD1* (Q684H) and *SYK* (R217L). These variants have not been adequately characterized in the scientific literature and their prognostic and therapeutic significance is unclear.

Discussion and conclusions

Thyroid carcinosarcoma is a very aggressive malignant tumor with a clinical course similar to that of anaplastic thyroid carcinoma [4]. All reported thyroid carcinosarcoma cases have resulted in patients only surviving a few months after initial diagnosis [1–8]. To our knowledge, there is no previously published molecular analysis of thyroid carcinosarcoma. This is the first report to describe potential gene alterations identified using next generation sequencing. The DICER1 protein is a member of the ribonuclease III (RNase III) family that plays an important role in the post-transcriptional regulation of gene expression. Heterozygous germline *DICER* mutations are described in the so-called DICER1 syndrome, which leads to a predisposition to develop a variety of tumors in children, including pleuropulmonary blastoma, cystic nephroma, rhabdomyosarcoma, ovarian Sertoli-Leydig tumors and multinodular goiter. A recent case study reported that a germline *DICER1* mutation (S1814 L) is associated with an increased risk of thyroid follicular carcinoma [11]. A somatic *DICER1* hotspot mutation at E1705K was reported in a case of anaplastic sarcoma of the kidney and in approximately 60% of Sertoli-Leydig cell tumors [12, 13]. The presence of this point mutation of *DICER1* at E1705K in thyroid carcinosarcoma has never been reported. The presence of a *DICER1* mutation in this case provides further evidence that development of the carcinosarcoma may not be a random occurrence, but is a likely due to a specific genetic alteration. Due to the highly aggressive nature of thyroid carcinosarcomas, the identification of specific genetic signatures for these tumors becomes critical in identifying effective treatments. However, there are still many questions regarding the pathogenesis and tumorigenesis of thyroid carcinosarcoma. Further studies will be of great benefit for the diagnosis and treatment.

Other mutations that were identified in this tumor include *POLD1* (Q684H), *FLCN* (R239H) and *SYK* (R217L). *POLD1* (Q684H) is a recently described mutation that had been reported in a patient with colorectal cancer [14]. Germline mutations in the folliculin (FLCN*)* gene, encoding the folliculin tumor-suppressor protein, are reported to be associated with Birt Hogg Dubé syndrome [15]. Spleen tyrosine kinase (SYK) is an essential enzyme required for signaling involving multiple classes of immune receptors [16]. SYK functions as a modulator of tumorigenesis and has been reported in association with leukemia and breast cancers [16]. The clinical significance of *FLCN* (R239H) and *SYK* (R217L) mutations in thyroid carcinosarcoma is unknown.

The differential diagnosis of thyroid carcinosarcoma includes anaplastic carcinoma. P53 point mutations are present in 60–80% of anaplastic thyroid carcinomas. Patients develop anaplastic carcinoma from a pre or coexistent differentiated carcinoma after a multistep process of dedifferentiation associated with loss of the p53 oncogene suppressor. Due to the similarities between anaplastic carcinoma and carcinosarcoma of the thyroid gland, it has been proposed that p53 mutation may contribute to the pathogenesis of carcinosarcoma. In our patient, a less than 1 cm focus within the anaplastic area showed p53 IHC positivity. No P53 mutation was detected by next generation sequencing. Molecular pathogenetic mechanisms of p53 involvement in the transformation of carcinosarcoma are not well understood. Other mutations reported in anaplastic thyroid carcinoma include *RAS, BRAF, PTEN, TERT,* and PIK3-kinase which were not identified in this patient. Thus, the diagnosis of anaplastic carcinoma is not supported by our studies.

The clinical course of thyroid carcinosarcoma is similar to anaplastic carcinoma. Some case reports have recommended following the standard treatment approach for anaplastic carcinoma. Multimodality treatment for anaplastic carcinoma, consisting of radical surgery followed by radiotherapy and chemotherapy is reported to be associated with better clinical outcomes. However, there is no uniform consensus about the treatment approach for thyroid carcinosarcoma due to its very low incidence, its aggressive nature with poor prognosis, and the consequent lack of large clinical series. Most reported cases were treated with total or subtotal thyroidectomy. Adjuvant chemotherapy, radiation therapy and immunotherapy have not proven to be beneficial. However, NGS performed on collected thyroid carcinosarcoma cases could be of great benefit for the identification of targeted treatments.

In conclusion, the present study reports a rare case of primary thyroid carcinosarcoma with metastasis to the lung in a 45-year-old female patient who ultimately succumbed to the disease after receiving surgeries for primary and metastatic tumors and adjuvant chemoradiation therapy. Her total survival time was 11 months from the time of diagnosis and her total disease free survival was 7 months. A *DICER1* (E1705K) gene mutation was identified in this patient. Primary thyroid carcinosarcoma is extremely rare and can be diagnostically challenging.

Immunohistochemical staining may be useful for establishing a diagnosis and for distinguishing the disease from anaplastic carcinoma. Although the overall survival is dismal despite aggressive treatment, careful evaluation and the use of NGS to detect specific gene alterations may lead to the development of effective targeted therapies.

Abbreviations

BRAF: B-Raf Proto-Oncogene; DICER1: Ribonuclease III; EGFR: Epidermal growth factor receptor; IHC: Immunohistochemical; NGS: Next generation sequencing; PAX8: Paired box gene 8; PIK3kinase: Phosphatidylinositol-4, 5-bisphosphate 3-kinase; RET: Proto-oncogene encodes a receptor tyrosine kinase; TTF1: Thyroid transcription factor 1; WHO: World health organization

Acknowledgements

Not applicable.

Funding

Not applicable.

Author's contributions

All authors were directly involved in the care of this patient. JY and QZ contributed to the acquisition of data, writing and revision of the manuscript; all authors have read and approved the final version of the manuscript for publication.

Consent for publication

Consent was not obtained from this deceased patient but the presented data are anonymized and risk of identification is minimal.

Competing interests

The authors declare that they have no competing interests.

References

1. Giuffrida D, Attard M, Marasa L, Ferrau F, Marletta F, et al. Thyroid carcinosarcoma, a rare and aggressive histotype: a case report. Ann Oncol. 2000;11:1497–9.
2. Donnell C, Pollock W, Sybers W. Thyroid carcinosarcoma. Arch Pathol Lab Med. 1987;111:1169–72.
3. Cooper K, Barker E. Thyroid carcinosarcoma. A case report. S. Afr J Surg. 1989;27:192–3.
4. Al-Sobhi S, Novosolov F, Sabançi U, et al. Management of thyroid carcinosarcoma. Surgery. 1997;122:548–52.
5. Naqiyah I, Zulkarnaen AN, Rohaizak M, Das S. Carcinosarcoma of the thyroid: a case report. Hippokratia. 2010;14:141–2.
6. Agrawal M, Uppin SG, Challa S, Prayaga AK. Carcinosarcoma thyroid: an unusual morphology with a review of the literature. South Asian J Cancer. 2013;2:226.
7. Ekici M, Kocak C, Bayhan Z, et al. Carcinosarcoma of the thyroid gland. Case Rep Surg; 2015. https://doi.org/10.1155/2015/494383.
8. Rasheed R, Saeed N, Naqvi A, Rasheed S, et al. Sporadic carcinosarcoma of thyroid gland resistant to chemotherapy: a case report. J Endocrinol. Thyroid Res. 2017;1:1–3.
9. El-Naggar A, Baloch Z, Eng C, et al. Anaplastic thyroid carcinoma. In: Lloyd RV, Osamura RY, Kloppel G, Rosai J, editors. World Health Organization classification of tumors, pathology and genetics of tumors of endocrine organs. Lyon, France: IARC Press; 2017. p. 104–6.
10. Xing M. Molecular pathogenesis and mechanisms of thyroid cancer. Nat Rev Cancer. 2013;13:184–99.
11. Rutter M, Jha P, Schultz K, et al. DICER1 mutations and differentiated thyroid carcinoma: evidence of a direct association. J Clin Endocrinol Metab. 2016; 101:1–5.
12. Yoshida M, Hamanoue S, Seki M, et al. Metachronous anaplastic sarcoma of the kidney and thyroid follicular carcinoma as manifestations of DICER1 abnormalities. Hum Pathol. 2017;61:205–9.
13. Conlon N, Schultheis A, Piscuoglio S, et al. A survey of DICER1 hotspot mutations in ovarian and testicular sex cord-stromal tumors. Mod Pathol. 2015;28:1603–12.
14. Raskin L, Guo Y, Du L, et al. Targeted sequencing of established and candidate colorectal cancer genes in the colon cancer family registry cohort. Oncotarget. 2017;8:93450–63.
15. Schmidt L, Linehan W. FLCN: the causative gene for Birt-Hogg-Dubé syndrome. Gene. 2018;640:28–42.
16. Krisenko M, Geahlen R. Calling in SYK: SYK's dual role as a tumor promoter and tumor suppressor in cancer. Biochim Biophys Acta. 1853;2015:254–63.

Association between iron status and thyroid function in Nepalese children

Saroj Khatiwada[1*], Basanta Gelal[2], Nirmal Baral[2] and Madhab Lamsal[2]

Abstract

Background: Deficiencies of iodine and iron may have adverse effect on thyroid function. This study was undertaken to investigate the association between iron status and thyroid function in Nepalese children living in hilly regions.

Methods: A cross-sectional study was conducted among 227 school children aged 6–12 years living in hilly regions of eastern Nepal. Urine and blood samples were analyzed for urinary iodine concentration, free thyroxine, free triiodothyronine, thyroid stimulating hormone, hemoglobin, serum iron and total iron binding capacity, and percentage transferrin saturation was calculated.

Results: The cohort comprised euthyroid (80.6 %, $n = 183$), overt hypothyroid (1.3 %, $n = 3$), subclinical hypothyroid (16.3 %, $n = 37$) and subclinical hyperthyroid (1.8 %, $n = 4$) children respectively. About 35.2 % ($n = 80$) children were anemic, 43.6 % ($n = 99$) were iron deficient and 19.8 % ($n = 45$) had urinary iodine excretion < 100 μg/L. Hypothyroidism (overt and subclinical) was common in anemic and iron deficient children. The relative risk of having hypothyroidism (overt and subclinical) in anemic and iron deficient children was 5.513 (95 % CI: 2.844–10.685, $p < 0.001$) and 1.939 (95 % CI: 1.091-3.449, $p = 0.023$) respectively as compared to non-anemic and iron sufficient children. Thyroid stimulating hormone had significant negative correlation with hemoglobin ($r = -0.337$, $p < 0.001$) and transferrin saturation ($r = -0.204$, $p = 0.002$).

Conclusions: Thyroid dysfunction, iron deficiency and anemia are common among Nepalese children. In this cohort, anemic and iron deficient children had poor thyroid function.

Keywords: Anemia, Iron deficiency, Nepal, School children, Thyroid dysfunction, Thyroid hormone

Background

Multiple micronutrient deficiencies are still a major public health problem faced by developing countries. Such deficiencies have adverse effects on growth and development, especially in vulnerable groups like pregnant women and children [1]. Deficiencies of trace elements like iodine, iron, zinc and selenium also impairs thyroid function [2]. Thyroid hormones influence a number of metabolic pathways and physiological components. Excess thyroid hormones cause hyperthyroidism whereas deficiency causes hypothyroidism [3]. Iodine deficiency and iron deficiency are considered as the most common cause of preventable brain damage and anemia respectively in developing countries like Nepal [4, 5]. Anemia and iron deficiency have been found to be highly prevalent among Nepalese school children, whereas iodine nutrition has been continuously improving in school children [6, 7]. Iron deficiency with or without anemia affects child development and also has multiple adverse effects on thyroid metabolism [8, 9].

Studies have reported the association of thyroid function with iron status [10–12]. In the study by Metwalley et al. in Egypt, it was found that primary school children with iron deficiency anemia were liable to develop subclinical hypothyroidism and intellectual dysfunction [12]. Since, iron deficiency and anemia are highly prevalent in the Nepalese population, assessment of thyroid function in such a population may help to determine the potential effects of iron deficiency on thyroid metabolism [6]. Thyroid dysfunction has been also been reported more frequently in Nepalese population although iodine nutrition has been improving continuously [13, 14]. It is however, unknown about the factors responsible for thyroid disorders in this region. It has been hypothesized that iron deficiency

* Correspondence: khatiwadasaroj22@gmail.com
[1]Department of Biochemistry, Modern Technical College, Lalitpur, Nepal
Full list of author information is available at the end of the article

negatively affects thyroid function leading to increased rate of thyroid disorders [10]. Thus, there might be potential link between iron deficiency and thyroid dysfunction in this population as well. Taking in to account of poor iron status and higher rates of thyroid dysfunction in Nepalese population, we tried to find the possible effects of iron deficiency on thyroid function in Nepalese children by conducting the present study.

Specifically, we selected school children aged 6–12 years randomly from hilly regions of eastern Nepal and analyzed urine and blood samples to assess iodine status, iron status and thyroid function, and determine their association.

Methods

A cross-sectional study was conducted among children of two hilly districts (Sankhuwasabha and Dhankuta) of eastern Nepal in 2014. We assessed iodine status, iron status and thyroid function to find the association between iron status and thyroid function in the cross sectional population. Six schools (three schools in each district) were picked randomly and school children aged 6–12 years whose parents gave consent were enrolled randomly in the study. A total of 227 children (124 from Sankhuwasabha and 103 from Dhankuta district) were selected for the study. The ethical clearance for this study was given by the Institutional Review Board of B P Koirala Institute of Health Sciences (BPKIHS), Dharan. Sample size estimation was done on the basis of approximate prevalence of iodine deficiency (15 %), iron deficiency (30 %) and thyroid dysfunction (20 %) in Nepalese children.

Demographic variables (age, gender), urine samples (10 ml) and venous blood samples (3 ml) were collected from each child. The samples were transported to biochemistry laboratory of B P Koirala Institute of Health Sciences under refrigeration. Hemoglobin (Hb) was measured within 24 h of sample collection by cyanmethemoglobin method, whereas other parameters were estimated within a week of sample collection [15]. Urinary iodine excretion (UIE) was measured by using ammonium persulphate digestion method (APDM) [16]. Serum iron and total iron binding capacity (TIBC) were measured by colorimetric methods using commercial kits (Roche Diagnostics). Transferrin saturation was calculated using serum iron and TIBC value [17]. Thyroid hormones (free triiodothyronine (fT3), free thyroxine (fT4) and thyroid stimulating hormone (TSH)) were measured by immunoassay methods using ELISA kits from HUMAN Diagnostics. Normal reference range provided by kits for serum iron was 37–145 μg/dl for women and 59–158 μg/dl for men and 274–385 μg/dl for TIBC. Similarly the normal reference range for thyroid hormones were fT3 (1.4–4.2 pg/ml), fT4 (0.8-2.2 ng/dl) and TSH (0.39-6.16 mIU/L) according to kit provider.

The data generated from the study were entered in ms-excel and analyzed using SPSS version 19 software. Continuous variables were expressed as mean ± SD, except for UIE and TSH (expressed as median) and categorical variables as number (percentage). Independent t test, one way ANOVA, Man whitney test and Kruskal Wallis test was applied for continuous variables and chi-square test for categorical variables at 95 % confidence interval. Pearson correlation and Spearman's rho correlation analysis was done among variables to see the association between iron status indicator and thyroid hormones at 95 % confidence interval. Relative risk for hypothyroidism in anemic and iron deficient as compared to non-anemic and iron sufficient was calculated at 95 % confidence interval.

Results

Among the study population, 55.5 % ($n = 126$) were males and 44.5 % ($n = 101$) were females. The median UIE and TSH with IQR was 222 μg/L (121 μg/L; 296 μg/L) and 4.0 mIU/L (2 mIU/L; 6 mIU/L) respectively. The mean level of Hb, serum iron, TIBC, transferrin saturation, fT3, fT4 and TSH were 12.2 ± 1.9 gm/dl, 70.5 ± 35.4 μg/dl, 382.8 ± 89.5 μg/dl, 20.1 ± 12.6 %, 2.7 ± 0.8 pg/ml, 1.2 ± 0.4 ng/dl and 4.4 ± 2.8 mIU/L respectively in the study population, which are all in normal range. No significant differences in UIE ($p = 0.98$), Hb ($p = 0.078$), serum iron ($p = 0.594$), TIBC ($p = 0.781$), transferrin saturation ($p = 0.766$), fT3 ($p = 0.912$), fT4 ($p = 0.842$) and TSH ($p = 0.383$) were observed among gender. On the basis of Hb cutoff value for anemia for different age group and transferrin saturation cutoff < 16 for iron deficiency, 35.2 % ($n = 80$) and 43.6 % ($n = 99$) children were anemic and iron deficient respectively [18]. About, 19.8 % ($n = 45$) children had UIE < 100 μg/L, which is considered as iodine deficiency on the basis of WHO criteria for iodine status [19]. Level of biochemical parameters according to anemia and iron status is shown in Table 1. Median TSH level was higher in anemic than non-anemic ($p < 0.001$), but similar in iron deficient and iron sufficient ($p = 0.05$). fT3 was significantly higher in iron sufficient than iron deficient ($p = 0.003$). Level of Hb, serum iron, TIBC and transferrin saturation was 12.3 ± 2.1 gm/dl versus 12.3 ± 1.9 gm/dl ($p = 0.924$), 81.4 ± 35.9 μg/dl versus 67.9 ± 34.9 μg/dl ($p = 0.022$), 371.7 ± 97.5 μg/dl versus 385.6 ± 87.6 μg/dl ($p = 0.354$), and 23.8 ± 12.8 % versus 19.3 ± 12.5 % ($p = 0.032$) among iodine deficient and iodine sufficient children respectively. Similarly, the mean level of fT3, fT4 and median TSH was 2.8 ± 0.9 pg/ml versus 2.7 ± 0.8 pg/ml ($p = 0.78$); 1.2 ± 0.5 ng/dl versus 1.2 ± 0.4 ng/dl ($p = 0.567$) and 4.0 mIU/L (2; 6) versus 4.0 mIU/L (2; 6) ($p = 0.953$) among iodine deficient and iodine sufficient respectively.

Table 1 Biochemical parameters in study population according to anemia and iron status

Variables	Total	Anemia status			Iron status		
		Anemic	Non-anemic	*P* value	Iron deficient	Iron sufficient	*P* value
	N = 227	*N* = 80	*N* = 147		*N* = 99	*N* = 128	
UIE (μg/L)	222 (121; 296)	225 (112.7; 303.5)	222 (125; 281)	0.788	228 (133; 307)	220 (119.5; 291)	0.428
Hemoglobin (gm/dl)	12.2 ± 1.9	10.3 ± 1.0	13.3 ± 1.3	<0.001	11.6 ± 1.8	12.7 ± 1.7	<0.001
Serum iron (μg/dl)	70.5 ± 35.4	55.4 ± 21.8	78.8 ± 38.6	<0.001	39.6 ± 12.9	94.4 ± 28.1	<0.001
TIBC (μg/dl)	382.8 ± 89.5	414.6 ± 81.5	365.4 ± 89.2	<0.001	433.2 ± 81.9	343.8 ± 74.8	<0.001
Transferrin saturation (%)	20.1 ± 12.6	14.2 ± 7.6	23.4 ± 13.6	<0.001	9.2 ± 2.5	28.6 ± 10.7	<0.001
Free T3 (pg/ml)	2.7 ± 0.8	2.6 ± 0.9	2.8 ± 0.7	0.13	2.6 ± 0.8	2.9 ± 0.7	0.003
Free T4 (ng/dl)	1.2 ± 0.4	1.2 ± 0.5	1.2 ± 0.4	0.526	1.2 ± 0.5	1.2 ± 0.4	0.531
TSH (mIU/L)	4.0 (2; 6)	5.0 (3; 8)	3.0 (2; 5)	<0.001	4.0 (3; 7)	4.0 (2; 6)	0.05

The data is expressed as mean ± SD except for UIE and TSH (expressed as median with IQR). *P* value was calculated at 95 % confidence interval

Among the study children, 80.6 % ($n = 183$), 1.3 % ($n = 3$), 16.3 % ($n = 37$) and 1.8 % ($n = 4$) were euthyroid, overt hypothyroid, subclinical hypothyroid and subclinical hyperthyroid respectively. Thyroid status according to anemia and iron deficiency is shown in Table 2. Similarly, level of UIE, Hb and iron status indicators in the study population according to thyroid function status is shown in Table 3. No significant difference in number of euthyroid (36 versus 147, $p = 1.0$), overt hypothyroid (2 versus 1, $p = 0.101$), subclinical hypothyroid (7 versus 30, $p = 1.0$) and subclinical hyperthyroid (0 versus 4, $p = 0.587$) was observed among iodine deficient and iodine sufficient children.

A significant positive correlation was observed between Hb level and transferrin saturation ($r = 0.411$, $p = <0.001$). Correlation of Hb and transferrin saturation with TSH level is shown in Figs. 1 and 2 respectively. Transferrin saturation was significantly negatively correlated with TSH ($r = -0.204$, $p = 0.002$), positively with fT3 ($r = 0.13$, $p = 0.051$) and weakly negatively with fT4 ($r = -0.089$, $p = 0.182$). Similarly, Hb was significantly negatively correlated with TSH ($r = -0.337$, $p < 0.001$), but weakly correlated with fT3 ($r = 0.077$, $p = 0.249$) and fT4 ($r = -0.018$, $p = 0.787$). UIE was very weakly correlated with TSH ($r = 0.031$, $p = 0.643$), fT3 ($r = -0.014$, $p = 0.832$) and fT4 ($r = 0.047$, $p = 0.484$). The risk of having hypothyroidism (overt and subclinical) in anemic and iron deficient children was 5.513 (95 % CI: 2.844-10.685, $p < 0.001$) and 1.939 (95 % CI: 1.091-3.449, $p = 0.023$) respectively as compared to non-anemic and iron sufficient children.

Discussion

Iodine and iron deficiencies are very common in the regions where adequate iodine and iron is not present in normal diet [20]. We observed anemia and iron deficiency in 35.2 % and 43.6 % children respectively. Anemia and iron deficiency have been found highly prevalent in Nepalese school children. Study by Khatiwada et al. reported anemia and iron deficiency in 34.5 % and 43.4 % school children respectively [6]. The anemia prevalence according to Nepal demographic and health survey, Baral et al. study and Khatiwada et al. study were 48 % (among age 6–59 months), 65.6 % (among age 10–19 years) and 37.9 % (among age 4–13 years) respectively [7]. Iron deficiency has been considered as the most common cause of anemia in developing countries [18]. Our findings further support that iron deficiency is the most common cause for anemia in Nepalese children as indicated by poor iron status indicators in anemic children. Besides the lack of adequate iron in diet, other chronic conditions like hook worm infestation, malaria and genetic factors also contribute to high prevalence of anemia in developing countries [18].

Table 2 Thyroid function status in study population according to anemia and iron status

Variables	Total	Anemia status			Iron status		
		Anemic	Non-anemic	*P* value	Iron deficient	Iron sufficient	*P* value
	N = 227	*N* = 80	*N* = 147		*N* = 99	*N* = 128	
Euthyroidism, n (%)	183 (80.6 %)	49 (21.6 %)	134 (59 %)	<0.001	72 (31.7 %)	111 (48.9 %)	0.011
Overt hypothyroidism, n (%)	3 (1.3 %)	3 (1.3 %)	-	0.043	3 (1.3 %)	-	0.082
Subclinical hypothyroidism, n (%)	37 (16.3 %)	27 (11.9 %)	10 (4.4 %)	<0.001	21 (9.3 %)	16 (7 %)	0.102
Subclinical hyperthyroidism, n (%)	4 (1.8 %)	1 (0.4 %)	3 (1.3 %)	1.0	3 (1.3 %)	1 (0.4 %)	0.32

The data is expressed as number (percentage). *P* value was calculated at 95 % confidence interval

Table 3 Biochemical parameters in study population according to thyroid function

Variables	Euthyroid N = 183	Hypothyroid* N = 40	Subclinical hyperthyroid N = 4	P value
UIE (μg/L)	213 (120; 290)	236.5 (155.5; 301.5)	219 (141.7; 295.5)	0.345
Hemoglobin (gm/dl)	12.6 ± 1.7	10.7 ± 2.0	13.9 ± 2.5	<0.001
Serum iron (μg/dl)	74.0 ± 36.7	57.0 ± 26.6	50.5 ± 23.3	0.012
TIBC (μg/dl)	374.7 ± 84.2	418.8 ± 104.8	393.4 ± 101.1	0.018
Transferrin saturation (%)	21.5 ± 13.2	14.6 ± 8.1	14.0 ± 8.7	0.004

The data is expressed as mean ± SD except for UIE (expressed as median with IQR). Asterik (*) indicates that hypothyroid group included both overt and subclinical hypothyroid. *P* value was calculated at 95 % confidence interval

Though, the median UIE (222 μg/L) in our study population was more than optimum, we found 19.8 % children had insufficient UIE, which is considered as iodine deficiency [19]. Our results suggest improvement on iodine status in Nepalese children. Higher median UIE than optimum as seen in our study also indicates excessive iodine intake and raises concern about the risk for iodine-induced hyperthyroidism [21]. The median UIE in the present study was slightly lower than in our previous study in Terai region where median UIE was 226.3 μg/L, but higher than in remote hilly regions where we reported median UIE of 187.52 μg/L [21, 22]. Since, soils in hills and mountains are reported to lack sufficient iodine and thus in the food derived from them, continuous provision of adequately iodized salt in such areas is necessary. Both, excess or insufficient intake of iodine adversely affects thyroid health, so optimum iodine intake should be maintained [23].

Present study reveals subclinical hypothyroidism (16.3 %) as the commonest thyroid dysfunction in Nepalese school children followed by overt hypothyroidism (1.3 %) and subclinical hyperthyroidism (1.8 %). In one community based study among school children in eastern Nepal, Chaudhari et al. reported that 31.8 % and 29.5 % children had subclinical hypothyroidism in Sunsari and Dhankuta districts respectively. However they did not reported any overt hypothyroidism or subclinical hyperthyroidism [24]. Study by Baral et al. at a hospital in eastern Nepal reported that 13.6 % population had hyperthyroidism and 17.1 % had hypothyroidism [13]. Previous studies in chronic disease patients like diabetes mellitus and chronic kidney diseases in eastern Nepal have reported thyroid dysfunction particularly subclinical hypothyroidism in large part of study patients [25, 26]. The high rate of hypothyroidism in the study subjects may be due to high rate of thyroid autoimmunity and deficiency of micronutrients like iron [25]. The most common cause of thyroid disorders worldwide is iodine deficiency, leading to goitre formation and hypothyroidism. In iodine-replete areas, most persons with thyroid disorders have autoimmune diseases

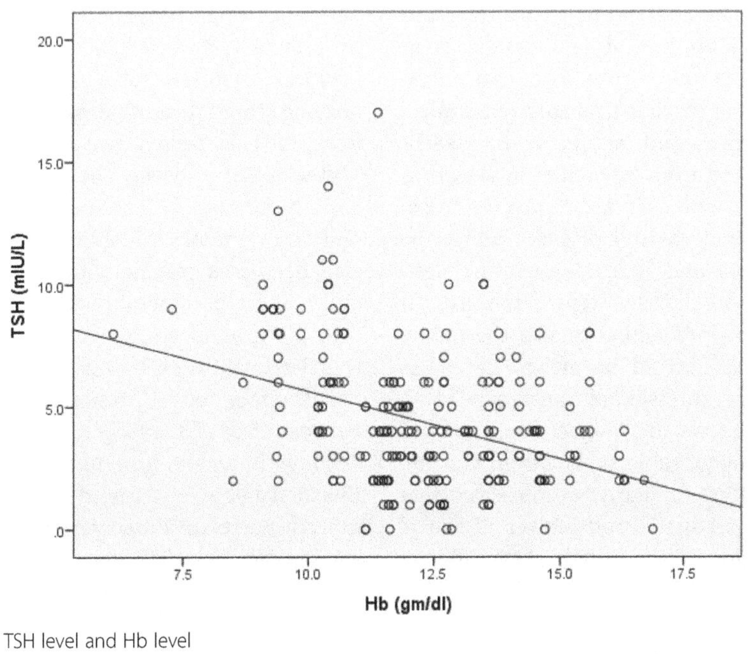

Fig. 1 Correlation between TSH level and Hb level

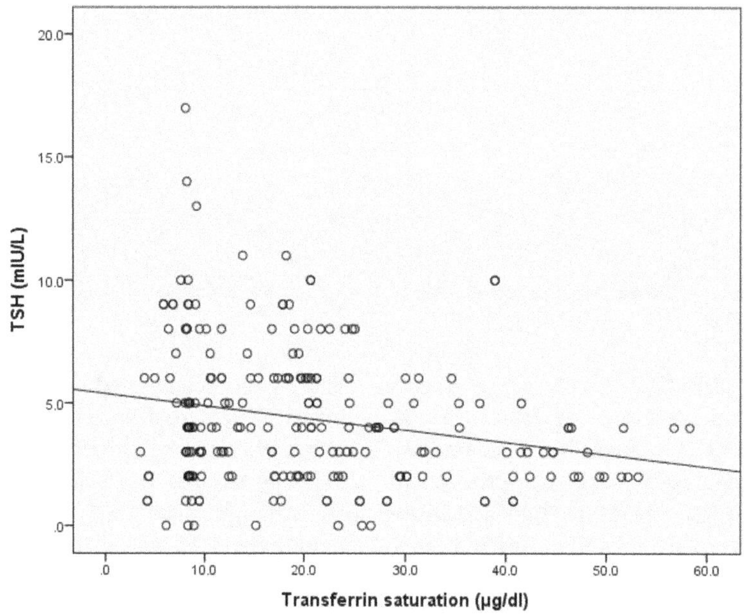

Fig. 2 Correlation between TSH level and transferrin saturation

like hashimoto's thyroiditis and Graves' disease [27]. The present study reveals no difference in thyroid function among iodine deficient and iodine sufficient children, and no association between UIE and thyroid hormones. Previous studies have also reported that there are usually no, or weak, associations between UIE and thyroid hormone concentrations [28].

In the present study, we observed significantly lower Hb level and iron status indicators in hypothyroids (overt and subclinical) than euthyroids, and iron deficiency and anemia in larger fraction of hypothyroid (both overt and subclinical) children. Our findings are in accord to results of previous studies by Bremner et al. and Banday et al. [29, 30]. Bremner et al. found serum iron concentrations significantly lower in participants with subclinical hypothyroidism than euthyroid subjects ($p = 0.001$), and Banday et al. reported iron deficiency in a significant portion of patients with primary hypothyroidism [29, 30]. It is believed that thyroid diseases affect the process of hematopoiesis and thyroid hormone deficiency may lead to bone marrow repression and/or decrease in erythropoietin production due to the reduction of O_2 requirements. Thyroid hormones have also found to regulate the gene expression of transferrin [31].

Our findings suggest that anemic subjects tend to have higher TSH than non-anemic subjects, however, fT3 and fT4 does not seem to differ. Similarly, we observed that iron deficient children had significantly lower fT3 level than iron sufficient children. In a study by Metwalley et al., iron deficient children with hemoglobin level 10.9-7 gm/dl had significantly higher levels of serum fT3 and fT4 ($p < 0.01$ for both) and significantly lower levels of serum TSH ($p < 0.05$) as compared to patients with Hb level < 7 gm/dl [12]. In another study in Bangladesh among general population, serum TSH level was significantly higher ($p < 0.05$) and serum fT4 was significantly lower ($p < 0.05$) in iron deficient subjects than healthy controls, however, serum fT3 was almost similar between iron deficient and healthy controls [32]. Our finding demonstrates that anemic and iron deficient children have high risk for hypothyroidism, and hypothyroidism is associated with anemic and iron deficient children. Thus our findings suggests for the possibility that iron deficiency might impair thyroid metabolism as reported in previous studies. The two initial steps of thyroid hormone synthesis are catalyzed by heme containing enzyme, thyroid peroxidase. Severe iron deficiency may lower thyroid peroxidase activity and interfere with the synthesis of thyroid hormones thereby leading to hypothyroidism [33]. Studies have revealed that iron deficiency anemia (IDA) impairs thyroid metabolism and also decreases plasma total T4 and T3 concentrations and reduces peripheral conversion of T4 to T3 [9].

In the present study, we observed negative relation of transferrin saturation and Hb with TSH. Previous study by Bremner et al. reported significant relationships between free T3 and Hb, and inverse relationship of TSH with serum iron and transferrin saturation [29]. Bivolarska et al. also found slight positive statistically significant correlative association between the levels of free T4 and Hb ($r = 0.217$, $p = 0.033$) [11]. While many studies have found that both iron metabolism and thyroid functions are interdependent and each one of them could have a regulatory role, some studies have reported no association between thyroid hormones and anemia or iron deficiency [31–34]. In the study in Bangladesh, Akhter et al. observed no significant correlation of Hb concentration with serum TSH, fT3 and fT4 concentrations both in iron deficient and healthy control group [32]. Similarly, in the study in an area of mild iodine deficiency in Turkey, thyroid hormone levels of children with anemia were not significantly different from those without anemia, and there was no significant correlation between thyroid hormones and iron status [34]. There are several limitations of the present study. The sample size was small. Also, because of its cross-sectional nature we cannot draw conclusion about cause and effect relation between iron deficiency and thyroid dysfunction. Since, anti-thyroid peroxidase antibody (anti-TPO) was not assayed in the population, high prevalence of thyroid autoimmunity may also contribute for high rate of thyroid dysfunction in the study population.

Conclusions

The study finds high prevalence of thyroid dysfunction, anemia and iron deficiency among Nepalese children and a significant association between iron status and thyroid function. Thus, anemia and iron deficiency seems to be associated with thyroid dysfunction particularly hypothyroidism. Future studies should be done in large samples and be directed toward finding the reasons for low thyroid hormones in anemic and iron deficient children.

Abbreviations

Anti-TPO: Anti-thyroid peroxidase antibody; APDM: Ammonium persulphate digestion method; Free T3: Free triiodothyronine; Free T4: Free thyroxine; Hb: Hemoglobin; IDA: Iron deficiency anemia; TIBC: Total iron binding capacity; TSH: Thyroid stimulating hormone; UIE: Urinary iodine excretion.

Competing interests

The authors declare that they have no competing interests.

Authors' contributions

SK, BG, NB and ML designed the study. SK performed laboratory analysis and wrote manuscript. BG, NB and ML reviewed manuscript. All authors read and approved the final version of manuscript.

Acknowledgements

We kindly acknowledge Institute advisory authority of B P Koirala Institute of Health Sciences for the financial assistance.

Source of funding

This study was supported by Nepal India Corpus fund through the Institute Advisory Authority of B P Koirala Institute of Health Sciences (BPKIHS).

Author details

[1]Department of Biochemistry, Modern Technical College, Lalitpur, Nepal. [2]Department of Biochemistry, B P Koirala Institute of Health Sciences, Ghopa, Dharan, Nepal.

References

1. Arlappa N, Laxmaiah A, Balakrishna N, Harikumar R, Kodavanti MR, Reddy CG, et al. Micronutrient deficiency disorders among the rural children of West Bengal, India. Ann Hum Biol. 2011;38(3):281–9.
2. Eftekhari MH, Eshraghian MR, Mozaffari-Khosravi H, Saadat N, Shidfar F. Effect of iron repletion and correction of iron deficiency on thyroid function in iron-deficient Iranian adolescent girls. Pak J Biol Sci. 2007;10(2):255–60.
3. Pucci E, Chiovato L, Pinchera A. Thyroid and lipid metabolism. Int J Obes Relat Metab Disord. 2000;24 Suppl 2:S109–12.
4. Kapil U. Health consequences of iodine deficiency. Sultan Qaboos Univ Med J. 2007;7(3):267–72.
5. Olivares M, Walter T, Hertrampf E, Pizarro F. Anaemia and iron deficiency disease in children. Br Med Bull. 1999;55(3):534–43.
6. Khatiwada S, Lamsal M, Gelal B, Gautam S, Nepal AK, Brodie D, et al. Anemia, Iron Deficiency and Iodine Deficiency among Nepalese School Children. Indian J Pediatr. 2015. doi: 10.1007/s12098-015-1924-y.
7. Khatiwada S, Gelal B, Gautam S, Tamang MK, Shakya PR, Lamsal M, et al. Anemia among school children in eastern Nepal. J Trop Pediatr. 2015;61(3): 231–3. doi:10.1093/tropej/fmv016.
8. World Health Organization. Assessing the iron status of populations. 2nd Ed. Geneva, Switzerland: World Health Organization/Centers for Disease Control and Prevention Technical Consultation on the Assessment of Iron Status at the Population Level; 2004. http://www.who.int/nutrition/publications/micronutrients/anaemia_iron_deficiency/9789241596107.pdf.
9. Hess SY, Zimmermann MB, Arnold M, Langhans W, Hurrell RF. Iron deficiency anemia reduces thyroid peroxidase activity in rats. J Nutr. 2002; 132(7):1951–5.
10. Kammal M, Abdrabo AA. Assessment of thyroid hormone levels in Sudanese females with iron deficiency. Sudan Med J. 2014;50(2):98–102.
11. Bivolarska A, Gatseva P, Maneva A. Association between thyroid and iron status of pregnant women in Southern Bulgaria. J Endocrinol Diabetes Mellit. 2013;1:15–21.
12. Metwalley KA, Farghaly HS, Hassan AF. Thyroid status in Egyptian primary school children with iron deficiency anemia: Relationship to intellectual function. Thyroid Res Pract. 2013;10:91–5.
13. Baral N, Lamsal M, Koner BC, Koirala S. Thyroid dysfunction in eastern Nepal. Southeast Asian J Trop Med Public Health. 2002;33:638–41.
14. Nepal AK, Khatiwada S, Shakya PR, Gelal B, Lamsal M, Brodie D, et al. Iodine status after iodized salt supplementation in school children of eastern Nepal. Southeast Asian J Trop Med Public Health. 2013;44(6):1072–8.
15. Bain BJ, Lewis SM, Bates I. Basic haematological techniques. In: Lewis SM, Bain BJ, Bates I, editors. Dacie and Lewis practical hematology. 10th ed. Germany: Churchill livingstone elsevier; 2006. p. 25–54.
16. Ohashi T, Yamaki M, Pandav CS, Karmarkar MG, Irie M. Simple microplate method for determination of urinary iodine. Clin Chem. 2000;46(4):529–36.
17. Worwood M. Iron deficiency anemia and iron overload. In: Lewis SM, Bain BJ, Bates I, editors. Dacie and Lewis practical hematology. 10th ed. Germany: Churchill livingstone elsevier; 2006. p. 132–60.
18. Zimmermann MB, Hurrell RF. Nutritional iron deficiency. Lancet. 2007;370: 511–20.
19. Zimmermann MB, Jooste PL, Pandav CS. Iodine-deficiency disorders. Lancet. 2008;372(9645):1251–62.
20. Mirmiran P, Golzarand M, Majem LS, Aziz F. Iron, iodine and vitamin A in the Middle East; a systematic review of deficiency and food fortification. Iranian J Publ Health. 2012;41(8):8–19.
21. Khatiwada S, Gelal B, Shakya PR, Lamsal M, Baral N. Urinary Iodine Excretion among Nepalese School Children in Terai Region. Indian J Pediatr. 2015; doi: 10.1007/s12098-015-1755-x
22. Khatiwada S, Gelal B, Gautam S, Lamsal M, Baral N. Iodine status among school children of remote Hilly regions of Nepal. Indian Pediatr. 2015;52(5): 436–7.
23. Khatiwada S, Gelal B, Tamang MK, Kc R, Singh S, Lamsal M, et al. Iodized salt use and salt iodine content among household salts from six districts of Eastern Nepal. J Nepal Health Res Counc. 2014;12(28):191–4.
24. Chaudhari RK, Gelal B, Brodie DA, Baral N. Thyroid function and urinary iodine status in primary school age children of the hills and the plains of Eastern Nepal. Indian Pediatr. 2012;49(4):332–3.
25. Khatiwada S, Kc R, Sah SK, Khan SA, Chaudhari RK, Baral N, et al. Thyroid dysfunction and associated risk factors among nepalese diabetes mellitus patients. Int J Endocrinol. 2015;2015:570198. doi:10.1155/2015/570198.

26. Khatiwada S, Kc R, Gautam S, Lamsal M, Baral N. Thyroid dysfunction and dyslipidemia in chronic kidney disease patients. BMC Endocr Disord. 2015; 15:65. doi:10.1186/s12902-015-0063-9.
27. Vanderpump MPJ. The epidemiology of thyroid disease. Br Med Bull. 2011; 99(1):39–51.
28. Zimmermann MB, Boelaert K. Iodine deficiency and thyroid disorders. Lancet Diabetes Endocrinol. 2015;3(4):286–95.
29. Bremner AP, Feddema P, Joske DJ, Leedman PJ, Leary PC O, Olynyk JK, et al. Significant association between thyroid hormones and erythrocyte indices in euthyroid subjects. Clin Endocrinol (Oxf). 2012;76(2):304–11.
30. Banday TH, Bhat SB, Bhat SB, Shah N, Bashir S. To study prevalence of incipient iron deficiency in primary hypothyroidism. Int J Res Med Sci. 2014;2(2):472–5.
31. Refaat B. Prevalence and characteristics of anemia associated with thyroid disorders in non-pregnant Saudi women during the childbearing age: a cross-sectional study. Biomed J. 2015;38(4):307–16.
32. Akhter S, Naher ZU, Parvin S, Nahar K, Ali M, Bashar T, et al. The status of thyroid hormones in iron deficient patients in Bangladesh. Medicine today. 2012;24(1):1–4.
33. Eftekhari MH, Keshavarz SA, Jalali M, Elguero E, Eshraghian MR, Simondon KB. The relationship between iron status and thyroid hormone concentration in iron-deficient adolescent Iranian girls. Asia Pac J Clin Nutr. 2006;15(1):50–5.
34. Yavuz O, Yavuz T, Kahraman C, Yesildal N, Bundak R. The relationship between iron status and thyroid hormones in adolescents living in an iodine deficient area. J Pediatr Endocrinol Metab. 2004;17(10):1443–9.

20

Malignant Struma ovarii in a 30-year old nulliparous patient

J. Colin Boyd[1*], Blair A. Williams[2], Matthew H. Rigby[2], Katharina Kieser[3], Saul Offman[4], Hemlata Shirsat[4], Jonathan R. B. Trites[2], S. Mark Taylor[2] and Robert D. Hart[2]

Abstract

Background: Struma ovarii is a rare monodermal germ cell tumor where the ovary is comprised of at least half thyroid tissue. This phenomenon may indicate an embryological origin.

Case presentation: A 30-year old nulliparous woman presented with acute right lower quadrant pain and underwent laparoscopic right salpingo-oophorectomy. The excised ovarian mass showed evidence of struma-derived papillary thyroid carcinoma. Ultrasound of the thyroid showed mild enlargement with two solid nodules. A fine needle aspirate of a thyroid nodule was positive for malignancy and a total thyroidectomy was performed. Microscopic features of the thyroid were consistent with papillary thyroid carcinoma. The two tumours were considered as synchronous independent primaries based on their histological presentation.

Conclusions: We believe that aggressive surgical management followed by radioiodine therapy is best to reduce recurrence risk and optimize survival. The broad scope of interventions needed to treat malignant struma ovarii require a strong interdisciplinary team.

Keywords: Thyroid carcinoma, Thyroidectomy, I-131, Radioiodine, Oncology

Background

Struma ovarii is a monodermal germ cell tumor first described by R. Boëttlin in 1889 [1]. It represents 2–3% of all ovarian tumours and by definition must be comprised of at least half thyroid tissue [2–4]. Struma ovarii is rare; less than 200 cases have been reported in the medical literature [3, 5]. Malignant struma ovarii is rarer still, with malignancy occurring in less than 5% of cases and metastases highly uncommon [6, 7]. However, recurrence rates vary widely and have been reported from 7.5–35% [4, 6, 8]. Goffredo et al. [3] report excellent survival rates for patients with malignant struma ovarii but emphasize the high risk of aggressive thyroid cancers, which occurred in 6 of their 68 patients.

Multifocal thyroid-type tumors that arise synchronously in separate locations may represent a common genetic predisposition for tumor formation, likely occurring in embryogenesis. These cells differentiate into thyroid-type tissue and, after exposure to carcinogens later in life, undergo distinct but parallel tumorigenesis [9]. This phenomenon may similarly be explained by "field cancerization", where exposure to carcinogens creates a carcinogen-damaged field of thyroid type tissue regardless of anatomic location [10].

Given its rarity, little is known about malignant struma ovarii and accordingly there are few guidelines to manage its treatment [4, 8, 9, 11, 12]. A significant issue for clinicians to consider is the intensity of treatment. This may include pelvic surgery, thyroidectomy and radioactive iodine (I-131), which must be balanced against the risks of infertility and the low rate of metastasis.

Here we present the case of a 30 year-old nulliparous patient with malignant struma ovarii and concomitant papillary thyroid carcinoma.

Case Presentation

A 30-year old nulliparous woman presented to her regional hospital with acute right lower quadrant pain. She was otherwise healthy with no significant past medical history. She reported smoking 10–15 cigarettes per day. A pelvic mass was palpated posteriorly and a pelvic ultrasound revealed a right adnexal mass suggestive of

* Correspondence: c.boyd@dal.ca
[1]Dalhousie Medical School, Dalhousie University, 5849 University Avenue, Halifax, NS B3H 4H7, Canada
Full list of author information is available at the end of the article

an ovarian cyst, with the possibility of torsion due to the patient's level of discomfort. The patient was taken to the operating room and underwent a laparoscopic right salpingo-oophorectomy.

The ovarian mass (8.5 x 5.0 x 4.0 cm) was solid and cystic, with cysts containing milky-mucoid material. The solid area had a characteristic red-brown cut surface and a tooth was also identified. Histologic sections showed struma ovarii (Fig. 1) with limited non-strumal teratomatous elements (i.e. epidermal derivatives). The thyroid-type tissue showed multiple zones of increased cellularity, crowding, and nuclear alteration (enlargement, clearing, grooves, and membrane irregularity) along with scattered mitotic figures (Fig. 2). The features were diagnostic of struma-derived papillary thyroid carcinoma. Positive immunohistochemical staining for HBME1, Galectin 3 and CK19 supported the histologic impression. Neither surface involvement nor lymphovascular space invasion was identified.

The patient was referred to the Gynecology Oncology Cancer Site Team at a tertiary care centre who also involved the care of a thyroid team including Otolaryngology and Radiation Oncology.

Workup for thyroglobulin, serum TSH, anti-thyroglobulin antibody, and free T4 were performed and were consistent with euthyroid status. Ultrasound of the thyroid showed a mildly enlarged gland with a 1.1 cm solid isoechoic nodule in the upper pole of the right thyroid gland and a 5 mm hypoechoic solid nodule in the interpolar region of the left thyroid gland. Colloid cysts bilaterally measured up to 1.7 cm. An 18 F-FDG PET scan was conducted from skull base to proximal thighs and identified two low-density lesions in the right lobe of the thyroid with otherwise unremarkable uptake throughout the thyroid gland. However, absence of uptake FDG on PET does not exclude thyroid malignancy as most are low-grade differentiated thyroid cancers which are not particularly FDG-avid.

The combined results of the ultrasound and PET scan prompted referral for an ultrasound guided aspiration biopsy. Cytology results of the fine needle aspiration on right lobe nodule of thyroid were positive for malignancy, consistent with papillary thyroid carcinoma. These findings were discussed with the patient and a recommendation of total thyroidectomy was made. The thyroid was resected without complication.

The thyroid showed multiple cysts in both lobes and a solid 1.0 cm lesion in the lower pole of the right lobe. The microscopic features were consistent with papillary thyroid carcinoma. Neither lymphovascular space invasion nor extra thyroidal extension was identified.

The two tumours were interpreted as synchronous independent primaries. The presence of admixed epidermal derivatives in the ovary reflected primary teratomatous origin. The thyroid carcinoma was likewise deemed to be a primary, due to the distinct histomorphology, lack of aggressive features, absence of lymphatic or capsular/surface invasion in either organ, and absence of metastases elsewhere.

Following thyroidectomy, the patient was seen by Radiation Oncology who recommended I-131 therapy. She was treated on an outpatient basis and received a 100 mCi dose of I-131. The procedure was tolerated well and there were no complications. The follow-up whole body I-131 scan detected no evidence of nodal or distant metastatic disease.

Discussion and Conclusions

Struma ovarii is a rare ovarian tumor, with malignancy reported in less than 5% of cases [3, 6]. Metastases are

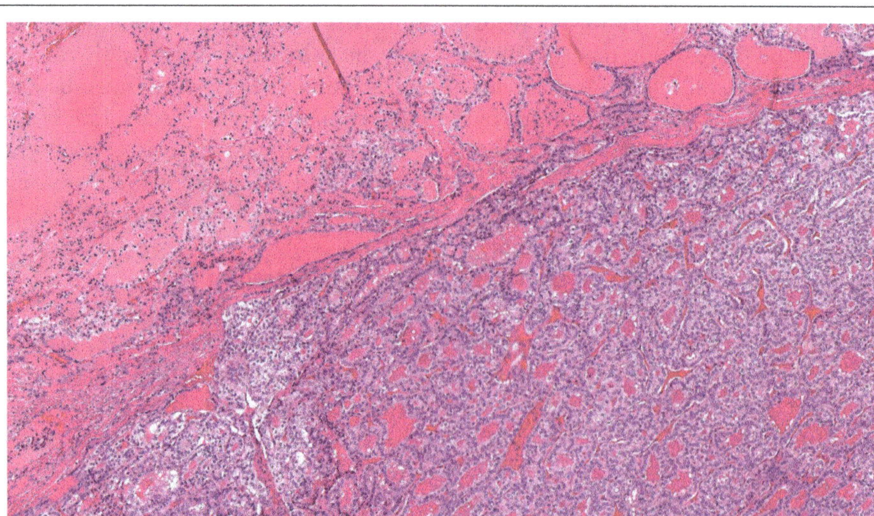

Fig. 1 Struma ovarii with papillary thyroid carcinoma (H&E 4X)

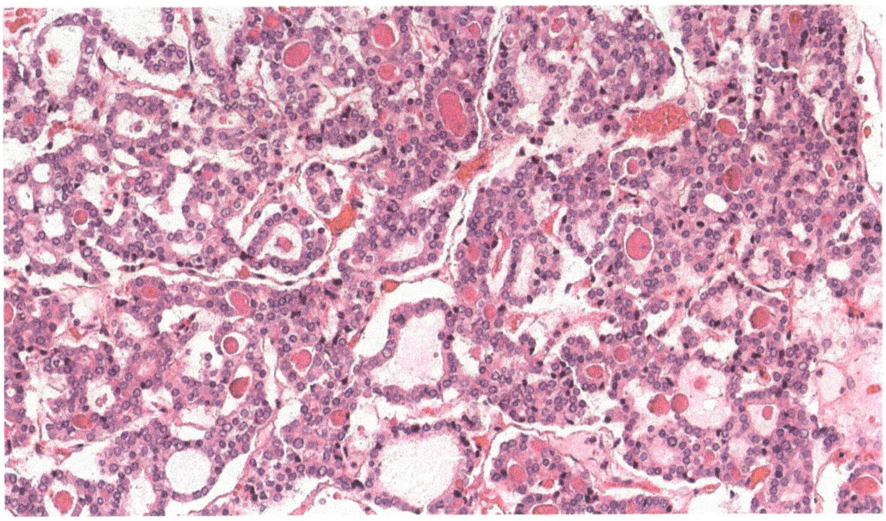

Fig. 2 Papillary thyroid carcinoma in ovary (H&E 20X)

uncommon, occurring in 5–23%, of cases and mostly contained within the abdomen [12, 13]. Long-term follow up is crucial, as recurrence rates range from 7.5 to 35% [4, 6, 8]. Fortunately, survival rates after malignant struma ovarii are high: 92–96.7% at 5-years, 85–94.3% at 10-years, 84.9% at 20-years, and 79% at 25 yrs [3, 14]. To date, there has been no evidence of metastasis in the current case and close follow-up will continue to ensure early detection of any potential recurrence.

The rarity of malignant struma ovarii has limited our understanding of the natural course of the disease and as such the best approach to treatment is unknown [9, 15]. Various treatment strategies have been suggested, but no diagnostic or treatment guidelines have been established [3, 4, 11].

An important consideration in treatment of struma ovarii, given its occurrence in a reproductive organ and often in a younger population, is the threat to fertility. While the most comprehensive treatment for malignant struma ovarii would be abdominal hysterectomy and bilateral salpingo-oophorectomy with omentectomy, some have cautioned against overtreatment given the significant implication of permanent infertility [3, 8, 11]. Gynecologic intervention in the case presented above was limited to a unilateral oophorectomy to preserve fertility [6, 11] in our 30 year-old nulliparous patient. A prophylactic contralateral procedure may be considered in the future should the preservation of fertility become unnecessary.

A particularly contentious issue in the treatment of struma ovarii has been at what point to consider the use of thyroidectomy and radioactive iodine ablation therapy. Some conservative approaches suggest that, in the absence of high-risk features, surgical resection of the ovarian tumor may be adequate [9] and that thyroidectomy and radioiodine therapy should be reserved for metastases or recurrent disease [14]. More aggressive recommendations have suggested thyroidectomy and ablation therapy for malignant struma ovarii tumors with the following characteristics: ≥ 1 cm [15], disease outside the ovary, or with aggressive histological features [8]. Further to that, Marcy et al. [5] have suggested thyroidectomy be mandatory and performed quickly following pelvic surgery to preclude potentially lethal metastatic outcomes.

Generally, thyroidectomy and radioablation iodine therapy appear to be well-accepted practices for malignant struma ovarii in the literature [6, 9]. Importantly, there is some evidence to suggest that aggressive therapy including radioablation may provide better long term outcomes in cases of malignant struma ovarii. DeSimone et al. [6] reviewed 24 cases of malignant struma ovarii and found those who had thyroidectomy and radioactive ablation had no recurrence of disease compared to 50% recurrence in those who had surgery alone. Management of the current case seems to be in keeping with previous cases [4, 9, 15]. We believe that care of our patient is greatly improved by involving an interdisciplinary team including Gynecologic-Oncology, Radiation-Oncology, Endocrinology, Pathology, and Otolaryngology-Head and Neck Surgery.

The phenomenon of thyroid cancer concurrent with malignant struma ovarii, as described in the current case, has been observed previously [3, 9, 16]. Leong et al. [9] hypothesized that early genomic instability may explain tumorgenesis in discrete sites of thyroid-type tissue and explain the different tissue histology between thyroid and ovary tumours. Similarly, it has been hypothesized that mutations in the BRAF gene may be responsible for the mutual pathogenesis for papillary thyroid cancers at distinct locations in the body [16]. Six of the ten individuals with a cancer diagnosis secondary to malignant struma ovarii were thyroid cancers as reported by Goffredo et al. [3]. The authors indicate that this is an above average proportion of thyroid malignancies compared to the general public and that these patients had more invasive disease than would typically be expected [3]. Taken together, it appears that malignant struma ovarii poses a significant risk of additional thyroid cancer and clinicians would be wise to investigate that possibility at their earliest opportunity.

In conclusion, though no guideline recommendations exist for management of malignant struma ovarii, a generally accepted approach involving thyroidectomy and radioactive iodine ablation is emerging. Based on our findings and reports in the literature we believe that aggressive surgical management followed by adjuvant radioiodine therapy is best to reduce recurrence risk and optimize survival. Gynecologic intervention was done cautiously to protect fertility in this young female patient. Physicians should be aware of the relationship between malignant struma ovarii and potential concomitant malignant disease in the thyroid.

Abbreviations
CK19: Cytokeratin 19; FDG: Fluorodeoxyglucose; mCi: Millicurie; PET: Positron emission tomography; TSH: Thyroid stimulating hormone

Acknowledgements
We would like to thank the patient described herein for agreeing to participate in this Case Report and for her contribution to medical literature on this subject.

Funding
Not applicable.

Authors' contributions
JCB, BAW, and RDH were responsible for literature review, synthesis of evidence, and editing of the manuscript. MHR, JRBT, and SMT provided expert advice on management of thyroid cancer and contributed to manuscript construction. KK provided expert advice on management of gynecologic cancer and contributed to manuscript construction. SO and HS performed histological examination of the ovarian and thyroid masses and contributed to manuscript construction. All authors read and approved the final manuscript.

Competing interests
The authors declare that they have no competing interests.

Consent for publication
The patient described in this report has given her express, informed consent for publication of this case and has completed our institutional consent form to that effect.

Author details
[1]Dalhousie Medical School, Dalhousie University, 5849 University Avenue, Halifax, NS B3H 4H7, Canada. [2]Division of Otolaryngology – Head and Neck Surgery, Department of Surgery, Dalhousie University, Halifax, NS, Canada. [3]Department of Obstetrics and Gynecology, Dalhousie University, Halifax, NS, Canada. [4]Department of Pathology, Dalhousie University, Halifax, NS, Canada.

References
1. Roth LM, Miller AW, Talerman A. Typical thyroid-type carcinoma arising in Struma ovarii: a report of 4 cases and review of the literature. Int J Gynecol Pathol. 2008;27(4):496–506.
2. Wirtz ED, Bothwell N, Klem C. Role of the otolaryngologist in the treatment of Struma ovarii. Laryngoscope. 2010;120:259–60.
3. Goffredo P, Sawka AM, Pura J, Adam MA, Roman SA, Sosa JA. Malignant Struma ovarii: a population-level analysis of a large series of 68 patients. Thyroid. 2015;25:211–5.
4. Marti JL, Clark VE, Harper H, Chhieng DC, Sosa JA, Roman SA. Optimal surgical management of well-differentiated thyroid cancer arising in Struma ovarii: a series of 4 patients and a review of 53 reported cases. Thyroid. 2012;22:400–6.
5. Marcy PY, Thariat J, Benisvy D, Azuar P. Lethal, malignant, metastatic Struma ovarii. Thyroid. 2010;20:1037–40.
6. DeSimone CP, Lele SM, Modesitt SC. Malignant Struma ovarii: a case report and analysis of cases reported in the literature with focus on survival and I131 therapy. Gynecol Oncol. 2003;89:543–8.
7. McGill JF, Sturgeon C, Angelos P. Metastatic Struma ovarii treated with total thyroidectomy and radioiodine ablation. Endocr Pract. 2009;15(2):167–73.
8. Yassa L, Sadow P, Marqusee E. Malignant Struma ovarii. Nat Clin Pract Endocrinol Metab. 2008;4:469–72.
9. Leong A, Roche PJ, Paliouras M, Rochon L, Trifiro M, Tamilia M. Coexistence of malignant Struma ovarii and cervical papillary thyroid carcinoma. J Clin Endocrinol Metab. 2013;98:4599–605.
10. Squire JA, Park PC, Yoshimoto M, Alami J, Williams JL, Evans A, et al. Prostate cancer as a model system for genetic diversity in tumors. Adv Cancer Res. 2011;112:183–216.
11. Brusca N, Del Duca SC, Salvatori R, D'Agostini A, Cannas P, Santaguida MG, et al. A case report of thyroid carcinoma confined to ovary and concurrently occult in the thyroid: is conservative treatment always advised? Int J Endocrinol Metab. 2015;13(1):e18220.
12. Makani S, Kim W, Gaba AR. Struma ovarii with a focus of papillary thyroid cancer: a case report and review of the literature. Gynecol Oncol. 2004;94:835–9.
13. McDougall IR, Krasne D, Hanbery JW, Collins JA. Metastatic malignant Struma ovarii presenting as paraparesis from a spinal metastasis. J Nucl Med. 1989;30(3):407–11.
14. Zhang X, Axiotis C. Thyroid-type carcinoma of Struma ovarii. Arch Pathol Lab Med. 2010;134:786–91.
15. Janszen EW, van Doorn HC, Ewing PC, de Krijger RR, de Wilt JH, Kam BL, et al. Malignant Struma ovarii: good response after thyroidectomy and I ablation therapy. Clin Med Oncol. 2008;2:147–52.
16. Schmidt J, Derr V, Heinrich MC, Crum CP, Fletcher JA, Corless CL, et al. BRAF in papillary thyroid carcinoma of ovary (Struma ovarii). Am J Surg Pathol. 2007;31(9):1337–43.

21

Ultrasound criteria for risk stratification of thyroid nodules in the previously iodine deficient area of Austria

Christina Tugendsam[1], Veronika Petz[2], Wolfgang Buchinger[3], Brigitta Schmoll-Hauer[1,4], Iris Pia Schenk[1,5], Karin Rudolph[1], Michael Krebs[1,6] and Georg Zettinig[1*]

Abstract

Background: We aimed to study the validity of six published ultrasound criteria for risk stratification of thyroid nodules in the former severely iodine deficient population of Austria.

Methods: Retrospective, single centre, observer blinded study design. All patients with a history of thyroidectomy due to nodules seen in the centre between 2004 and 2014 with preoperative in-house sonography and documented postoperative histology were analyzed ($n = 195$). A board of five experienced thyroidologists evaluated the images of 45 papillary carcinomas, 8 follicular carcinomas, and 142 benign nodules regarding the following criteria: mild hypoechogenicity, marked hypoechogenicity, microlobulated or irregular margins, microcalcifications, taller than wide shape, missing thin halo.

Results: All criteria but mild hypoechogenicity were significantly more frequent in thyroid cancer than in benign nodules. The number of positive criteria was significantly higher in cancer (2.79 ± 1.35) than in benign nodules (1.73 ± 1.18; $p < 0.001$). Thus, with a cut-off of two or more positive criteria, a sensitivity of 85% and a specificity of 45% were reached to predict malignancy in this sample of thyroid nodules. As expected, the findings were even more pronounced in papillary cancer only (2.98 ± 1.32 vs. 1.73 ± 1.18, $p < 0.001$). The six ultrasound criteria could not identify follicular cancer.

Conclusion: Our findings support the recently published EU-TIRADS score. Apart from mild hypoechogenicity, the analyzed ultrasound criteria can be applied for risk stratification of thyroid nodules in the previously severely iodine deficient population of Austria.

Keywords: TIRADS, Sonography, Ultrasound, Nodule, Hypoechogenicity, Microcalcifications, Halo

Background

Thyroid nodules are a common finding in any given population, with an estimated prevalence of 20-76% on ultrasound examination [1]. The vast majority of these nodules – regardless of whether they were initially palpable or incidental findings (e.g. upon carotid artery sonography) – are benign [2].

Therefore it is of high importance to discern truly benign thyroid nodules from those at higher risk [3]. Thyroid cancer is a tumor entity with steep increase in incidence, albeit with the majority of new cases belonging to the group of low risk tumor stages [4]. How to select the thyroid nodules for further assessment by fine needle aspiration is currently still a matter of debate [5]. Especially with the widespread use of high resolution neck ultrasound, many thyroid nodules are detected as incidentalomas [1, 2].

There is no typical sonographic pattern of thyroid cancer. Various sonographic criteria have been proposed to estimate the risk of malignancy in thyroid nodules. In 2009, two different proposals for a so-called TIRADS

* Correspondence: georg.zettinig@meduniwien.ac.at
[1]Schilddruesenpraxis Josefstadt, Laudongasse 12/8, Vienna AT-1080, Austria
Full list of author information is available at the end of the article

scoring system based on ultrasound nodule patterns were published [6, 7]. The concept was inspired by the widely used BIRADS system for assessing breast lesions, but partly been criticized for its complexity. It is still under debate whether this system can easily be applied to routine clinical use [5], and several modifications have been proposed during the last years [8–10].

In August 2017, the European Thyroid Association Guidelines for Ultrasound Malignancy Risk Stratification of Thyroid Nodules in Adults have been published [11]. Prior to this, the British Thyroid Association has published ultrasound features indicative of malignant nodule in its Guidelines for the management of thyroid cancer in 2014 [12], and the American Thyroid Association presented sonographic patterns suspicious for thyroid cancer in their 2015 guidelines [13], leading to some modifications of the Korean Thyroid Association guidelines in 2016 [14].

A number of studies evaluated the sensitivity and specificity of various criteria in patient samples from e.g. Korea [8, 15, 16], France [9, 10], or Poland [17]. We selected the following six criteria: mild hypoechogenicity [7–9, 11, 12], marked hypoechogenicity [7–9, 11, 12], microlobulated or irregular margins [7, 8, 9, 11, 12,], microcalcifications [7–9, 11, 12], taller than wide shape [7–9, 11, 12], and the absence of a thin halo [7, 12].

The presence of two or more of the six ultrasound criteria mild hypoechogenicity, marked hypoechogenicity, microlobulated or irregular margins, microcalcifications, taller than wide shape, and a solid component have been proposed to identify nodules at risk in a large Korean study evaluating more than 1600 patients including follow-up data which was the basis for the TIRADS Kwak score [8]. In the TIRADS French score system the four criteria irregular shape, irregular margins, microcalcifications, and marked hypoechogenicity are classified as highly suspect whereas mild hypoechogenicity in the absence of any of the four high suspicious features is the criterion for intermediate risk [11].

Comparable to France and several other European countries, Austria has been a moderately to even severely iodine depleted area with a high prevalence of endemic goiter, functional autonomies and cretinism, especially in the alp regions, for a long time [18]. In Austria, table salt has been iodized by federal law since 1963. The initial concentration of 10 mg KI per kg salt was increased to 20 mg/kg in 1990 when urine iodine secretion was still found to be in the mildly deficient range, currently it is 15-20 mg/kg. This strategy proved to be successful in greatly reducing the incidence of the above mentioned consequences of iodine deficiency [19].

Yet recent data indicate that iodine intake is still insufficient in at least part of the Austrian population, especially in pregnant women [20]. Due to decreased intake of table salt (as advocated for preventing hypertension) and the widespread use of not iodinated industrial salt, iodine intake might be insufficient even in the general population [20, 21].

The aim of our study was to assess six ultrasound criteria indicating thyroid cancer mainly published in the TIRADS Kwak score [8] and the TIRADS French score [9, 10] in the former iodine deficient Greater Vienna area. The study was conducted as a single centre, retrospective analysis of all nodules with postoperative histologic data available over the time course of 10 years (2004-2014). Five blinded experts rated the sonographic images according to the presence of published criteria. Diagnostic values of these criteria were then determined and compared to the published literature.

Methods

Setting and Study sample

The thyroid centre "Schilddruesenpraxis Josefstadt" is the largest private thyroid centre in Vienna and has been founded in 2004. We analysed all patients who were seen in this secondary care centre between October 2004 and December 2014 and identified all patients with the diagnosis of "history of thyroidectomy". Among these 491 patients, 47 were operated due to Graves' disease and excluded from analysis. There were 91 patients with thyroid cancer and 353 with benign thyroid nodules. Of the 444 patients seen postoperatively, 223 had preoperative thyroid sonography at the centre. From this sample another 28 patients were excluded due to the following reasons: poor image quality (12), very small microcarcinoma (14), original histological data not available (2).

Thus the initial study sample consisted of 195 patients: 45 papillary thyroid carcinomas (PTC), 8 follicular thyroid carcinomas (FTC), and 142 benign nodules (BN). Considering the medical history of each patient, the two unblinded investigators (GZ and VP) assigned all preoperative ultrasound images either to the thyroid cancer group or to the benign nodules group and anonymized all ultrasound images using the individual patient numbers given to all patients at the initial visit at the centre. GZ also selected the nodule that led to surgery in all patients with multinodular goitre. Images were available as electronic files since 2009, and before 2009 as prints.

Retrospective expert review of the ultrasound images

Five experienced Austrian thyroidologists (CT, WB, BSH, KR, MK) met in April 2016 to review all preoperative sonographic patterns in a single session. They all have their focus on treating thyroid patients for many years, and their experience in thyroid sonography is up to 27 years.

Table 1 Detailed characteristics of the subgroups

	BN	PTC	FTC
Females	127/142 (89%)	36/45 (80%)	6/8 (75%)
Age (mean ± SD)	49 ± 11 years	42 ± 12 years	36 ± 11 years
Date of birth after 1 January 1963	63/142 (44%)	36/45 (80%)	6/8 (75%)
Maximum diameter of the nodule (mean ± SD)	28 ± 11 mm	20 ± 12 mm	31 ± 7 mm

The experts reviewed each nodule regarding the presence or absence of six ultrasound criteria given below. In a second step, they ranked the nodule as benign or malignant. Each expert wrote his or her assessment in an evaluation form (criterion 1-6 present or absent, nodule benign or malignant). Thereafter, the experts decided on the presence or absence of all six criteria and categorized the nodule as benign or malignant together. In case of disagreement between the experts, consensus was reached by discussion.

Definition of ultrasound criteria of suspicion

The study was designed to evaluate the presence or absence of the following six criteria:

Mild hypoechogenicity

The nodule was classified as mildly hypoechogenic if the echogenicity was less than the thyroid parenchyma but more than the surrounding strap muscle.

Marked hypoechogenicity

The nodule was classified as marked hypoechogenic if the echogenicity was less than that of the surrounding strap muscle.

Microlobulated or irregular margins

The margin had many small lobules on the surface of a nodule or was infiltrative.

Microcalcifications

Defined as calcifications that were equal to or less than 1 mm in diameter and visualized as tiny punctate hyperechoic foci, either with or without acoustic shadows.

Taller than wide shape

The nodule was greater in its anteroposterior dimension than in its transverse dimension.

No thin halo

Absence of a thin hypoechoic rim around the nodule.

In partly cystic lesions, always the solid component was evaluated. Mild hypoechogenicity excluded marked hypoechogenicity and vice versa. Therefore, a maximum number of five criteria were possible in a single nodule.

Statistics

Demographic data and nodule size are presented as mean ± standard deviation (SD). We compared them by chi-square statistics for categorical data and unpaired students t-test for continuous variables. The number of positive criteria was added for all nodules resulting in a minimum score of 0 and a maximum of 5 positive criteria (with mild hypoechogenicity and marked hypoechogenicity being mutually exclusive). Mean number of positive criteria in benign versus malignant lesions were compared by unpaired student's t-test. A $p < 0.05$ was considered statistically significant. One-way ANOVA, followed by multiple t-tests with Bonferroni correction as post-hoc test (if appropriate), was used to compare mean numbers of positive criteria in the three subgroups of BN, PTC, and FTC.

The ability of the six ultrasound criteria to significantly discriminate between benign and malignant lesions was assessed by chi-square tests with Bonferroni correction for multiple testing. Thus, a *p*-value of < 0.0083 (0.05/6) was considered statistically significant.

Additionally the diagnostic values sensitivity, specificity, positive and negative predictive values (together with their respective 95% intervals) for each parameter and the expert opinion were calculated to predict the

Table 2 Chi-square statistics: Number (%) of positive criteria - BN versus cancer

BN vs. cancer:	BN	Cancer	X^2	*p*-value
Mild hypoechogenicity	55/142 (39%)	19/53 (36%)	0.136	0.712
Marked hypoechogenicity	26/142 (18%)	22/53 (42%)	11.194	0.001
Microlobulated/ irregular margins	39/142 (27%)	29/53 (55%)	12.621	0.0004
Microcalcifications	10/142 (7%)	16/53 (30%)	17.894	0.00002
Taller than wide	17/142 (12%)	15/53 (28%)	7.503	0.006
No thin halo	99/142 (70%)	47/53 (89%)	7.375	0.007

Table 3 Chi-square statistics: Number (%) of positive criteria - BN versus PTC

BN vs.PTC:	BN	PTC	X^2	*p*-value
Mild hypoechogenicity	55/142 (39%)	17/45 (38%)	0.013	0.909
Marked hypoechogenicity	26/142 (18%)	20/45 (44%)	12.583	0.0004
Microlobulated/ irregular margins	39/142 (27%)	27/45 (60%)	15.839	0.00007
Microcalcifications	10/142 (7%)	15/45 (33%)	20.394	0.00001
Taller than wide	17/142 (12%)	15/45 (33%)	10.993	0.001
No thin halo	99/142 (70%)	40/45 (89%)	6.582	0.010

risk of cancer and PTC. The same diagnostic values were also calculated to compare the risk of malignancy in nodules with less than 2 vs. 2 or more criteria and less than 3 vs. 3 or more criteria, respectively. Statistical analysis was performed using SPSS Version 24 statistic software package.

Results

Demographic characteristics

Patients with cancer were significantly younger compared to the BN group (41 ± 11.9 vs. 49 ± 11.4 years; $p < 0.001$), and there was a lower rate of females among the cancer patients (79% vs. 89%, $p = 0.063$). An overview of the demographic characteristics of the subgroups (BN, PTC, FTC) is given in Table 1. PTC were significantly smaller than the nodules from the other groups.

The study sample included 103 patients (53%) born after 1963 (the year when iodization of table salt became mandatory in Austria). All but one patient were born before 1990 (when iodine content of table salt was increased from 10 to 20 mg/kg salt).

Ultrasound criteria

Of the investigated malignancy suspicious criteria, all but mild hypoechogenicity were statistically different between benign and malignant lesions when compared by chi-square statistics. When comparing subgroups, the criterion no thin halo reached only borderline significance to predict PTC after Bonferroni correction for multiple comparisons ($p = 0.01$). Table 2 and 3 provide a detailed overview. Noteworthy, 23% of the carcinomas were isoechogenic.

The sensitivity, specificity, positive predictive value, and negative predictive value of each of the six criteria is given in Table 4 and 5 for both analyses (BN vs. cancer and the subgroup analysis). Sensitivity for the criterion no thin halo was 89%, all other criteria showed sensitivities of 60% and less. Several criteria showed a specificity of > 80%, whereas the most sensitive criterion no thin halo showed a specificity of only 30%.

Mean number of positive criteria

Mean number of positive criteria were statistically different between BN and cancer (1,73 ± 1,18 versus 2,79 ± 1,35, respectively; $p < 0.001$, unpaired student's t-test). There was also a significant difference between the three subgroups BN, PTC, and FTC ($p < 0.001$, one-way ANOVA). In the post-hoc tests (multiple t-tests with Bonferroni correction), PTC were statistically significantly different from BN ($p < 0.001$) as well as from FTC ($p = 0.026$), while mean number of criteria were comparable in BN and FTC. See Table 6 for details.

Calculated sums of positive criteria

Three out of 45 PTC (6.6%) did not show any of the criteria published in the literature. Of those, two were T1b and one was T1a. All three were labelled benign by the expert panel.

With a cut-off value of two or more positive criteria, 45 out of 53 malignant lesions (89%) were labelled correctly and 78 out of 142 benign lesions (55%) incorrectly as cancer. Thus, this cut-off resulted in a sensitivity of 89%[76-96], specificity of 45%[37-55], PPV of

Table 4 Diagnostic parameters for cancer

Cancer	Sensitivity	Specificity	PPV	NPV
Mild hypoechogenicity	36%	61%	26%	72%
Marked hypoechogenicity	42%	82%	46%	79%
Microlobulated/ irregular margins	55%	73%	43%	81%
Microcalcifications	30%	93%	62%	78%
Taller than wide	28%	88%	47%	77%
No thin halo	89%	30%	32%	88%

Table 5 Diagnostic parameters for PTC

PTC	Sensitivity	Specificity	PPV	NPV
Mild Hypoechogenicity	38%	61%	24%	76%
Marked hypoechogenicity	44%	82%	44%	82%
Microlobulated/ irregular margins	60%	73%	41%	85%
Microcalcifications	33%	93%	60%	82%
Taller than wide	33%	88%	47%	81%
No thin halo	89%	30%	29%	90%

Table 6 Mean number of positive ultrasound criteria in BN and in all cancer patients as well as in the subgroups of PTC and FTC

	BN (n = 142)	Cancer (n = 53)	PTC (n = 45)	FTC (n = 8)
Mean number of criteria	1.73 ± 1.18	2.79 ± 1.35*	2.98 ± 1.32*	1.75 ± 1.04 **

* BN vs. Cancer: p < 0.001
* PTC vs. BN: p < 0.001, PTC vs. FTC: p = 0.026
** FTC vs. BN: p > 0.99, FTC vs. PTC: p = 0.026

34%[30-38], and NPV of 93%[85-97] to detect cancer based on ultrasound criteria when compared to benign lesions.

When increasing the threshold to three or more criteria, correct assignment of cancer to benign decreased while incorrect labelling of benign lesions as cancer dropped. See Tables 7, 8, 9, and 10 for details for both the PTC as well as the cancer group.

With this criterion, 16 nodules with a postoperative diagnosis of PTC were rated as benign. Those nodules were staged pT1a (7 nodules), pT1a(m) (2 nodules), pT1b (5 nodules), pT2 (1 nodule), pT3 (1 nodule).

Pooled expert opinion

The experts diagnosed cancer with a specificity of 84%[76-90] and a sensitivity of 52%[38-65]. PPV was 58%[47-69] and NPV 80%[75-84]. The diagnostic values of the pooled expert opinion for PTC were: sensitivity 64%[49-78], specificity 78%[70-85], PPV 48%[39-58], NPV 87%[82-91]. Of the 16 PTC falsely labelled as benign by the experts staging was pT1a in 7, pT1b in 5, pT1b(m) in 1, and pT3 in 1 lesion. 6 fulfilled 3 or more positive ultrasound criteria. On the other hand experts rated 7 lesions fulfilling only 2 ultrasound criteria correctly as carcinomas. 8 lesions were missed by both methods (5 fulfilling 1 and 3 fulfilling 2 ultrasound criteria).

Discussion

In light of the widespread use of ultrasonography and frequent findings of thyroid incidentalomas, strategies that systematically and reliably identify those thyroid nodules with a higher risk of malignancy are highly warranted.

In iodine deficient areas like Austria the spectrum of thyroid malignancies differs from iodine sufficient areas with a relatively higher proportion of follicular carcinomas and the occurrence of anaplastic carcinomas in multinodular goiters (which almost disappeared after the introduction of iodization of table salt) [22].

We therefore conducted a retrospective analysis of sonographic images from thyroid nodules with available postoperative histological data from Austrian patients (mainly from Vienna and surroundings). Since the published sonographic criteria relate to papillary carcinomas only, we also calculated a statistical analysis restricted to PTC vs. benign lesions.

At the time the study was designed, several criteria were repeatedly studied and published [7–9, 12]. According to previously published reports, we analyzed mild hypoechogenicity, marked hypoechogenicity, microlobulated or irregular margins, microcalcifications, and a taller than wide shape. As retrospective assessment of the composition of a nodule (solid, mainly solid, mainly cystic) in two dimensional images seemed problematic to us, we decided not to include this criterion in our analysis. These five criteria are also among the proposals for the TIRADS French [9] and the recently published EU-TIRADS scoring system [11] and are included in the system proposed in the recently published ATA 2015 guidelines [13]. Due to the rather small sample size, however, we decided to restrict our analysis to applying the most widely used criteria without applying a formal scoring system. In addition, we evaluated the absence of a thin perinodular halo. There is no hard evidence from studies, but the halo sign traditionally has been regarded as an important ultrasound sign for the risk stratification of thyroid nodules in central Europe [23, 24] and is still discussed as a suggested feature for thyroid cancer in several diagnostic algorithms [12, 25, 26]. Noteworthy, the halo sign has also recently been discussed also in the European Thyroid Association Guidelines for Ultrasound Malignancy Risk Stratification of Thyroid Nodules in Adults [11] and is one of the nine sonographic features initially identified in the white paper

Table 7 Chi-square statistics of calculated sums of positive criteria – BN vs. cancer

BN vs. cancer	BN	Cancer	X^2	p-value
≥1 criterion	120/142 (85%)	49/53 (93%)	2.10869	0.14646
≥2 criteria	78/142 (55%)	45/53 (85%)	14.89056	0.00011
≥3 criteria	36/142 (25%)	31/53 (59%)	18.79224	0.00001
≥4 criteria	10/142 (7%)	19/53 (36%)	25.29781	0.0000005
5 criteria	2/142 (1%)	4/53 (8%)	4.87687	0.02722

Table 8 Chi-square statistics of calculated sums of positive criteria – BN vs. PTC

BN vs. PTC	BN	PTC	X^2	p-value
≥1 criterion	120/142 (85%)	42/45 (93%)	2.29850	0.12950
≥2 criteria	78/142 (55%)	40/45 (89%)	16.92502	0.00004
≥3 criteria	36/142 (25%)	29/45 (64%)	23.02780	0.000002
≥4 criteria	10/142 (7%)	19/45 (42%)	32.27589	0.00000001
5 criteria	2/142 (1%)	4/45 (9%)	6.15697	0.01309

Table 9 Sensitivity, specificity, PPV, and NPV of the number of criteria for cancer

Cancer	≥1 criterion	≥2 criteria	≥3 criteria	≥4 criteria	5 criteria
Sensitivity	93%	85%	59%	36%	8%
Specificity	16%	45%	75%	93%	99%
PPV	29%	37%	46%	66%	67%
NPV	85%	89%	83%	80%	74%

of the ACR TIRADS Committee [26]. Our findings indicate that the absence of a thin halo is also helpful for the diagnosis of thyroid cancer, at least in the former severely iodine depleted population of Austria.

Overall we found a good accordance of the published risk markers with the lesions evaluated in this sample. Our findings support the validity of the TIRADS Kwak criteria [8], the ATA 2015 criteria [13] as well as the TIRADS French [10] and the EU-TIRADS [11] criteria for the former severely iodine deficient area of Austria. One notable exception is the criterion of mild hypoechogenicity. In contrast to marked hypoechogenicity, mild hypoechogenicity could not discriminate between benign and malignant lesions in our sample. This is different to TIRADS Kwak [8]. ATA 2015 does not discriminate between mild and marked hypoechogenicity. In EU-TIRADS, mild hypoechogenicity indicates intermediate risk but no high risk for thyroid cancer [11], indicating that also in the previously iodine deficient population of France, mild hypoechogenicity is not that strict criterion for malignancy as in iodine sufficient regions such as Korea.

There are several possible reasons for this finding. Firstly, all the nodules included in this sample were considered to be reason enough to operate on the patient. Reasons leading to the operation decision were not systematically recorded, but included suspicious results in fine needle aspiration, nodule size, local complaints, patient's wish, and also suspicion of malignancy in ultrasound. Thus, unambiguously benign lesions were underrepresented or (e.g. simple cysts) even absent from the study sample.Yet another possible reason for this finding is the effect of iodine deficiency that might results in changes in thyroid tissue that are only partially reversible upon iodine supplementation. In a large French sample (France being a formerly iodine deficient region), mild hypoechogenicity conferred only intermediate risk for thyroid cancer [27], in contrast to the iodine sufficient region of Korea.

Table 10 Sensitivity, specificity, PPV, and NPV of the number of criteria for PTC

PTC	≥1 criterion	≥2 criteria	≥3 criteria	≥4 criteria	5 criteria
Sensitivity	93%	89%	64%	42%	9%
Specificity	16%	45%	75%	93%	99%
PPV	26%	34%	45%	66%	67%
NPV	88%	93%	87%	84%	77%

Of note, 48% of the patients included in the study were born before the year 1963, when iodization of table salt was introduced in Austria and therefore spent at least parts of their early lives in severe iodine deficiency. Only one of the patients was born after 1990 when iodization of table salt in Austria was doubled to 20 mg/kg, because iodine supplementation was still considered insufficient [27]. The different iodine status in Austria and France could also be the explanation mild hypoechogenicity being classified as an intermediate risk factor in the TIRADS French study, but not discriminating in our sample.

A third European country with former iodine deficiency is Poland [28]. Recently an evaluation of four TIRADS classification systems in Polish multinodular goiter patients was published suggesting TIRADS Kwak as a suitable and practicable tool for this patient group. [17].

There is no single ultrasound feature which could reliably distinguish benign from malignant lesions. Some markers (e.g. microcalcifications) have a high specificity but insufficient sensitivity and vice versa. Thus, the combination of several features enhances the diagnostic value of sonography. In a recent Korean study [15], performed on a very large sample of thyroid nodules 10-19 mm in size, a head to head comparison of six risk stratification systems proposed in the literature was performed and yielded, as would be expected, different diagnostic values. Application of TIRADS French (using the number of positive criteria with a cut-off of two or more criteria being present for proposing fine needle aspiration) resulted in a sensitivity of 95% and a specificity of 52%, respectively. In the sample presented here, the cut-off value of two or more positive criteria for PTC resulted in a roughly comparable diagnostic performance (with slightly lower sensitivity of 89% and specificity of 45%). Other stratification systems resulted in even higher sensitivity at the cost of lower specificity.

On the other hand, the pooled expert estimation of malignancy risk yielded sensitivity and specificity very similar to the 3 criteria cut-off condition. Thus, 35% of PTC were mislabelled as benign from the expert panel (although the PTC misjudged as benign were all but one postoperatively staged as pT1).

The experts diagnosed cancer with a specificity of 84%, but the sensitivity was only 52%. For the diagnosis of PTC, the expert's sensitivity of 64% was only slightly higher. These findings indicate that in real life setting, the accurate differential diagnosis of nodules still remains difficult. Our five thyroidologists, who have long-time experience in interpreting thyroid ultrasound, did not predict malignancy accurately. Using a number of at least two positive ultrasound criteria to define the risk of malignancy yields a higher sensitivity but a lower specificity than expert judgement.

Our findings suggest that mild hypoechogenicity should be clearly differentiated from marked hypoechogenicity. The role of mild hypoechogenicity as a malignancy marker has to be clarified in relation to iodine status: In the sample studied here, in opposition to marked hypoechogenicity - which was significantly more frequent in PTC - mild hypoechogenicity didn't even show a trend towards higher frequency in PTC. On the other hand, the absence of a thin halo added diagnostic value in the sample presented here and might be worthy of consideration when evaluating nodules for possible malignancy.

The 2015 American Thyroid Association Management Guidelines for Adult Patients with Thyroid Nodules and Differentiated Thyroid Cancer [13] have been published after a long debate including a revised concept for ultrasonographic risk stratification of thyroid nodules. These guidelines do not distinguish between mild and marked hypoechogenicity. Hypoechogenic solid nodules without other risk patterns are classified as intermediately suspicious with a malignancy risk of 10-20%. In our study sample, however, the criterion hypoechogenicity was not found more often in cancer than in benign lesions.

The six criteria were not helpful for diagnosing follicular cancer. As presented in Table 6, the mean number of ultrasound criteria of FTC did not differ from BN, but from PTC. In these patients, the "nodule in nodule sign" could be a criterion for future studies [29]. If, as sometimes is suggested, the scintigraphic pattern (with reduced versus isointense activity) would be helpful in risk stratification of those nodules, is currently unclear. The sample did not include any patient with medullary thyroid cancer. Most probably this is because in Vienna nearly all patients with medullary thyroid cancer are followed up in a single tertiary centre after surgery.

Strengths of the study include the assessment by five thyroid experts in a systematic way and the availability of histological data of all the included nodules. Limitations of the study include the retrospective study design, that only B-mode images were used, the lack of information on the actual iodine status of the patients, the rather small sample size and the single center study design.

Conclusions

In conclusion, we report validity of published ultrasound malignancy risk markers of thyroid nodules in the formerly severely iodine deficient area of Austria for the first time. Our findings support the EU-TIRADS scoring system. With the exception of hypoechogenicity, ultrasound criteria as described in the literature were applicable with good sensitivity for risk adjustment of thyroid nodules in this secondary care setting. Additionally, the missing halo sign was a sensitive malignancy marker in this sample, which might be useful in a screening setting.

Abbreviations

BN: Benign nodules; FTC: Follicular thyroid cancer; PTC: Papillyry thyroid cancer; SD: Standard deviation

Authors' contributions

CT was involved in the study design, analysis, and writing of the manuscript, and reviewed all preoperative sonographic patterns. VP collected the data and was involved in the study design and analysis. WB reviewed all preoperative sonographic patterns and was involved in the study design and writing of the manuscript. BSH and KR reviewed all preoperative sonographic patterns. IPS was involved in collecting the data. MK was involved in the study design, analysis, and writing of the manuscript, and reviewed all preoperative sonographic patterns. GZ was involved in the study design, analysis, and writing of the manuscript, and reviewed all preoperative sonographic patterns. All authors read and approved the final manuscript.

Consent for publication

All authors gave their approval for the final version to be published and agree to be accountable for this work.

Competing interests

The authors declare that they have no competing interests.

Author details

[1]Schilddruesenpraxis Josefstadt, Laudongasse 12/8, Vienna AT-1080, Austria. [2]Division of Nuclear Medicine, Department of Biomedical Imaging and Image-guided Therapy, Medical University of Vienna, Vienna, Austria. [3]Schilddrueseninstitut Gleisdorf, Gleisdorf, Austria. [4]Department of Nuclear Medicine, Krankenanstalt Rudolfstiftung, Vienna, Austria. [5]Department of Nuclear Medicine, Sozialmedizinisches Zentrum Hietzing, Vienna, Austria. [6]Clinical Division of Endocrinology, Department of Medicine III, Medical University of Vienna, Vienna, Austria.

References

1. Russ G, Leboulleux S, Leenhardt L, Hegedues L. Thyroid incidentalomas: epidemiology, risk stratification with ultrasound and workup. Eur Thyroid J. 2014;3:154–63.
2. Buchinger W, Petnehazy E, Pap A, Kaserer K, Zettinig G. Der Schilddrüsenfall: Leitliniengerechte Knotenabklärung. J Klin Endokrinol Stoffw. 2016;9:16–17.
3. Zafon C, Díez JJ, Galofré JC, Cooper DS. Nodular Thyroid Disease and Thyroid Cancer in the Era of Precision Medicine. Eur Thyroid J. 2017;6:65–74.
4. Lim H, Devesa SS, Sosa JA, Check D, Kitahara CM. Trends in Thyroid Cancer Incidence and Mortality in the United States, 1974-2013. JAMA. 2017;317:1338–48.
5. Negro R, Attanasio R, Grimaldi F, Frasoldati A, Guglielmi R, Papini E. A 2016 Italian Survey about Guidelines and Clinical Management of Thyroid Nodules. Eur Thyroid J. 2017;6:75–81.
6. Horvath E, Majlis S, Rossi R, Franco C, Niedmann JP, Castro A, Dominguez M. An ultrasonogram reporting system for thyroid nodules stratifying cancer risk for clinical management. J Clin Endocrinol Metab. 2009;94:1748–51.
7. Park JY, Lee HJ, Jang HW, Kim HK, Yi JH, Lee W, Kim SH. A proposal for a thyroid imaging reporting and data system for ultrasound features of thyroid carcinoma. Thyroid. 2009;19:1257–64.

8. Kwak JY, Han KH, Yoon JH, Moon HJ, Son EJ, Park SH, Jung HK, Choi JS, Kim BM, Kim EK. Thyroid imaging reporting and data system for US features of nodules: a step in establishing better stratification of cancer risk. Radiology. 2011;260:892–9.
9. Russ G, Royer B, Bigorgne C, Rouxel A, Bienvenu-Perrard M, Leenhardt L. Prospective evaluation of thyroid imaging reporting and data system on 4550 nodules with and without elastography. Eur J Endocrinol. 2013; 168:649–55.
10. Russ G, Bigorgne C, Royer B, Rouxel A, Bienvenu-Perrard M. Le système TIRADS en échographie thyroïdienne. J Radiol. 2011;92:701–13.
11. Russ G, Bonnema SJ, Erdogan MF, Durante C, Ngu R, Leenhardt L. European Thyroid Association Guidelines for Ultrasound Malignancy Risk Stratification of Thyroid Nodules in Adults: The EU-TIRADS. Eur Thyroid J. 2017;6:225–37.
12. Perros P, Colley S, Boelaert K, Evans C, Evans RM, Gerrard GE, Gilbert JA, Harrison B, Johnson SJ, Giles TE, Moss L, Lewington V, Newbold KL, Taylor J, Thakker RV, Watkinson J, Williams GR. British Thyroid Association Guidelines for the Management of Thyroid Cancer. Clin Endocrinol. 2014;81(1):1–122.
13. Haugen BR, Alexander EK, Bible KC, Doherty GM, Mandel SJ, Nikiforov YE, Pacini F, Randolph GW, Sawka AM, Schlumberger M, Schuff KG, Sherman SI, Sosa JA, Steward DL, Tuttle RM, Wartofsky L. 2015 American Thyroid Association Management Guidelines for Adult Patients with Thyroid Nodules and Differentiated Thyroid Cancer: The American Thyroid Association Guidelines Task Force on Thyroid Nodules and Differentiated Thyroid Cancer. Thyroid. 2016;26:1–133.
14. Yi HK. The Revised 2016 Korean Thyroid Association Guidelines for Thyroid Nodules and Cancers: Differences from the 2015 American Thyroid Association Guidelines. Endocrinol Metab (Seoul). 2016;31:373–8.
15. Yoon JH, Han K, Kim EK, Moon HJ, Kwak JY. Diagnosis and Management of Small Thyroid Nodules: A Comparative Study with Six Guidelines for Thyroid Nodules. Radiology. 2017;283:560–9.
16. Yoon JH, Lee HS, Kim EK, Moon HJ, Kwak JY. Malignancy Risk Stratification of Thyroid Nodules: Comparison between the Thyroid Imaging Reporting and Data System and the 2014 American Thyroid Association Management Guidelines. Radiology. 2016;278:917–24.
17. Migda B, Migda M, Migda AM, Bierca J, Slowniska-Srzednicka J, Jakubowski W, Slapa RZ. Evaluation of Four Variants of the Thyroid Imaging Reporting and Data System (TIRADS) Classification in Patients with Multinodular Goiter. Endokrynol Pol. 2018;69:142–9.
18. Weissel M. Legal augmentation of iodine content in table salt from 10 to 20 mg KI/kg: documented effects a decade later. Exp Clin Endocrinol Diabetes. 2003;111:187–90.
19. Heinisch M, Kumnig G, Asböck D, Mikosch P, Gallowitsch HJ, Kresnik E, Gomez I, Unterweger O, Lind P. Goiter prevalence and urinary iodide excretion in a formerly iodine-deficient region after introduction of statutory Iodization of common salt. Thyroid. 2002;12:809–14.
20. Lindorfer H, Krebs M, Kautzky-Willer A, Bancher-Todesca D, Sager M, Gessl A. Iodine deficiency in pregnant women in Austria. Eur J Clin Nutr. 2015; 69:349–54.
21. Buchinger W, Lorenz-Wawschinek O, Semlitsch G, Langsteger W, Binter G, Bonelli RM, Eber O. Thyrotropin and thyroglobulin as an index of optimal iodine intake: correlation with iodine excretion of 39,913 euthyroid patients. Thyroid. 1997;7:593–7.
22. Passler C, Scheuba C, Prager G, Kaczirek K, Kaserer K, Zettinig G, Niederle B. Prognostic factors of papillary and follicular thyroid cancer: differences in an iodine-replete endemic goiter region. Endocr Relat Cancer. 2004;11:131–9.
23. Zettinig G, Buchinger W, Gessl A. Schilddruesen Ultraschall Kursbuch. 1st ed. Vienna: facultas.wuv; 2013. p. 50–1.
24. Dietlein M, Kobe C, Schmidt M, Schicha H. The incidentaloma of the thyroid. Over- or underuse of diagnostic procedure for an epidemiologic finding? Nuklearmedizin. 2005;44:213–24.
25. Andrioli M, Carzaniga C, Persani L. Standardized Ultrasound Report for Thyroid Nodules: The Endocrinologist's Viewpoint. Eur Thyroid J. 2013;2:37–48.
26. Grant EG, Tessler FN, Hoang JK, Langer JE, Beland MD, Berland LL, Cronan JJ, Desser TS, Frates MC, Hamper UM, Middleton WD, Reading CC, Scoutt LM, Stavros AT, Teefey SA. Thyroid Ultrasound Reporting Lexicon: White Paper of the ACR Thyroid Imaging, Reporting and Data System (TIRADS) Committee. J Am Coll Radiol. 2015;12:1272–9.
27. Lind P, Kumnig G, Heinisch M, Igerc I, Mikosch P, Gallowitsch HJ, Kresnik E, Gomez I, Unterweger O, Aigner H. Iodine supplementation in Austria: methods and results. Thyroid. 2002;12:903–7.
28. Zygmunt A, Lewinski A. Iodine prophylaxis in pregnant women in Poland - where we are? (update 2015). Thyroid Res. 2015;8:17.
29. Kobayashi K, Ota H, Hirokawa M, Yabuta T, Fukushima M, Masuoka H, Higashiyama T, Kihara M, Ito Y, Miya A, Miyauchi A. "Nodule in Nodule" on Thyroid Ultrasonography. Possibility of Follicular Carcinoma Transformed from Benign Thyroid Tumor. Eur Thyroid J. 2017;6:101–7.

Metastatic carcinoma to the thyroid gland from renal cell carcinoma: role of ultrasonography in preoperative diagnosis

Kaoru Kobayashi*, Mitsuyoshi Hirokawa, Tomonori Yabuta, Mitsuhiro Fukushima, Hiroo Masuoka, Takuya Higashiyama, Minoru Kihara, Yasuhiro Ito, Akihiro Miya, Nobuyuki Amino and Akira Miyauchi

Abstract

Background: Patients with metastases to the thyroid from renal cell carcinoma (RCC) that need surgical management are not many and unfamiliar to clinicians and thyroid endocrinologists. Therefore, little information is available on ultrasonographic features of metastatic carcinoma in the thyroid. The strategic value of ultrasound in preoperative surgical planning for patients with thyroid nodules has become increasingly appreciated. The purposes of this article are to clarify the ultrasound characteristics of metastatic carcinoma to the thyroid from RCC by evaluating many patients in one institute, and to investigate the role of ultrasonography in preoperative diagnosis.

Methods: Ten patients with these carcinomas who had undergone surgical management were investigated clinically and ultrasonographically. Ultrasonographic features to be evaluated were the form of involvement in the thyroid, size, shape, pattern, calcifications, vascularity, and tumor thrombus. Clinical features were previous history of RCC, serum thyroglobulin levels, cytology, preoperative diagnosis, and surgery.

Results: Ultrasonographic features of these carcinomas were more likely to involve a solitary, irregular, and solid without calcifications, and prominent intra-tumoral vascularity and tumor thrombus in the vein. These patients tended to be older, and to have relatively late recurrence in the thyroid, RCC in the right kidney as the primary site, and relatively low serum thyroglobulin levels.

Conclusions: Metastatic carcinomas to the thyroid from RCC presented highly characteristic features on ultrasonography. These ultrasonographic features combined with cytological findings and previous medical history of RCC can provide the optimal process for the preoperative diagnosis of such patients.

Keywords: Thyroid, Ultrasonography, Metastatic carcinoma, Renal cell carcinoma, Diagnosis, Tumor thrombus

Background

Metastases of renal cell carcinoma to multiple sites occur in the course of the disease and are generally regarded as the result of spread by a hematogenous route [1]. The thyroid gland is one of the metastatic sites from the primary lesion [1-3], but metastases to the thyroid that need surgical management are infrequent. It is reported that a surgical approach for such patients is associating with a favorable prognosis, when metastatic tumors are confined within the thyroid [1,3-6]. Therefore, preoperative diagnosis has clinical significance. Needless to say, previous medical history of renal cell carcinoma and fine-needle aspiration cytology of thyroid tumors of such patients are important for preoperative diagnosis.

The strategic value of ultrasound in preoperative surgical planning of patients with thyroid nodules has become increasingly appreciated [7,8]. The ultrasonogaphic features of a metastatic tumor to the thyroid from renal cell carcinoma are unfamiliar to clinicians and thyroid endocrinologists because of the rarity of such patients. It is unclear whether the ultrasonogaphic features can be helpful in the preoperative diagnosis, in addition to characteristic findings of cytology and previous medical history of renal cell carcinoma.

In this article, we focus on the ultrasonographic features of metastatic carcinomas to the thyroid from renal

* Correspondence: kobayashi@kuma-h.or.jp
Kuma Hospital, 8-2-35 Shimoyamate-dori, Chuo-ku, Kobe-City 650-0011, Japan

cell carcinoma, and discuss the significance of ultrasound for the preoperative diagnosis of such patients.

Methods

We retrospectively reviewed the medical database of patients with thyroid malignancies who underwent surgery between January 1998 and December 2013 in Kuma Hospital. A total of 10 patients with metastatic carcinoma to the thyroid from renal cell carcinoma undergoing thyroid surgery were included in this study. Preoperative ultrasonography was performed in all patients who had thyroid surgery during this time period. The ultrasound readings that were used in this study were made as part of the care of the patients. Surgical samples of the thyroid, tumor thrombi, and lymph nodes were cut before fixation. Specimens were fixed in buffered formalin and embedded in paraffin, and HE and immunohistochemical staining was performed. All related pathological specimens were reviewed (by M.H.), and the histopathological diagnosis was included in this study. The preoperative ultrasound readings were confirmed visually by surgeons at surgery and histopathological examination postoperatively. The surgical findings and histopathological diagnosis were recorded in the medical database of the hospital. The ethics committee of Kuma Hspital approved the study protocol (US-RCC meta), which was in adherence to the Declaration of Helsinki.

Ultrasonographic examination was performed by well-trained, registered ultrasonographers, using a TOSHIBA Aplio SSA-770A ultrasound system with PLT-1204AX (7–14 MHz) and PLT-805AT (5–12 MHz) linear probes. We used both grayscale and power Doppler ultrasonography. Power Doppler ultrasonography was used predominantly to assess the vascularity of the thyroid tumor and to identify the presence or absence of tumor thrombus in the vein.

Age at thyroid surgery, sex, previous history of renal cell carcinoma, serum thyroglobulin level, anti-thyroglobulin autoantibody, and ultrasonographic findings of the thyroid tumor, fine-needle aspiration cytology, preoperative diagnosis, and surgery were investigated.

The ultrasonographic features of metastatic carcinomas to the thyroid from renal cell carcinoma to be estimated were as follows:

(1) Form of involvement in the thyroid
Tumor formation or diffuse involvement in the thyroid gland was estimated.

(2) Location in the thyroid gland and size of tumors
In terms of the right or left lobe, or the isthmus of the thyroid gland, the site where the tumor was located was estimated. The size of the tumor was recorded in mm.

(3) Shape of tumor, tumor pattern, and strong echoes (calcifications)
The shape of the tumor was classified into regular or irregular. The tumor pattern was classified into solid, mixed, or cystic. The presence or absence of strong echoes with acoustic shadowing (calcifications) was estimated within the tumor lesion.

(4) Vascularity and distribution of blood signals
The intensity of blood signals in the tumor was estimated by Doppler ultrasonography, and classified into -, ±, +, or ++. The distribution of blood signals was classified into intra-tumoral or peripheral dominant.

(5) Extrathyroidal spread (swollen lymph node and tumor thrombus)
The presence or absence of swollen lymph nodes in the neck and tumor thrombus in the thyroid veins and the internal jugular vein adjacent to the thyroid tumor was estimated.

Results

Clinical findings

There were 10 surgical patients with metastatic carcinoma to the thyroid from renal cell carcinoma in this period (Table 1). The histopathological diagnosis of the thyroid tumors was the clear cell variant of renal cell carcinoma in all of the 10 patients. One patient (Patient 7) revealed metastatic carcinoma in benign adenomatous nodule. The patients were 4 men and 6 women, and the age at thyroid surgery was 67.8 ± 7.3 years old (range, 57–79 years old; median, 68.5 years old). Eight patients presented with a previous medical history of nephrectomy for renal cell carcinoma 13.4 ± 8.4 years earlier (range, 2–30 years; median, 12.5 years). In two patients (Patients 9 and 10), renal cell carcinoma in the right kidney was discovered as a primary carcinoma after the thyroid surgery and the histopathological diagnosis of metastatic carcinoma to the thyroid gland. The side of renal cell carcinoma was the right in nine patients (Patients 1–6, and 8–10) and the left in one patient (Patient 7). One patient (Patient 5) revealed positivity for anti-thyroglobulin auto-antibody. Serum thyroglobulin (normal range, < 40 ng/ml) was 136. 9 ± 285.2 ng/ml (range, 9.3-894.6 ng/ml; median, 30.2 ng/ml) in the other 9 patients without auto-antibody.

Ultrasonographic features

Form of involvement in the thyroid

Metastatic carcinomas showed tumor formation in the thyroid in all 10 of the patients (Figures 1, 2 and 3), and did not show diffuse involvement in the thyroid.

Table 1 Patients with metastatic carcinoma to the thyroid from renal cell carcinoma and ultrasonographic features

Patient		History, Side of RCC	Serum Tg, TgAb	Ultrasonographic features of metastatic carcinoma				FNAC	Pre-op. DX	Surgery
No	Age, Sex			Location, Size (mm)	Shape, Pattern, Calc.	Intra-tumoral vascularity	Tumor thrombus			
1	70F	8 yr, Right	81.3 (-)	Rt, 36x19x36	irregular solid, (-)	++	(-)	malignant, meta/RCC	meta/RCC	LO
2	77M	9 yr, Right	9.3 (-)	Rt, 56x35x48	irregular solid, (-)	++	(-)	indeterminate	meta/RCC	LO
3	72M	30 yr, Right	27.4 (-)	Lt, 31x19x24	irregular solid, (-)	++	(-)	benign, AN	meta/RCC	LO
4	58F	10 yr, Right	68.2 (-)	Rt, 39x23x36	irregular solid, (-)	++	(+) TV-IJV	indeteminate	meta/RCC	LO+RTV+RIJV
5	67F	18 yr, Right	128.5 (+)	Rt, 81x41x70	irregular solid, (-)	++	(+)	malignant, meta/RCC	meta/RCC	TT+RTV+RIJV
				Lt, 27x16x18		++	TV-IJV			
6	63F	2 yr, Right	894.6 (-)	Rt, 48x29x30 +LNS	irregular solid, (-)	++	(-)	malignant, meta/RCC	meta/RCC	LO+MND
7*	57M	15 yr, Left	26.1 (-)	Rt, 48x40x43	irregular solid, (-)	+	(+) TV	malignant, meta/RCC	meta/RCC	LO+RTV
8	79F	15 yr, Right	24.5 (-)	Rt, 45x33x34	irregular solid, (-)	++	(-)	benign, AN	AN	LO
9	65F	(-)** Right	70.7 (-)	Rt, 23x20x21	regular solid, (-)	+	(-)	fol. tumor, FT	FT	LO
10	70M	(-)** Right	30.2 (-)	Rt, 25x19x19	irregular solid, (-)	++	(+)	benign, AG	AG or PC?	TT+CND+RTV
				Lt, 12x5x10			TV			

A previous history of renal cell carcinoma was recognized in 7 patients (Patients 1-7) before surgery, and in 3 patients (Patients 8-10) it was not. Age: age at thyroid surgery, F: female, M: male, Rt: right, Lt: left, History: previous history of nephrectomy for renal cell carcinoma, RCC: renal cell carcinoma, Tg: thyroglobulin (normal range: < 40 ng/ml), TgAb: anti-thyroglobulin autoantibody. Shape of the tumor was classified into regular or irregular. Pattern of the tumor was classified into solid, mixed, or cystic. Calc.: intra-tumoral calcification; (+) or (-). Intra-tumoral vascularity was classified into -, +, or ++ according to the intensity of blood signals by Doppler ultrasonography. FNAC: fine-needle aspiration cytology, Pre-op. DX: preoperative diagnosis, meta/RCC: metastatic carcinoma to the thyroid from renal cell carcinoma, LO: lobectomy of the thyroid, TT: total thyroidectomy, MND: modified neck dissection, CND: central node dissection, TV: thyroid vein, IJV: internal jugular vein RIJV: partial resection of internal jugular vein, RTV: resection of thyroid vein, LNS: lymph node swelling in the neck, FT: follicular tumor, AN: adenomatous nodule, AG: adenomatous goiter, PC; papillary carcinoma. Patient 7*: Metastatic renal cell carcinoma in benign adenomatous nodule. The benign part of the tumor could not be detected on ultrasonography because of small size. (-)**: Existence of renal cell carcinoma was recognized after the thyroid surgery and the histopathological diagnosis of thyroid tumor.

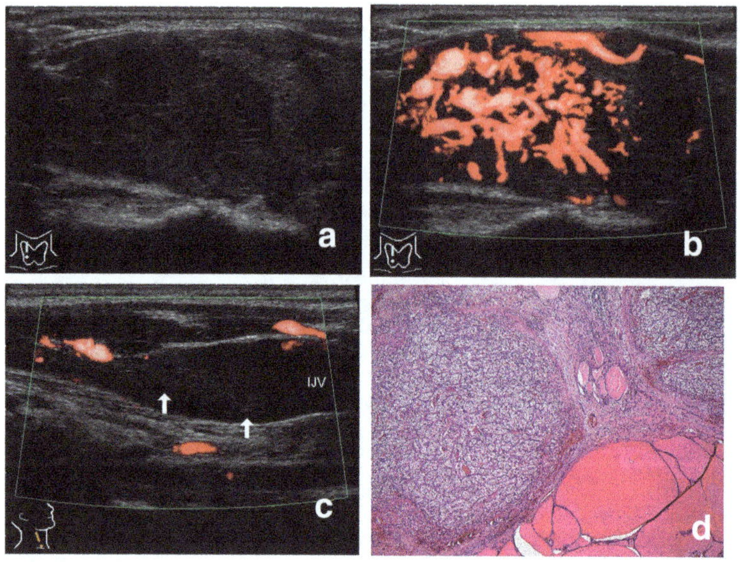

Figure 1 (Patient 4). a. Ultrasonography of the right lobe. A solid tumor. The margins are well demarcated and irregular, and the internal echo is predominantly hypoechoic and partially anechoic. Strong echoes with acoustic shadowing (calcifications) are not present. **b**. Power Doppler ultrasonography of the same section as in Figure 1a. Marked chaotic vascularity is predominantly shown in the intra-tumoral lesions. **c**. Power Doppler ultrasonography of the right internal jugular vein. A solid mass (arrows), that is, tumor thrombus, is shown as an "echogenic tongue" in the lumen. **d** Hematoxylin & eosin staining. Metastatic carcinoma of the clear cell variant of renal cell carcinoma and normal thyroid tissue are shown. Tissue of the tumor histopathogically demonstrates a pseudo-alveolar or pseudo-follicular structure and no calcifications.

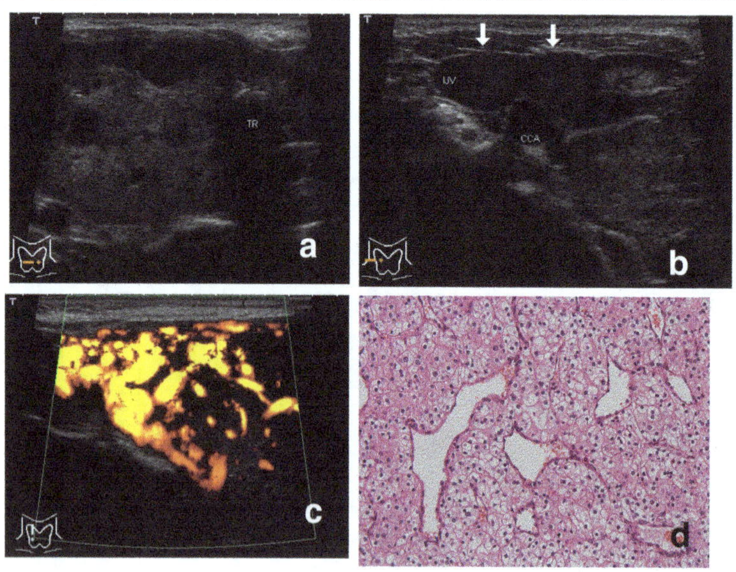

Figure 2 (Patient 5). a. Ultrasonography of the right lobe. A predominantly solid tumor. Internal echo shows homogenity in the solid area and interspersed cystic-like areas. (Power Doppler showed intense blood signals in these cystic-like areas). **b** Ultrasonography of the right lobe and the jugular vein. A solid mass (arrow on the left), that is, tumor thrombus, is shown in the lumen of the jugular vein. The lumen of the middle thyroid vein is completely occupied with tumor thrombus (arrow on the right). **c**. Power Doppler ultrasonography. Marked chaotic vascularity. **d** Hematoxylin & eosin staining. A rich vascular network.

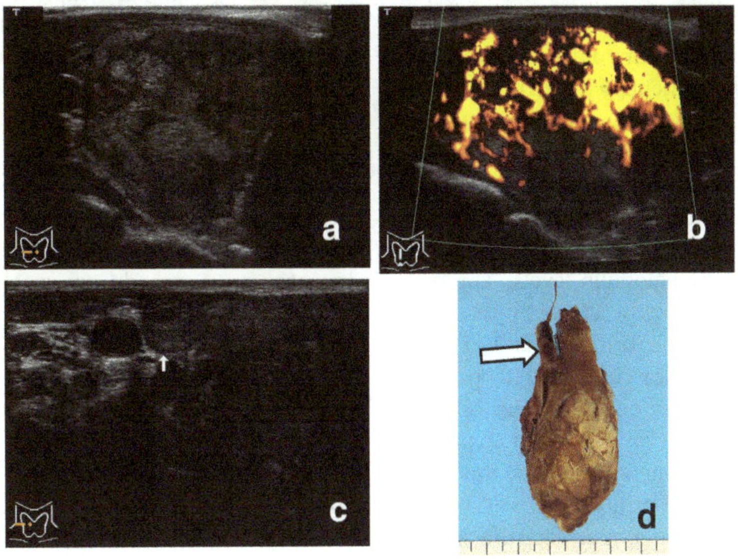

Figure 3 (Patient 7). a. Ultrasonography of the right lobe. A solid tumor. The internal echo is iso- to hypo-echoic and heterogeneous, and appears to show multiple small masses in the tumor. **b**. Power Doppler ultrasonography. **c**. Ultrasonography of the right lobe. Tumor thrombus (arrows) is observed in the superior thyroid vein. **d**. Gross resected specimen. Solid tumor in the right lobe of the thyroid and bulbous intravascular component, tumor thrombus (arrow), are shown.

Location and size of thyroid tumor

The location of metastatic tumors was the right lobe of the thyroid gland in 9 patients, and the left lobe in 3 patients (Patients 3, 5, and 10). Two patients (Patients 5 and10) presented two tumors in the right and left lobes of the thyroid gland. The maximum size of the tumors was 39.3 ± 18.2 mm (range, 12–81 mm; median, 37.5 mm).

Shape of tumor, tumor pattern, and calcifications

The shapes of the tumors were irregular and well demarcated, and the tumor pattern showed a solid and hypoechoic level without a capsule-like structure and direct contact to the normal thyroid tissue in all 10 of the patients. None of the tumors demonstrated strong echoes with acoustic shadowing (calcifications) within them.

Vascularity and distribution of blood signals

The intensity of vascularity in the tumors by Doppler ultrasonography was ++ in 8 patients (Figures 1b, 2c, 3b) and + in 2 patients. Blood signals were more dominant in intra-tumoral lesions than in peripheral lesions of the tumors in all of the patients.

Extrathyroidal spread (swollen lymph node and tumor thrombus)

One patient (Patient 6) showed swollen lymph nodes in the neck in addition to the thyroid tumor. Direct tumor extension into the adjacent veins, that is, tumor thrombi, was detected in 4 patients preoperatively. Tumor thrombi within the internal jugular vein via the thyroid vein ("echogenic tongue") were demonstrated in two patients (Patients 4 and 5) (Figures 1c, 2b), and those within the thyroid veins in two patients (Patienta 7 and 10) (Figure 3c). Intravascular components of the lesions appeared as a solid and hypoechoic mass without calcifications (Figures 1c, 2b, 3c).

Fine-needle aspiration cytology (FNAC)

FNAC showed metastatic carcinoma to the thyroid from renal cell carcinoma in 4 patients, indeterminate in 2 patients (Patients 2 and 4), benign in 3 patients (Patients 3, 8, and 10), and follicular neoplasm in one patient (Patient 9).

Preoperative diagnosis

Among the eight patients who had a previous history of nephrectomy for renal cell carcinoma, seven patients were accurately diagnosed with metastatic carcinoma to the thyroid from renal carcinoma preoperatively, and one patient (Patient 8) was diagnosed with a benign thyroid tumor. Two patients (Patients 9 and 10) who did not have a previous history of nephrectomy for renal cell carcinoma were misdiagnosed with follicular tumor and benign tumor, or papillary carcinoma preoperatively as the primary tumors.

Surgery

Total thyroidectomy was performed in 2 patients and lobectomy in 8 patients. Resection of thyroid veins or partial resection of internal jugular veins was performed in 4 patients because of tumor thrombi in the veins (Patients 4, 5, 7, and 10). Central and modified neck lymph node dissections in addition to thyroid lobectomy were performed in two patients (Patients 6 and 10).

Discussion

Table 1 reveals that these patients tend to be older, and to have relatively late recurrence in the thyroid, renal cell carcinoma in the "right" kidney as a primary site, and relatively low serum thyroglobulin levels. Three patients (Patients 8–10) could not be correctly diagnosed preoperatively, although 7 patients (Patients 1–7) were identified to have metastatic carcinoma. The previous history of renal cell carcinoma could not be obtained preoperatively in one patient (Patient 8). In 2 patients (Patients 9 and 10), thyroid metastasis was the initial presentation of the renal cell carcinoma. It is of interest that ultrasonography played an important role in preoperative diagnosis.

Thyroid ultrasound is particularly useful for estimating the location of a nodule, its size, and its solid or cystic nature, and also for guiding the performance of fine-needle aspiration biopsies. Therefore, it has already become established as the diagnostic procedure of choice in guidelines [7,8] for the management of thyroid nodules by every professional organization of endocrinologists. Papillary thyroid carcinoma is the most common and primary malignancy, and ultrasound features of such patients, for example, a predominantly solid, hypoechoic, ill-circumscribed nodule and lymph node swelling in the neck [9], have already become familiar. On the other hand, patients with metastases to the thyroid from renal cell carcinoma that need surgical management are not many and unfamiliar to clinicians and endocrinologists. It is reported that a surgical procedure for thyroid metastasis from renal cell carcinoma has benefits for the prognosis of such patients [1,3-6]. Little information is available on the ultrasonographic features of metastatic tumor to the thyroid from renal cell carcinoma [2,10-13]. For the reasons mentioned above, ultrasound features of metastatic carcinoma to the thyroid from renal cell carcinoma should be clarified by the evaluation of many patients. A full understanding of ultrasound features is clinically important and essential for such patients' care.

The most common primary site from which metastasis to the thyroid gland occurs is reported to be the kidney in a clinical series [1,2]. Renal cell carcinoma arises from the renal tubular epithelial cells, and the clear cell type is the most common variant [14]. Histopathologically, clear cell carcinoma shows polygonal cells with clear cytoplasm, distinct cell membranes, and small compact eccentric nuclei, and a rich vascular network [14]. The propensity of primary renal cell carcinoma in the kidney to spread to regional lymph nodes and virtually every organ site is well recognized [14]. Furthermore, this carcinoma often invades regional veins and forms tumor thrombus in the lumen of the renal veins or the inferior vena cava. In addition, this carcinoma behaves unpredictably and its recurrence after nephrectomy is highly variable, presenting as late metastases several years after the initial surgery [1-3,5,10,12,13]. In this situation, metastatic carcinomas in the thyroid occur as a result of hematogenous spread from renal cell carcinoma [14].

A pseudo-alveolar or pseudo-follicular pattern of clear cell carcinoma may resemble the clear cell variant of thyroid carcinoma and adenoma histopathologically. Recently, it has been described that metastatic tumor in the thyroid should be diagnosed based on rich vascularity, abundant extravasated erythrocytes, pseudofollicular spaces filled with blood, negativity for thyroglobulin, and positivity for CD10 and positivity for the renal cell carcinoma marker carbonic anhydrase IX [15]. Histopathological features of the thyroid tumors inevitably reflect ultrasound images of these tumors. Sonographers and endocrinologists must be aware that the ultrasound images of thyroid tumors should be read and understood on the basis of the histopathological features of the tumors.

According to our series (Table 1), metastatic carcinomas to the thyroid from renal cell carcinoma formed one or two nodules within any portion of the thyroid glands in all 10 of the patients. No patients revealed diffuse involvement in the thyroid such as diffuse sclerosing variant of papillary thyroid carcinoma or diffuse swelling of Hashimoto's thyroiditis on histopathology. Furthermore, these tumors did not form a distinct capsule of the tumor histopathologically, and neoplastic cells of these tumors were directly exposed to the normal thyroid tissue and showed invasiveness to adjacent tissue (Figure 1d). For that reason, these tumors showed an irregular margin without a capsule-like structure and directly contacted the normal thyroid region on ultrasonography (Figures 1, 2 and 3).

The tissue of these tumors histopathologically demonstrated a pseudo-alveolar or pseudo-follicular structure (Figures 1d, 2d), and cystic degeneration did not occur within the tumor. Additionally, calcifications did not form within these tumors, and there was a very rich vascular network in the tumor parenchyma (Figure 2d). In terms of the echogenicity of the internal echo of these tumors, they were hypoechoic compared with normal thyroid tissue, which reflected the homogenity of the tissue of these tumors on histopathology. These tumors did not demonstrate cystic anechoic lesions with posterior acoustic enhancement, or any type of echogenic foci with acoustic shadowing, that is, calcifications, on ultrasonography. Doppler ultrasonography showed intensive blood signals or prominent chaotic vascularity in the intra-tumoral area, but did not show prominent vascularity in the peri-tumoral area (Figures 1b, 2c, 3b).

Neoplastic cells of these tumors directly invaded intra-tumoral vessels and formed tumor thrombi in the lumen of the vessels. Grayscale and Doppler ultrasonography showed an "echogenic tongue", that is, tumor thrombus, in the lumen of the thyroid vein or the internal jugular vein (Figures 1c, 2b, 3c) in 4 of the 10 patients. We previously reported on tumor thrombus in surgical patients with thyroid malignancies [16]. Of the 5507 patients with thyroid malignancies, there were 9 patients with tumor thrombi. (Two of these previously reported patients are Patients 4 and 5 in Table 1 of this article.) It can be said that metastases to the thyroid from renal cell carcinoma have a high frequency of tumor thrombus as extrathyroidal spread on ultrasonography. In the literature, tumor thrombi were also reported in a small number of patients with metastatic carcinoma from renal cell carcinoma [4,10,17]. Tumor thrombi in veins adjacent to the thyroid gland can be described as a noteworthy ultrasonographic feature because they are highly suggestive of malignancy. We believe that the detection of tumor thrombus by ultrasonography is useful for preoperative determination of the surgical procedure for such patients [4,10,17] as well as for the diagnosis of metastasis from renal cell carcinoma.

In one patient (Patient 7), small nest of benign adenomatous nodule were demonstrated in the peripheral tissue of the tumor histopathologically, although the majority of the tumor was occupied with clear cell carcinoma. This tumor revealed metastatic renal cell carcinoma in benign adenomatous nodule. The benign part of the tumor could not be detected on ultrasonography preoperatively because of small size. It is reported that renal cell carcinoma rarely metastasized to primary thyroid tumors [18].

There are some ultrasonographic classification systems for thyroid nodules. Among them, Kuma Hospital's ultrasound classification system (Kuma's USC, USC 1–5) [19,20] and the Thyroid imaging reporting and date system (TIRADS, TIRADS 1–6) [21] are popular and useful for clinical management at present. These ultrasound classification systems represent the risk of malignancy of thyroid nodules. When these two ultrasound classification systems are applied to the tumors in these 10 patients, they are classified in USC 4 (probably malignant) and 5 (malignant) on Kuma's USC, and TIRADS 5 (probably malignant) and 6 (malignant) on the TIRADS classification. In particular, tumors with tumor thrombi (Patients 4, 5, 7, and 10) can be easily classified into USC 5 and TIRADS 6.

Quasi-static and shear-wave elastography now become available for diagnostic ultrasonic procedures in addition to conventional grayscale and Doppler ultrasonography. Quasi-static elastography is a relatively new technology that maps the relatively elastic properties of soft tissues, and shear-wave elastography is a new technology that shows quantitative stiffness value of tissues by measuring the velocity of wave propagation. Currently, Adamczewski et al. reported the findings of these two different elastography techniques in a patient with metastases of renal clear-cell carcinoma to the thyroid [22]. Both techniques revealed differences in relative stiffness (strain ratio) between the normal tissue and metastases. However, the absolute stiffness values for metastases in shear-wave elastography were within the range characteristic benign lesions. The data accumulation of these new techniques will add to the interpretation of conventional ultrasound images, and be helpful for ultrasonic diagnosis.

Thyroid metastasis from renal cell carcinoma has some characteristic ultrasonographic findings, such as prominent chaotic intra-tumoral vascularity and tumor thrombus as mentioned above; however, these findings are not specific to this disease. It is thus necessary to perform ultrasonography and fine-needle aspiration biopsy and to obtain information on the previous history of renal cell carcinoma in order to make a correct diagnosis preoperatively. It is reported that fine-needle aspiration cytology can suggest the possibility of metastatic tumor from renal cell carcinoma, and is essential for preoperative diagnosis [1,3,23]. Cytological findings of thyroid metastasis from renal cell carcinoma tend to be bloody, a lack of colloid, and striped nuclei with only occasional cells showing clear cytoplasm [23]. When clear cells are identified within the thyroid gland, primary tumors with clear cell features including papillary, follicular, and medullary thyroid carcinoma, and secondary tumor such as those from lung and salivary gland also need to be considered.

When a previous history of nephrectomy for renal cell carcinoma is recognized in such a patient, ultrasound examination as well as cytology is effective and helpful in order to diagnose it preoperatively. Actually, three patients (Patients 2, 3, and 4) showed an "indeterminate" or "benign" status because of too many blood cells and no neoplastic cells in cytology. However, these patients had a previous history of nephrectomy for renal cell carcinoma and demonstrated characteristic ultrasonographic findings for metastatic carcinoma from renal cell carcinoma. Therefore, we could make the correct preoperative diagnosis. In contrast, when we do not recognize a previous history of renal cell carcinoma, or thyroid metastasis is the first symptom as renal cell carcinoma in a patient, it seems to be difficult to diagnose it preoperatively because of the rarity of the disease. Unfortunately, two patients (Patients 9 and 10) who had no previous history of renal cell carcinoma were not correctly diagnosed preoperatively in spite of the existence of characteristic features on ultrasonography. Preoperative recognition of a previous history of renal cell carcinoma in a patient must be the most important clue for the correct diagnosis of the disease, which many articles in the literature have emphasized [1,2,6].

Cytology was falsely negative in four patients with previous history of renal cell carcinoma (Patients 2, 3, 4, and 8). We should have measured thyroglobulin in the washout of fine-needle aspiration cytology. When thyroglobulin was low or detectable, clinical suspicion of metastatic nodule would become more definitely.

Conclusions

Comprehensive judgment of ultrasonographic findings of thyroid tumor, cytological findings, and previous medical history of renal cell carcinoma are suggested to lead to the correct diagnosis of patients with metastases to the thyroid from renal cell carcinoma. In this situation, ultrasound is the initial examination and such characteristic features on ultrasonography mentioned above can be clues to the correct diagnosis.

Consent

Written informed consent was obtained from the patient's guardian/parent/next of kin for the publication of this report and any accompanying images.

Competing interests

The authors declare that they have no competing interests.

Authors' contributions

All authors read and approved the final manuscript.

References

1. Chung AY, Tran TB, Brumund KT, Weisman RA, Bouvet M. Metastases to the thyroid: a review of the literature from the last decade. Thyroid. 2012;22:258–68.
2. Sindoni A, Rizzo M, Tuccari G, Ieni A, Barresi V, Calbo L, et al. Thyroid metastases from renal cell carcinoma: review of the literature. Scientific World Journal. 2010;10:590–602.
3. Hegerova L, Griebeler ML, Reynolds JP, Henry MR, Gharib H: Metastasis to the thyroid gland: Report of a large series from the Mayo Clinic. *Am J Clin Oncol* doi: [10.1097/COC.0b013e31829d1d09]
4. De Stefano, Carluccioo R, Zanni E, Marchiori D, Cicchetti G, Bertaccini A, et al. Management of thyroid nodules as secondary involvement of renal cell carcinoma: case report and literature review. Anticancer Res. 2009;29:473–6.
5. Assouad J, Banu E, Brian E, Pham DN, Dujon A, Foucault C, et al. Strategies and outcomes in pulmonary and extrapulmonary metastases from renal cell cancer. Eur J Cardiothorac Surg. 2008;33:794–8.
6. Duggal NM, Horattas MC. Metastatic renal cell carcinoma to the thyroid gland. Endocr Pract. 2008;4:1040–6.
7. Gharib H, Papini E, Paschke R, Duick DS, Valcavi R, Hegedues L, et al. AACE/AME/ETA Task Force on Thyroid Nodules: American Association of Clinical Endocrinologists and Associazione Medici Endocrinologi for clinical practice for the diagnosis an management of thyroid nodules. Endocrine Pract. 2006;12:63–102.
8. American Thyroid Taskforce on Thyroid Nodules and Differentiated Thyroid Cancer, Cooper DS, Doherty GM, Haugen BR, Kloos RT, Lee SL, et al. Revised American Thyroid Association management guideline for patients with and differentiated thyroid cancer. Thyroid. 2009;19:1167–214.
9. Ahuja AT: Head and Neck. Differentiated thyroid carcinoma; In *Diagnostic Imaging: Ultrasound*, ed 1, Salt Lake City, Utah. AMIRSYS: 2007; 6–11.
10. Pickhardt PJ, Pickard RH. Sonography of delayed thyroid metastasis from renal cell carcinoma with jugular vein extension. Am J Roentgenol. 2003;81:272–4.
11. Kim AY, Park SB, Choi HS, Hwang JC. Isolated thyroid metastasis from renal cell carcinoma. J Ultrasound Med. 2007;26:1799–802.
12. Kihara M, Yokomise H, Yamauchi. Metastasis of renal cell carcinoma to the thyroid gland 19 years after nephrectomy: a case report. Auris Nasus Larynx. 2004;31:95–100.
13. Wada N, Hirakawa S, Rino Y, Hasuo K, Kawachi K, Nakatani Y, et al. Solitary metachronous metastasis to the thyroid from renal clear cell carcinoma 19 years after nephrectomy: report of a case. Surg Today. 2005;35:483–7.
14. Russo P. Renal cell carcinoma: presentation, staging, and surgical treatment. Semin Oncol. 2000;27:160–76.
15. Cimino-Mathew A, Sharma R, Netto GJ. Diagnostic use of PAX8, CAIX, TTF-1, and TGB in metastatic renal cell carcinoma of the thyroid. Am J Surg Pathol. 2011;35:757–61.
16. Kobayashi K, Hirokawa M, Yabuta T, Fukushima M, Kihara M, Higashiyama T, et al. Tumor thrombus of thyroid malignancies in veins: Importance of detection by ultrasonography. Thyroid. 2011;21:527–31.
17. Matei DV, Brescia A, Nordio A, Spinelli MG, Melegari S, Cozzi G, et al. Renal cell carcinoma and synchronous thyroid metastasis with neoplastic thrombosis of the internal jugular vein: report of a case. Arch Ital Urol Androl. 2001;3:203–6.
18. Bohn OL, De las Casas LE, Leon ME. Tumor-to-tumor metastasis: Renal cell carcinoma metastatic to papillary carcinoma of thyroid-report of a case and review of the literature. Head Neck Pathol. 2009;3:327–30.
19. Yokozawa T, Miyauchi A, Kuma K, Sugawara M. Accurate and simple method of diagnosing nodules the modified technique of ultrasound-guided fine needle aspiration biopsy. Thyroid. 1995;5:141–5.
20. Ito Y, Amino N, Yokozawa T, Ota H, Ohshita M, Murata N, et al. Ultrasonographic evaluation of thyroid nodules in 900 patients: comparison among ultrasonographic, cytological, and histological findings. Thyroid. 2007;17:1269–76.
21. Horvath E, Majlis S, Rossi R, Franco C, Niedmann JP, Castro A, et al. An ultrasonogram reporting system for thyroid nodules stratifying cancer risk for clinical management. J Clin Endoccrinol Metab. 2009;94:1748–4751.
22. Adamczewski Z, Dedecjus M, Skowronska-Jozwiak E, Lewinski A. Metastases of renal clear-cell carcinoma to the thyroid: a comparison of shear-wave and quasi-static elastograhy. Pol Arch Med Wewn. 2014;124:485–6.
23. Bhalla R, Popp A, Nassar A. Case report: metastatic renal carcinoid to the thyroid diagnosed by fine needle aspiration biopsy. Diagn Cytopathol. 2007;35:597–600.

23

Synergistic inhibition of MEK/ERK and BRAF V600E with PD98059 and PLX4032 induces sodium/iodide symporter (NIS) expression and radioiodine uptake in BRAF mutated papillary thyroid cancer cells

Honglai Zhang[1] and Dong Chen[2*]

Abstract

Background and Aims: The activating mutation BRAF^{V600E} is a frequent genetic event in papillary thyroid carcinomas (PTC). Mutation BRAF^{V600E} is associated with the loss of a sodium/iodine symporter (NIS), and subsequent radioiodide-refractory (RAI) metastatic disease. Use of BRAF V600E inhibitors could partly restore NIS expression and Iodide uptake by inhibition of mitogen-activated protein kinase (MAPK) pathway. Previous study has reported that the BRAF V600E inhibitors could re-activate MAPK signals. In the present study, we investigated whether the combination treatment of BRAF V600E inhibitor and MAPK signal inhibitor could more effectively increase NIS expression and RAI uptake, and explore the mechanisms.

Methods: BCPAP and K1 cells were exposed to increasing concentrations of BRAF V600E inhibitor PLX4032 (0.01 μM, 0.1 μM, 1 μM) or MEK/ERK inhibitor PD98059 (0.01 μM, 0.1 μM, 1 μM) or with their association or/and in the presence of 3 mM perchlorate ($ClO^-{}_4$) for 0–72 h. Iodide uptake and expression of BRAF, phosphorylated (p) ERK1/2, NIS were detected.

Results: PLX4032 or PD98059 alone did not induce NIS expression and increase Iodide uptake in BCPAP and K1 cells. But combined treatment of PLX4032 and PD98059 significantly induce NIS expression and increase Iodide uptake in BCPAP and K1 cells. PLX4032 alone inhibited p-ERK expression at early time, and re-activated p-ERK expression at late time. However, combined treatment of PLX4032 and PD98059 completely inhibited p-ERK expression.

Conclusion: Simultaneously suppressing BRAF V600E and p-ERK restored NIS expression and increase Iodide uptake in PTC cells, which was associated the inhibition of p-ERK expression. The results warrants clinical trials to confirm.

Keywords: Papillary thyroid carcinoma, Assodium/iodide symporter, Mutation BRAF^{V600E}, Mitogen-activated protein kinase

* Correspondence: chendd820@126.com
[2]Department of General Surgery, the affiliated Hospital of Qingdao University, Qingdao, Shandong, China
Full list of author information is available at the end of the article

Background

Differentiated thyroid cancer follicular cells have the ability to absorb iodine, which is the theoretical basis for radioactive iodine (RAI) treatment of differentiated thyroid cancer [1]. RAI is the standard treatment for differentiated thyroid cancer at present. If patients with RAI-ineffective thyroid cancer have lost surgical indications, any other method currently used clinicall cannot be curing. This is the main cause of thyroid cancer-related morbidity and mortality. Sodium iodide cotransporter (NIS) mediates the active iodide uptake at the basolateral membrane of the thyroid follicular cell, plays a crucial role in the success of radioiodine therapy [2]. Thyroid-stimulating hormone receptor (TSHR) up-regulates NIS and related molecular processes [2]. The main mechanism of RAI-refractory thyroid cancer is the abnormal silencing of NIS and TSHR gene in the thyroid cancer cells [2]. NIS is negatively regulated by the MAPK pathway in thyroid cancer, in which the BRAF V600E mutation plays an important role [3].

BRAF600E (valine-to-glutamate, position 600) is the second most common mutation in human cancer, and the most common oncogenic mutation in thyroid cancer [4]. Mutated BRAF600E protein results in increased mitogen-activated protein kinase (MAPK) activity (MEK1/2/ERK1/2) [5]. It has previously reported that targeting MAPK pathway using MEK inhibitors could increased thyroid gene expression and radioiodine uptake in thyroid cancer cells [6, 7] and melanoma [8]. We therefore suggested that targeting BRAF/MAPK or MEK/ERK pathway could be clinically effective in restoring RAI avidity in RAI-refractory thyroid cancer.

It has been recently found that using dabrafenib, the BRAF V600E inhibitor could partially induce radioiodine uptake in RAI-refractory thyroid cancer in patients [9], suggesting that the therapeutic effectiveness of RAI treatment using single agents was limited. PLX4032 (vemurafenib) is a selective small molecule inhibitor of BRAF V600E, showing a preferential inhibition of BRAF V600E-positive metastatic melanoma [10-12]. Data from preliminary studies suggest that PLX4032 might have activity in BRAFV600E-positive papillary thyroid cancer [13, 14]. Brose et al. has recently reported that Vemurafenib showed antitumour activity in patients with progressive, BRAFV600E-positive papillary thyroid cancer refractory to radioactive iodine who had never been treated with a multikinase inhibitor [15]. The mutation of the BRAFV600E gene is related with greater resistance to postoperative treatment with 131I since the onset of the disease [16]. A new study suggests that the PLX4032 may be effective in the 25 to 50% of patients with papillary thyroid cancer who develop resistance to radioactive iodine, a standard treatment. This image illustrates a multimodal therapeutic strategy for an iodine-refractory BRAF-mutated metastatic papillary thyroid carcinoma with reversed radioiodine resistance using BRAF inhibitors. As such, this agent represents a potential new treatment option for these patients.

We have recently found that treatment of thyroid cancer cells with PLX4032 alone resulted in a transient inhibition of pERK1/2 expression at 4–6 h, but quickly lead to paradoxically increased ERK signalingat 24–48 h, which maked the thyroid cancer cells resistant to PLX4032 treatment [17]. Therefore, we hypothesize that simultaneously suppressing BRAF V600E and ERK1/2 signaling could suppress the re-activation of ERK1/2 signaling by PLX4032, which may likely have a synergistic effect on thyroid gene expression and RAI uptake in thyroid cancer cells with BRAF V600E mutation.

In our study, we tested the effect of BRAF V600E inhibitor PLX4032 or in combination of the MEK/ERK inhibitor PD98059 on RAI uptake and NIS expression, in papillary thyroid cancer cell (PTC) with mutated BRAF600E.

Methods

Cell cultures

$BRAF^{V600E}$-positive papillary thyroid cancer cell BCPAP and K1 cells were obtained from the German Collection of Microorganisms and Cell Culture (DSMZ, Braunschweig, Germany). They were authenticated by short tandem repeat profiling, as previously described [18]. Cells were grown in humidified incubator at 37 °C with 5% CO_2, 6H hormone (1 mU/ml bovine TSH, 10 μg/ml bovine insulin, 10 nM hydrocortisone, 5 μg/ml transferrin, 10 ng/ml somatostatin, and 2 ng/ml L-glycyl-histidyllysine) and 10% fetal bovine serum in RPMI 1640 medium. Cells were expanded to 70–80% confluence and then used for the experiments described below.

Western blot

BCPAP and K1 cells (1.5×10^5 cells per well) were seeded in 96-well cell culture plates and harvested at 70 to 80% confluence. Then the cells were exposed to increasing concentrations of the BRAF V600E inhibitor PLX4032 (0.01 μM, 0.1 μM, 1 μM) or the ERK inhibitor, PD98059 (0.01 μM, 0.1 μM, 1 μM) or with their association for 2, 6, 12, 24, 48, 72 h. Cell lysates were prepared in 0.5% Triton X-100, 150 mM NaCl, 5 mM Tris supplemented with 1 × Halt protease inhibitor cocktail and 1 × Halt phosphatase inhibitor cocktail (Pierce, Rockford, IL), centrifuged at 3500 r.p.m. for 10 min at 4 °C. Protein concentration was measured using a Bio-Rad protein assay (Bio-Rad Laboratories, Hercules, CA). Proteins resolved by SDS–PAGE were electrophoretically transferred to polyvinylidene difluoride membrane and Western blots were carried out using standard techniques. The primary antibodies were as below: phosphorylated (p) ERK1/2 and ERK antibody (Santa Cruz Biotechnology, Shanghai, China); BRAF (sc-5284) (Santa Cruz Biotechnology); NIS (Protein tech). Anti-β-actin (Santa Cruz Biotechnology).

Primary antibody was incubated overnight at 4 °C in 5% milk/PBST. Membranes were washed with PBST and incubated with HRP-conjugated secondary antibodies diluted in 5% milk/PBST. Bands were visualised with enhanced chemiluminescence developed with X-ray film. Densitometry was performed (Kodak MI SE software, Carestream Health), and protein quantities recorded relative to anti-β-actin. All samples were analysed at least in triplicate.

Iodide uptake assays

Iodide uptake was measured as previously described [19]. Briefly, cells (1.5×10^5) were seeded in 6-well plates and then incubated with PLX4032 or PD98059 alone or their combination at 0.1 μM for 24–72 h. Then the cells were incubated with 2 μCi NaI125 in 5 μM nonradioactive NaI for 30 min at 37 °C with 5% CO2. Cells were then washed with cold Hank's Balanced Salt Solution two times and then lysed in cold 95% ethanol for 20 min at room temperature. Cell lysate was collected and counted for radioactivity by the gamma-counter (Packard Instruments, Waltham, MA, USA). Radioiodide uptake not mediated by NIS was excluded by performing the assay in the presence of 3 mM perchlorate (ClO – 4), a competitive inhibitor of iodide uptake by NIS. Experiments were performed in triplicates.The uptake was normalized to the cellular protein concentration measured with Bio-Rad protein assay.

Statistical analysis

Statistical analysis was performed by SPSS22.0. Data are presented as mean ± SEM. For comparison among two groups, Student's t test was used. For multiple comparisons, ANOVA was used for initial analyses followed by Fisher's protected least significant difference for post hoc analyses. Differences with $P < 0.05$ were determined as statistically significant.

Results

Effects of PLX4032 and PD98059 on NIS expression

BCPAP and K1 cells were exposed to increasing concentrations of PLX4032 (0.001 μM,0.01 μM, 0.1 μM) or PD98059 (0.001 μM, 0.01 μM, 0.1 μM) or with their association for 24 h, 48 h and 72 h. NIS protein was detected by western blot (Fig. 1a and b). The results

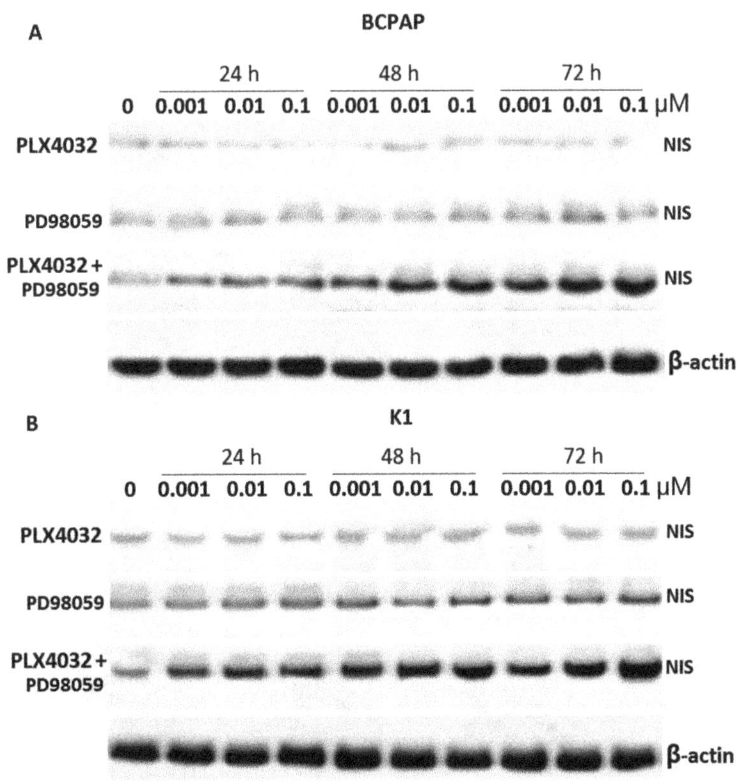

Fig. 1 Western blot of NIS in lysates of BCPAP cells (**a**) and K1 cells (**b**) treated with PLX4032 (0.001–0.1 μM) or PD98059 (0.001–0.1 μM) or their combination for indicated times

showed that PLX4032 alone did not significantly increase NIS protein levels, and PD98059 alone slightly increased NIS protein levels, especially in K1 cells. However, combined treatment significantly increased NIS protein in a dose- and time- dependent way.

Effects of PLX4032 and PD98059 on radioiodine uptake

As shown in Fig. 2, radioiodine uptake was not significantly increased in the BCPAP and K1 cells with PLX4032 (0.001–0.1 μM) treatment for 24–72 h, but slightly increased in BCPAP and K1 cells with PD98059 (0.001–0.1 μM) treatment. However, combination of PLX4032 and PD98059 significantly increased radioiodine uptake in both of the two cell lines respectively, but suppressed iodide uptake by 3 mM perchlorate ($ClO^{-}{}_{4}$), a competitive inhibitor of iodide uptake by NIS. It is suggested that Iodine uptake was specifically dependent on NIS because it was blocked by NaClO4 (Fig. 2).

PLX4032 failed to increase NIS and NIS-mediated radioiodine uptake due to its activation of ERK signaling

PLX4032 (0.1 μM) treatment alone resulted in completely inhibition of BRAF in 6–8 hs by western blot assay (Fig. 3a) in BCPAP cells. But PLX4032 (0.1 μM) treatment resulted in a transient inhibition of pERK expression, but quickly recovery from ERK1/2 activation inhibition by PLX4032 treatment in 8 h, and gradually reached the high levels at 24 hs and matained this levels for 72 h (Fig. 3a). However, combined treatment of PLX4032 and PD98059 completely inhibited ERK1/2

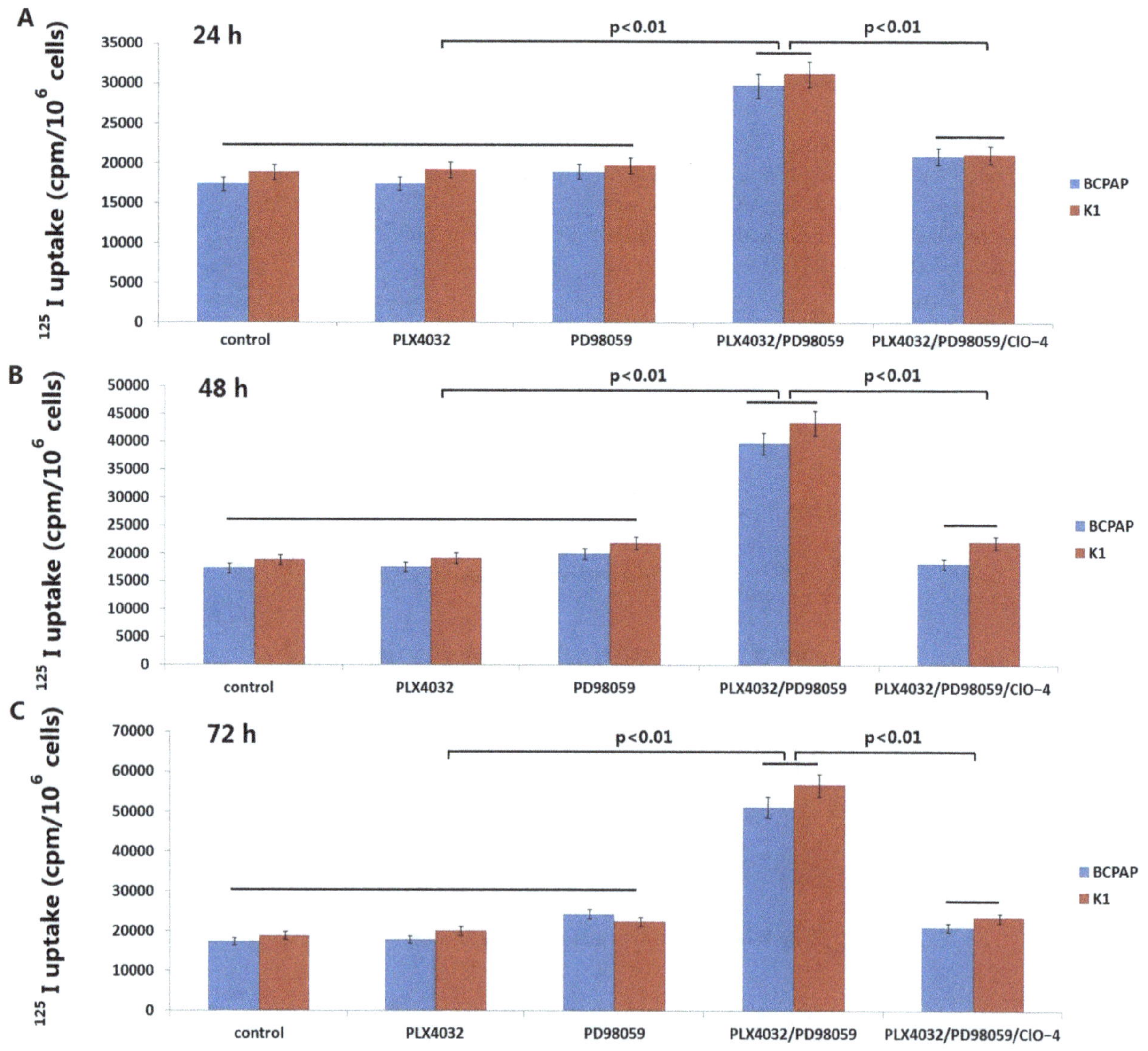

Fig. 2 ^{125}I accumulation in BCPAP and K1 cells. BCPAP and K1 cells were treated with PLX4032 (0.001–0.1 μM) or PD98059 (0.001–0.1 μM) or their combination or/and NaClO4 for 24 hs (**a**), 48 hs (**b**) and 72 hs (**c**)

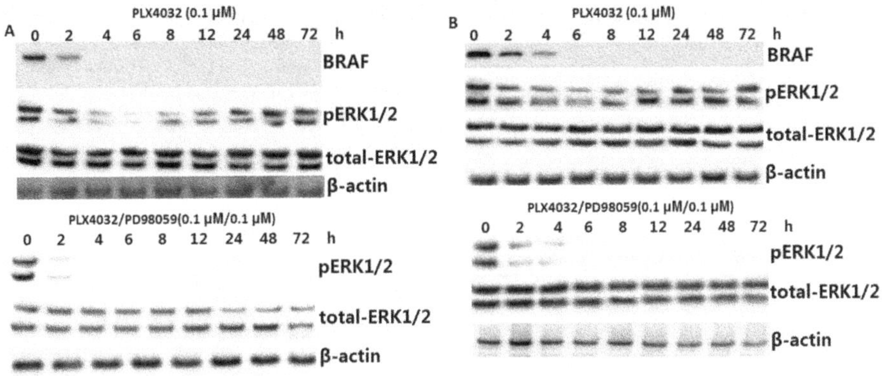

Fig. 3 Western blot of BRAF and pERK levels in lysates of BCPAP cells (**a**) and K1 cells (**b**) treated with PLX4032 (0.1 μM) or PLX4032 (0.1 μM)/PD98059 (0.1 μM) for indicated times

activation in BCPAP cells (Fig. 3a). PLX4032 or PD98059 (0.1 μM) treatment has the same results on K1 cells (Fig. 3b).

Discussion

Radioiodine ablation is the classical and standard treatments for thyroid cancer, which takes advantage of the unique iodide-transporting function of NIS in the thyroid cell membrane. However, the expression of iodide-metabolizing gene NIS is reduced in thyroid cancer, resulting in the reduction of iodide accumulation in the thyroid cells, particularly in dedifferentiated carcinoma. The decrease of NIS expression level directly leads to the reducion of iodine accumulation capacity in thyroid gland cells and the resistance to radioiodine therapy, leading to the treatment failure [20]. Therefore, understanding the mechanism of NIS and iodine treatment resistance is very important to overcome the radioiodine therapy resistance.

The BRAF^{V600E} mutation is the most common genetic change in thyroid cancer, particularly in papillary thyroid cancer (PTC) [4]. BRAF V600E mutation could abnormaly activate RAS-BRAF-MEK-MAP kinase (MAPK) pathway, leading to the thyroid tumorigenesis [19]. Several studies have demonstrated that B-RafV600E represses NIS expression [21, 22], but restoring NIS expression in thyroid cells when inhibiting the BRAFV600E/MEK pathway or silencing of BRAFV600E expression [7]. Clinical small sample size trials with MEK or BRAF inhibitors unfortunately failed to meet high expectations [23].

In our study, we demonstrated that inhibition of BRAF/MEK by PLX4032 alone did not significantly induce NIS expression and increase radioiodine uptake in both of the two cell lines, and PD98059 alone slightly increased NIS protein levels and radioiodine uptake in both of the two cell lines, especially in K1 cells. However, combination of PLX4032 and PD98059 significantly increased NIS protein levels and radioiodine uptake in both of the two cell lines, suggesting that inhibiting both BRAF/MEK and ERK1/2 can produce stronger redifferetiation effect.

Previous studies have found that PLX4032 treatment can cause a transient decrease of ERK1/2 activity in BRAFV600E-positive PTC cells, followed by the rebound of ERK1/2 activity in a time-dependent manne [17]. In our study, we found that PLX4032 (0.1 μM) treatment resulted in completely inhibition of pERK expression in 6–8 hs, but rebound from 8 h, and gradually reached the high levels at 24 hs and retained this levels for 72 h. However, PLX4032 combined with PD98059 completely prevented the reactivation of ERK1/2 in both of the cells. Our data shows that combination therapy by inhibiting the rebound of ERK1/2 activation induced NIS expression and increased radioiodine uptake in the two PTC cells.

Conclusion

In conclusion, our study showed that PLX4032 combined with PD98059 can induce NIS expression and increase radioiodine uptake in PTC cells harboring *BRAF*^{V600E} though effectively preventing ERK1/2 activity rebound. Our study provides a theoretical basis for combining PLX4032/PD98059 and ^{131}I treatment in in vivo expriments and clinical studies, which is also a promising treatment protocol for BRAF ^{V600E} positive PTC.

Abbreviations

NIS: Sodium/iodide symporter; RAI: Radioiodide-refractory; MAPK: Mitogen-activated protein kinase; TSHR: Thyroid-stimulating hormone receptor.

Funding

This work was founded by Shandong Natural Scientific Fund (funding reference no. ZR2016HM046).

Authors' contributions
ZHL and CD designed the project and performed all the experiments. ZHL wrote the article. Both authors read and approved the final manuscript.

Consent for publication
Not applicable.

Competing interests
The authors declare that they have no competing interests.

Author details
[1]Department of Thyroid Surgery, the affiliated Hospital of Qingdao University, Qingdao, Shandong, China. [2]Department of General Surgery, the affiliated Hospital of Qingdao University, Qingdao, Shandong, China.

References
1. Maxon HR, Thomas SR, Hertzberg VS, Kereiakes JG, Chen IW, Sperling MI, Saenger EL. Relation between effective radiation dose and outcome of radioiodine therapy for thyroid cancer. N Engl J Med. 1983;309:937–41.
2. Spitzweg C, Morris JC. The sodium iodide symporter: its pathophysiological and therapeutic implications. Clin Endocrinol. 2002;57:559–74.
3. Xing M, Haugen BR, Schlumberger M. Progress in molecular-based management of differentiated thyroid cancer. Lancet. 2013;381:1058–69.
4. Xing M. BRAF mutation in thyroid cancer. Endocr Relat Cancer. 2005;12:245–62.
5. Davies H, Bignell GR, Cox C. Mutations of the BRAF gene in human cancer. Nature. 2002;417:949–54.
6. Hou P, Bojdani E, Xing M. Induction of thyroid gene expression and radioiodine uptake in thyroid cancer cells by targeting major signaling pathways. J Clin Endocrinol Metab. 2010;95:820–8.
7. Liu D, Hu S, Hou P, Jiang D, Condouris S, Xing M. Suppression of BRAF/MEK/MAP kinase pathway restores expression of iodide-metabolizing genes in thyroid cells expressing the V600E BRAF mutant. Clin Cancer Res. 2007;13:1341–9.
8. Hou P, Liu D, Ji M, Liu Z, Engles JM, Wahl RL, Xing M. Induction of thyroid gene expression and radioiodine uptake in melanoma cells: novel therapeutic implications. PLoS One. 2009;4:e6200.
9. Rothenberg SM, McFadden DG, Palmer EL, Daniels GH, Wirth LJ. Redifferentiation of iodine-refractory BRAF V600E-mutant metastatic papillary thyroid cancer with dabrafenib. Clin Cancer Res. 2015;21(5):1028–35.
10. Yang H, Higgins B, Kolinsky K, et al. RG7204 (PLX4032) a selective BRAFV600E inhibitor, displays potent antitumor activity in preclinical melanoma models. Cancer Res 2010;70:9527–9527.
11. Kim G, McKee AE, Ning YM, et al. FDA approval summary: vemurafenib for treatment of unresectable or metastatic melanoma with the BRAFV600E mutation. Clin Cancer Res. 2014;20(19):4994–5000.
12. Flaherty KT, Puzanov I, Kim KB, Ribas A, McArthur GA, Sosman JA, O'Dwyer PJ, Lee RJ, Grippo JF, Nolop K, Chapman PB. Inhibition of mutated, activated BRAF in metastatic melanoma. N Engl J Med. 2010;363(9):809–19.
13. Kim KB, Cabanillas ME, Lazar AJ, Williams MD, Sanders DL, Ilagan JL, Nolop K, Lee RJ, Sherman SI. Clinical responses to vemurafenib in patients with metastatic papillary thyroid cancer harboring BRAF(V600E) mutation. Thyroid. 2013;23(10):1277–83.
14. Dadu R, Shah K, Busaidy NL, Waguespack SG, Habra MA, Ying AK, Hu MI, Bassett R, Jimenez C, Sherman SI, Cabanillas ME. Efficacy and tolerability of vemurafenib in patients with BRAF(V600E) -positive papillary thyroid cancer: M.D. Anderson Cancer center off label experience. J Clin Endocrinol Metab. 2015;100(1):E77–81.
15. Brose MS, Cabanillas ME, Cohen EE, Wirth LJ, Riehl T, Yue H, Sherman SI, Sherman EJ. Vemurafenib in patients with BRAF (V600E)-positive metastatic orunresectable papillary thyroid cancer refractory to radioactive iodine: anon-randomised, multicentre, open-label, phase 2 trial. Lancet Oncol. 2016;17(9):1272–82.
16. Domínguez Ayala M, Expósito Rodríguez A, Bilbao González A, Mínguez Gabiña P, Gutiérrez Rodríguez T, Rodeño Ortiz de Zarate E, García Carrillo M, Barrios T, Reviño B. BRAF V600E mutation in papillary thyroid cancer and its effect on postoperative radioiodine ($_{131}$I) therapy: should we modify our therapeutic strategy? Cir Esp. 2018;96(5):276–82.
17. Song H, Zhang J, Ning L, Zhang H, Chen D, Jiao X, Zhang K. The MEK1/2 inhibitor AZD6244 sensitizes BRAF-mutant thyroid Cancer to Vemurafenib. Med Sci Monit. 2018;24:3002–10.
18. Schweppe RE, Klopper JP, Korch C, Pugazhenthi U, Benezra M, Knauf JA, Fagin JA, Marlow LA, Copland JA, Smallridge RC, Haugen BR. Deoxyribonucleic acid profiling analysis of 40 human thyroid cancer cell lines reveals cross-contamination resulting in cell line redundancy and misidentification. J Clin Endocrinol Metab. 2008;93(11):4331–41.
19. Kogai T, Kanamoto Y, Li AI, Che LH, Ohashi E, Taki K, Chandraratna RA, Saito T, Brent GA. Differential regulation of sodium/iodide symporter gene expression by nuclear receptor ligands in MCF-7 breast cancer cells. Endocrinology. 2005;146:3059–69.
20. Xing M. Molecular pathogenesis and mechanisms of thyroid cancer. Nat Rev Cancer. 2013;13:184–99.
21. Mitsutake N, Miyagishi M, Mitsutake S, Akeno N, Mesa C Jr, Knauf JA, Zhang L, Taira K, Fagin JA. BRAF mediates RET/PTC-induced mitogen-activated protein kinase activation in thyroid cells: functional support for requirement of the RET/PTC-RAS-BRAF pathway in papillary thyroid carcinogenesis. Endocrinology. 2006;147:1014–9.
22. Riesco-Eizaguirre G, Gutiérrez-Martínez P, García-Cabezas MA, Nistal M, Santisteban P. The oncogene BRAF V600E is associated with a high risk of recurrence and less differentiated papillary thyroid carcinoma due to the impairment of Na+/I- targeting to the membrane. Endocr Relat Cancer. 2006;13:257–69.
23. Ho AL, Grewal RK, Leboeuf R, Sherman EJ, Pfister DG, Deandreis D, Pentlow KS, Zanzonico PB, Haque S, Gavane S, Ghossein RA, Ricarte-Filho JC, Dominguez JM, Shen R, Tuttle RM, Larson SM, Fagin JA. Selumetinib-enhanced radioiodine uptake in advanced thyroid cancer. N Engl J Med. 2013;368:623–32.

24

A retrospective review of the multidisciplinary management of medullary thyroid cancer: eligibility for systemic therapy

Georgia Geller[1], Janessa Laskin[1], Winson Y. Cheung[2] and Cheryl Ho[1*]

Abstract

Background: Medullary thyroid carcinoma (MTC) accounts for 1-2% of all thyroid cancers. The clinical course of metastatic disease can be indolent. Our aim was to characterize the natural history of disease to evaluate the true proportion of patients who would be eligible for the currently available systemic therapies.

Methods: The British Columbia Cancer Agency (BCCA) provides cancer care to a population of 4.6 million. A retrospective chart review was conducted of all patients with MTC referred to the BCCA from 1991 to 2013. Clinical characteristics, pathology, treatment and outcome data were collected. Relapse free survival and overall survival was determined for patients based on staging at the time of diagnosis.

Results: Of the 98 patients referred to the BCCA during the study period, inherited mutations were found in 6% though 60% did not undergo genetic testing. Based on clinical SEER staging at diagnosis 50% had localized disease, 38% regional, and 12% had distant metastasis. 77% had complete surgical resection of which 25% received adjuvant radiation therapy. Five year relapse free survival (RFS) for localized and regional disease was 75% and 66%, respectively ($p = 0.006$). Initial treatment of 23 patients with locally unresectable and metastatic disease predominantly involved multiple modalities. Of the 37 patients with relapsed or metastatic MTC only 7 (19%) patients received one or more course of chemotherapy for metastatic disease: 1 temsirolimus, 2 adriamycin, 3 sunitinib, 3 sorafenib, and 3 vandetanib. Five year OS based on clinical SEER stage: localized 93%, regional 72% and distant 33% ($p < 0.001$).

Conclusion: Localized and regional MTC treatment patterns reflect multidisciplinary management based on disease characteristics. Patients with distant disease had poor outcomes with 28% of patients dying from disease. In our cohort the minority of patients ultimately received systemic therapy due to timing and lack of TKI availability.

Keywords: Medullary thyroid carcinoma, Vandetinib, Cabozantinib, Population-based, Tyrosine kinase inhibitors

Background

Medullary thyroid cancer (MTC) is a neuroendocrine malignancy of the parafollicular cells of the thyroid [1]. These cells are responsible for secreting calcitonin, a hormone involved in calcium homeostasis. MTC currently accounts for 2% of all thyroid malignancies [2].

MTC can be associated with an inherited predisposition, with 20-25% of all cases due to mutations in the rearranged during transfection (RET) proto-oncogene. Mutations in RET are associated with autosomal dominant syndromes including MEN2A, MEN2B, familial MTC and are found in approximately 50% of sporadic cases [3].

The cornerstone of local treatment of MTC is surgical resection consisting of total thyroidectomy with dissection of central lymph node compartment and resection of the involved lateral compartment. Radiation has a limited role with little randomized control data supporting its use; however, adjuvant radiation is recommended for microscopic or macroscopic residual disease, extra-thyroidal

* Correspondence: cho@bccancer.bc.ca
[1]Medical Oncology, British Columbia Cancer Agency, 600 W 10th Avenue, Vancouver, BC V5Z 4E6, Canada
Full list of author information is available at the end of the article

extension or extensive lymph node metastases and in cases where there is a concern for airway obstruction [4].

Recurrent or metastatic MTC may not be amenable to localized treatment options. The course of disease may also vary significantly with many patients having an indolent course despite metastases. A select group of patients, however, may have more aggressive disease, which may be predicted by the type of RET mutation and the calcitonin doubling time [5, 6].

Up until recently there were no standard first line systemic therapies for inoperable MTC. There is now phase III evidence supporting the use of tyrosine kinase inhibitors (TKIs), vandetanib and cabozantinib, for patients with metastatic disease [7, 8]. Decision-making regarding systemic therapy incorporates not just biochemical parameters but include radiographic findings and the anticipated natural history of the disease.

Our objective was to review the multidisciplinary treatment and outcomes of patients referred to the BC Cancer Agency (BCCA) with MTC to determine the natural history of the disease in our population and the effect of different treatment modalities including surgery, radiation and systemic therapies on patients' outcomes. With the introduction of systemic therapy into the treatment algorithm, we sought to determine the proportion of patients who would clinically warrant therapy with a TKI.

Methods

A retrospective review of all patients referred to the BCCA between January 1, 1991 and December 31, 2013 for management of pathologically confirmed MTC was performed.

Patient and tumor characteristics were abstracted from the Outcomes and Surveillance Integrated System (OaSIS) and chart review, including age at diagnosis, gender, RET testing, history of associated MEN2 conditions, presenting symptoms, histology and staging information. The 7th edition TNM system was used for staging. Surveillance Epidemiology and End Results (SEER) program definitions included localized - tumor confined entirely to the thyroid gland, regional -extension beyond the thyroid directly into surrounding tissues or regional lymph node metastases and distant - metastasis to extracervical lymph nodes or organs [9].

Initial and subsequent management including type of surgery, dose, fraction and location of radiation and use of systemic therapy were collected. The disease status at last follow-up, date of death, and cause of death were recorded.

Kaplan-Meier curves for relapse free survival and overall survival were calculated and compared using the log rank test. Relapse free survival was defined as date of complete surgical resection to date of clinical, radiographic or pathologic evidence of recurrence with patients censored for death or date of last follow-up. Overall survival was defined as date of diagnosis to date of death from any cause, with living subjects censored at last follow-up. Cox regression was used to conduct multivariate analysis for OS.

The study was approved by the BC Cancer Agency research ethics board.

Results

Ninety-eight patients with pathology confirmed MTC were referred to the BCCA during the study period.

Table 1 outlines patient characteristics of the 98 patients. The median age of diagnosis was 54 (range 10-95). The majority of patients were female 53 (54%). Thirty nine patients (40%) had RET testing, with 6 patients (6%) having MEN2 or familial MTC syndrome. Eighty five patients presented with documented localized symptoms which included a neck mass, hoarseness, dysphagia or dyspnea. Twenty patients (20%) had systemic symptoms at presentation including constitutional symptoms, diarrhea, bone pain, or flushing. At baseline 50% of the patients presented with clinically localized disease, 37 patients (38%) with

Table 1 Baseline MTC patient characteristics

Patient Characteristics	*n* = 98
Male	45 (46)
Age at diagnosis – median (range)	54 (10-95)
Genetic Mutation – no. (%)	
FMTC or MEN 2	6 (6)
Sporadic	33 (34)
Unknown	59 (60)
Local symptoms at presentation – no. (%)	
Present	85 (87)
Not present	12 (12)
Unknown	1 (1)
Systemic symptoms at presentation – no. (%)	
Present	20 (20)
Not present	77 (79)
Unknown	1 (1)
Clinical Stage at presentation - no. (%)	
Stage I	19 (19)
Stage II	26 (27)
Stage III	11 (11)
Stage IVa	25 (26)
Stage IVb	0 (0)
Stage IVc	12 (12)
Unknown	5 (5)
Clinical SEER at presentation- no. (%)	
Localized	49 (50)
Regional	37 (38)
Distant	12 (12)

regional disease and 12 patients (12%) presented with metastatic disease based on the SEER classification system.

The initial management of patients is outlined in Fig. 1. Of the 86 patients with locoregional disease 75 were resected without evidence of gross residual disease. Surgical intervention included 1 lobectomy, 2 lobectomy with isthmusectomy and 72 total/subtotal thyroidectomy. Nodal management of disease included: 9 no nodal surgery, 31 limited and 35 modified radical/radical neck dissection. Nineteen of these patients also received adjuvant radiation. Sixty nine patients had post-operative calcitonin levels available and of these, 38 patients (55.1%) had normalization of calcitonin and 31 (44.9%) had persistently elevated calcitonin despite resection. The initial treatment of 23 patients with unresectable or metastatic disease were: 2 palliative debulking only, 4 radiation only, 11 palliative debulking and radiation, 3 all 3 modalities and 3 best supportive care alone.

The delivery of systemic treatment is outlined in Table 2. Thirty seven patients either presented with metastatic disease or developed recurrence or metastatic disease. Seven patients received one or more course of systemic therapy and 5 of these patients received one or more TKIs. Of the 27 patients who died from metastatic MTC, 19 died prior to the availability of TKIs.

RFS and OS are shown in Figs 2 and 3. Five year RFS for localized and regional disease was 75% and 66%, respectively ($p = 0.006$). Five year OS rates and medians based on clinical SEER stage: localized 93%/19.9 years, regional 72%/16.1 years, and distant 33%/0.9 years ($p < 0.001$). Median OS for all patients at diagnosis was 16.1 years.

Univariate and multivariate analysis showed that older age, systemic symptoms at presentation and more advanced SEER stage were associated with poorer OS (Table 3).

Discussion

This study confirms the typically indolent nature of MTC with the median OS of all patients being 16.1 years. On multivariate analysis patient age at diagnosis, systemic symptoms at presentation and more advanced stage were associated with poor overall survival. Following the natural history of disease over multiple years demonstrates that 38% of patients would be ultimately eligible for systemic therapy for disease based on the patterns of recurrence and the cause of death.

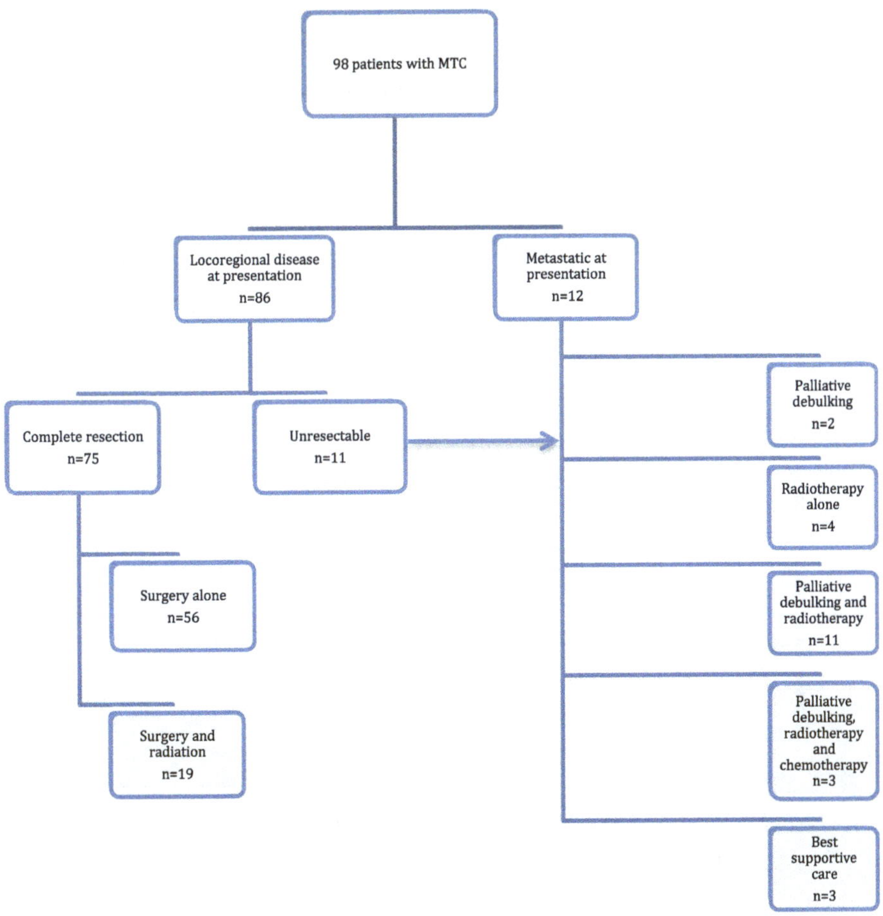

Fig. 1 Initial management of MTC

Table 2 Systemic treatment of unresectable or metastatic medullary thyroid carcinoma

Systemic therapy for MTC n = 98	n (%)
Metastatic disease at presentation (%)	12 (12)
Developed unresectable recurrence or metastatic disease (%)	25 (26)
Received systemic therapy for unresectable or metastatic MTC (%)	7/37 (19)
Systemic therapy given[a] – no.	
Sunitinib	3
Sorafenib	2
Vandetanib	3
Temsirolimus	1
Doxorubicin	2
Death due to MTC – no. (%)	27 (28)
Prescribed TKI	2
Prescribed doxorubicin	2
Discussed TKI but did not receive therapy	5
TKI available but never discussed	1
TKI not available	17

[a]Some patients received 2 or more lines of systemic therapy and are still alive on treatment

In our study, similar to other groups, negative prognostic indicators included advanced age, systemic symptoms at presentation and more advanced stage at presentation. The SEER database analysis of over 1200 patients with MTC identified that age > 65 and advanced stage were associated with worse survival outcomes [10]. Two Korean studies also noted that distant metastases portended a reduction in survival [11, 12]. T stage and age were noted in an Irish population to have poorer overall survival [13]. Beyond baseline characteristics, Barbet et al. found that a calcitonin doubling time over 2 years had a 10 y survival over 100%, compared to those with a doubling time less than 0.5 years being only 8% [6]. These variables can help provide some insight into prognosis and may facilitate selection of MTC patients for consideration of therapy.

With the introduction of new systemic therapies for management and the understanding that MTC can often be an indolent disease, our goal was to determine the proportion of patients truly eligible for systemic treatment based on recurrence and death from MTC. The BC Cancer Agency collects all malignant diagnoses in the province as part of our responsibilities for reporting to the Canadian Cancer Registry and provides all of the radiotherapy for a population of 4.6 million. This unique registry organization enables a true population based overview of the natural history of many cancers including MTC.

In our cohort, 38% of patients ultimately would have been eligible for systemic therapy based on disease aspects alone. The true number, however, would likely be lower due to comorbidities and patient preferences based on the side effect profiles of therapy. Due to timing and lack of availability, only 19% of patients had received systemic therapy, these patients were most commonly treated with multi-targeted tyrosine kinase inhibitors (TKIs) focused on vascular endothelial growth factor (VEGF) that were available off-label through a government funded compassionate access program. The positive phase III data for vandetinib and cabozantinib now offer symptomatic patients therapeutic options that improve

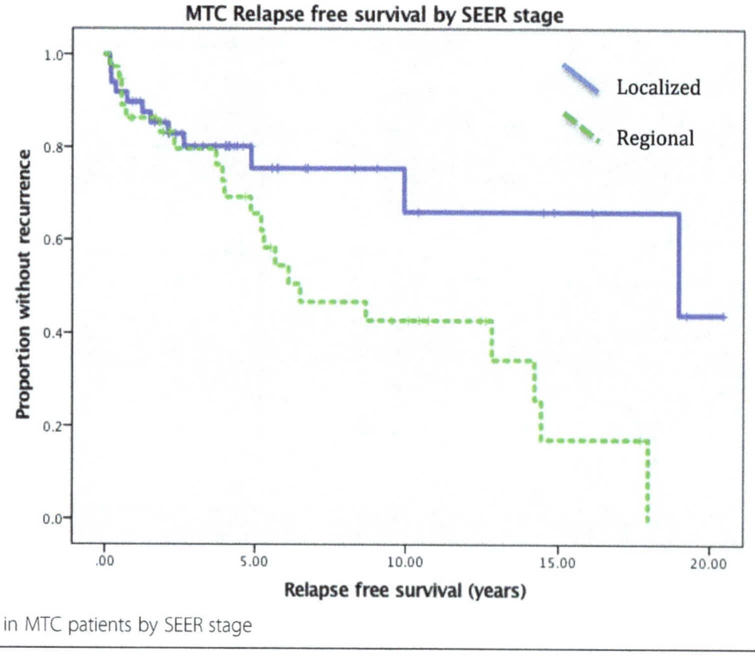

Fig. 2 Relapse free survival in MTC patients by SEER stage

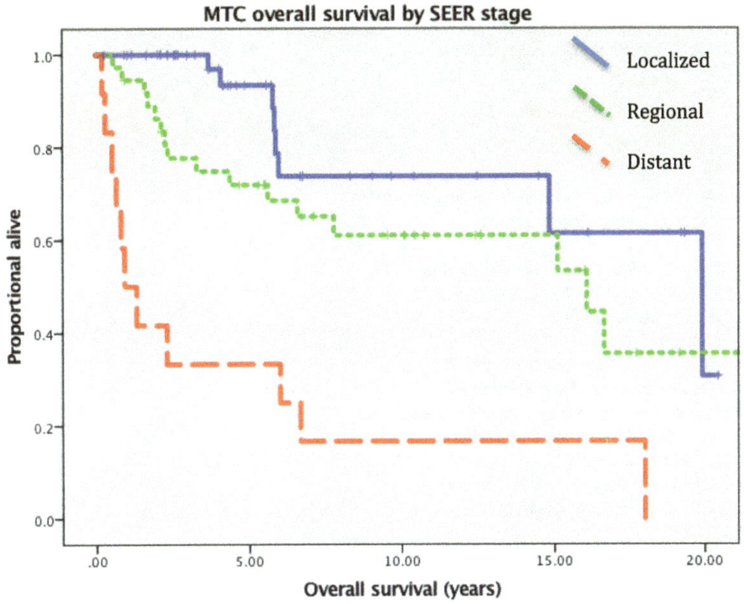

Fig. 3 Overall survival for MTC patients by SEER stage

progression free survival with an acceptable toxicity profile [7, 8].

There are several limitations to this study. It is retrospective in nature and despite serving a large population over a long duration of time there were only 98 patients. Several data points were not available because the data are based on physicians' usual patterns of practice; they included testing for RET mutations and calcitonin doubling time. While many patients did have serial calcitonin levels it was difficult to calculate a meaningful doubling time due to transition between 3 different laboratory tests over the study period. Our strengths include the population-based nature of the study that allows a longitudinal view of the natural history of disease.

Table 3 Univariate and multivariate analysis of the impact of baseline characteristics on overall survival

	Univariate HR	*P* value	Multivariate HR	*P* value
Female	1.58	0.19		
Older age	1.04	<0.001	1.06	<0.001
Local symptoms at presentation	0.54	0.27		
Systemic symptoms at presentation	3.68	<0.001	3.42	0.002
SEER stage				
Regional vs localized	2.19	0.07	3.55	0.007
Distant vs localized	7.76	<0.001	7.15	<0.001

Conclusions

The natural history of localized and regional MTC is generally indolent with many patients having excellent long-term outcomes. Our population-based study suggests that only a small proportion of MTC patients will require treatment with systemic therapy for palliation over the course of their disease. Baseline factors that may enable appropriate patient selection for systemic treatment are limited and it is the likely the behavior of disease over time with biochemical and radiologic changes being the best means of correctly selecting patients for therapy.

Acknowledgements
The OaSIS database system was developed with the financial assistance of Boehringer Ingelheim, Bristol Myer Squibb, Eli Lilly, Roche and the BC Cancer Foundation.

Funding
This research was conducted with financial support from Astra Zeneca.

Authors' contributions
GG collected the data for the study and was involved in the study design, analysis and writing of the manuscript. JL and WC were involved in study design and writing of the manuscript. CH was involved in the study design, analysis and writing of the manuscript. All authors read and approved the final manuscript.

Consent for publication
Not applicable.

Competing interests
The authors declare that they have no competing interests.

Author details
[1]Medical Oncology, British Columbia Cancer Agency, 600 W 10th Avenue, Vancouver, BC V5Z 4E6, Canada. [2]Medical Oncology, Tom Baker Cancer Centre, Calgary, AB, Canada.

References

1. Hazard JB, Hawk WA, Crile G Jr. Medullary (solid) carcinoma of the thyroid; a clinicopathologic entity. J Clin Endocrinol Metab. 1959;19:152–61. doi:10.1210/jcem-19-1-152.
2. Enewold L, Zhu K, Ron E, Marrogi AJ, Stojadinovic A, Peoples GE, Devesa SS. Rising thyroid cancer incidence in the United States by demographic and tumor characteristics, 1980-2005. Cancer Epidemiol Biomark Prev. 2009;18: 784–91. doi:10.1158/1055-9965.EPI-08-0960.
3. Hofstra RM, Landsvater RM, Ceccherini I, Stulp RP, Stelwagen T, Luo Y, Pasini B, Hoppener JW, van Amstel HK, Romeo G. A mutation in the RET proto-oncogene associated with multiple endocrine neoplasia type 2B and sporadic medullary thyroid carcinoma. Nature. 1994;367:375–6. doi:10.1038/367375a0.
4. Wells SA Jr, Asa SL, Dralle H, Elisei R, Evans DB, Gagel RF, Lee N, Machens A, Moley JF, Pacini F, et al. Revised American Thyroid Association guidelines for the management of medullary thyroid carcinoma. Thyroid. 2015;25:567–610. doi:10.1089/thy.2014.0335.
5. Machens A, Gimm O, Hinze R, Hoppner W, Boehm BO, Dralle H. Genotype-phenotype correlations in hereditary medullary thyroid carcinoma: oncological features and biochemical properties. J Clin Endocrinol Metab. 2001;86:1104–9. doi:10.1210/jcem.86.3.7290.
6. Barbet J, Campion L, Kraeber-Bodere F, Chatal JF, GTE Study Group. Prognostic impact of serum calcitonin and carcinoembryonic antigen doubling-times in patients with medullary thyroid carcinoma. J Clin Endocrinol Metab. 2005;90:6077–84. doi:10.1210/jc.2005-0044.
7. Wells SA Jr, Robinson BG, Gagel RF, Dralle H, Fagin JA, Santoro M, Baudin E, Elisei R, Jarzab B, Vasselli JR, et al. Vandetanib in patients with locally advanced or metastatic medullary thyroid cancer: a randomized, double-blind phase III trial. J Clin Oncol. 2012;30:134–41. doi:10.1200/JCO.2011.35.5040.
8. Elisei R, Schlumberger MJ, Muller SP, Schoffski P, Brose MS, Shah MH, Licitra L, Jarzab B, Medvedev V, Kreissl MC, et al. Cabozantinib in progressive medullary thyroid cancer. J Clin Oncol. 2013;31:3639–46. doi:10.1200/JCO.2012.48.4659.
9. National Cancer Institute D, Surveillance Research Program, Cancer Statistics Branch. Available at URL: http://seer.cancer.gov/about/. [Accessed February 2017].
10. Roman S, Lin R, Sosa JA. Prognosis of medullary thyroid carcinoma: demographic, clinical, and pathologic predictors of survival in 1252 cases. Cancer. 2006;107:2134–42. doi:10.1002/cncr.22244.
11. Lee CR, Lee S, Son H, Ban E, Kang SW, Lee J, Jeong JJ, Nam KH, Chung WY, Park CS. Medullary thyroid carcinoma: a 30-year experience at one institution in Korea. Ann Surg Treat Res. 2016;91:278–87. doi:10.4174/astr.2016.91.6.278.
12. Jung KY, Kim SM, Yoo WS, Kim BW, Lee YS, Kim KW, Lee KE, Jeong JJ, Nam KH, Lee SH, et al. Postoperative biochemical remission of serum calcitonin is the best predictive factor for recurrence-free survival of medullary thyroid cancer: a large-scale retrospective analysis over 30 years. Clin Endocrinol. 2016;84:587–97. doi:10.1111/cen.12852.
13. Lennon P, Deady S, White N, Lambert D, Healy ML, Green A, Kinsella J, Timon C, O'Neill JP. Aggressive medullary thyroid cancer, an analysis of the Irish National Cancer Registry. Ir J Med Sci. 2016. doi: 10.1007/s11845-016-1455-1

25

Correlation between anti-thyroid peroxidase antibody levels and diffuse thyroid uptake of ^{18}F-fluorodeoxyglucose in Hashimoto's thyroiditis

Naoki Edo[1], Koji Morita[1*], Miki Sakamoto[1], Tatsuro Kaminaga[2], Hiromi Edo[3], Erina Okamura[1], Masumi Ogawa[1], Kazuhisa Tsukamoto[1], Hiroko Okinaga[1] and Toshio Ishikawa[1]

Abstract

Background: On ^{18}F-fluorodeoxyglucose (FDG)-positron emission tomography (PET), diffuse uptake in the thyroid gland is often observed in patients with Hashimoto's thyroiditis. In this study, we evaluated the factors associated with diffuse uptake by comparing Hashimoto's thyroiditis patients with or without diffuse uptake in the thyroid.

Methods: A retrospective study was conducted of 18 patients with Hashimoto's thyroiditis who underwent blood tests, thyroid ultrasonography, and FDG-PET during the period from 2014 to 2015. The patients were divided into two groups: one with diffuse thyroid uptake (group 1, $n = 13$) and one without diffuse thyroid uptake (group 2, $n = 5$). Clinical and laboratory parameters, including maximum standardized uptake in the thyroid (SUVmax), which was defined as the higher value obtained in either the right or left thyroid lobe, were compared in the two groups.

Results: The frequency of abnormal findings, such as a rough or heterogeneous pattern, was significantly higher in group 1 ($p < 0.01$), as were anti-thyroid peroxidase (TPO) antibody titers, anti-thyroglobulin (Tg) antibody titers, and SUVmax ($p < 0.01$). The frequency of hypothyroidism did not differ significantly in the two groups. Anti-TPO and anti-Tg titers were positively correlated with SUVmax ($r = 0.856$, $p < 0.01$ and $r = 0.821$, $p < 0.01$, respectively); in univariate analysis, anti-TPO titer was predictive of SUVmax ($p < 0.01$).

Conclusions: The results of the current study suggest that Hashimoto's thyroiditis patients with high titers of anti-thyroid antibodies are likely to exhibit intense diffuse FDG uptake in the thyroid, and that thyroid function may be clearly impaired, even in the presence of mild FDG uptake in the thyroid.

Keywords: Anti-thyroid antibody, Diffuse uptake, FDG-PET, Hashimoto's thyroiditis

Background

Positron emission tomography (PET) with ^{18}F-fluorodeoxyglucose (FDG) is a functional imaging technique known as FDG-PET that exploits the typically increased rate of glycolysis in specific cell types, such as malignant tumors and inflammatory tissue [1, 2]. Its use as a method of detecting malignant tumors and foci of infection has recently become more frequent.

With regard to the thyroid, a normal thyroid gland is not visible or shows only low-grade FDG uptake on FDG-PET [3, 4]. However, the increasing use of FDG-PET has led to incidental identification of patients with increased FDG uptake in the thyroid gland. FDG uptake in the thyroid predominantly conforms to one of two patterns: focal and diffuse. The prevalences of incidental focal and diffuse uptake in the thyroid reportedly vary from 0.1 to 4.8% and 0.1 to 4.5%, respectively [5]. Focal

* Correspondence: kmorita@med.teikyo-u.ac.jp
[1]Department of Internal Medicine, Teikyo University School of Medicine, 2-11-1, Kaga, Itabashi, Tokyo 173-0003, Japan
Full list of author information is available at the end of the article

uptake in the thyroid suggests the possibility of a malignant tumor, such as papillary thyroid carcinoma, although most well-differentiated thyroid carcinomas are relatively slow-growing and can be FDG-negative [6, 7]. In contrast, diffuse FDG uptake is typically considered to be a result of benign conditions, such as Hashimoto's thyroiditis or Graves' disease, among others [8, 9]; however, there have been few reports of diffuse uptake. Furthermore, among patients with Hashimoto's thyroiditis, not all patients exhibit diffuse uptake.

In the current study, we evaluated the factors associated with diffuse uptake by comparing Hashimoto's thyroiditis patients with or without diffuse uptake in the thyroid.

Methods

Patients

Records of 18 consecutive attendees (five men, 13 women) with Hashimoto's thyroiditis who underwent blood tests, thyroid ultrasonography (US), and FDG-PET at our hospital during the period from 2014 to 2015 were examined retrospectively. Clinical diagnosis of Hashimoto's thyroiditis was made based on the elevation of either anti-thyroid peroxidase (TPO) antibody titer or anti-thyroglobulin (Tg) antibody titer. Additionally, the possibility of neoplastic diseases was considered highly unlikely based on clinical symptoms and ultrasonographic findings, although we did not perform histopathological examinations. Details of the subjects are presented in Table 1. The patients were divided into two groups, one with diffuse thyroid uptake (group 1, $n = 13$) and one without diffuse thyroid uptake (group 2, $n = 5$). Clinical and laboratory parameters were investigated, including the maximum standardized uptake value (SUVmax) in the thyroid. The study was approved by the institutional review board of Teikyo University Hospital, Japan (18–036), and the need for written informed consent was waived.

Data analysis

Serum levels of thyroid stimulating hormone (TSH), free T4, Tg, anti-Tg antibody, and anti-TPO antibody were measured. Thyroid US was performed close to the time of FDG-PET examination. SUVmax in the thyroid was recorded as the higher value obtained from either the right or the left thyroid lobe.

PET/computed tomography

All PET scans were performed on a PET/computed tomography (CT) system (Biograph 40 True Point, Siemens Health Care, Erlangen, Germany). FDG was supplied via

Table 1 Details of the subjects

Subject number	Age, sex	Findings in thyroid ultrasonography	TSH (μIU/mL)	FT4 (ng/dL)	FT3 (pg/mL)	L-T4 replacement dose (μg/day)	Tg-Ab (IU/mL)	TPO-Ab (IU/mL)	SUV max	Interval Between FDG-PET and thyroid test (days)
Diffuse uptake										
1	51 F	Hetero, Hypo	22.43	1.06	2.20	0	143	22	3.322	13
2	78 F	Hetero	6.73	0.78	2.08	0	> 4000	487	8.125	11
3	68 F	Hetero, Hypo	73.06	0.57	2.37	25	> 4000	16	3.741	28
4	59 F	Hetero	6.43	0.93	3.21	0	n.a.	184	6.070	64
5	80 M	Rough, Hetero	28.59	1.07	2.56	0	> 4000	> 600	5.714	3
6	86 F	Hetero	21.04	0.68	1.75	12.5	476	53	3.354	1
7	64 F	Hetero	3.79	1.32	1.16	0	122	29	2.923	1
8	66 M	Hetero, Hypo	8.45	0.93	2.64	0	> 4000	> 600	6.165	21
9	78 F	Rough, Hetero	87.87	0.50	1.50	25	n.a.	> 600	12.023	4
10	41 F	Rough, Homo	46.21	0.94	1.58	125	626	> 600	9.985	3
11	43 F	Hetero	3.24	1.31	2.49	0	537	332	4.113	7
12	67 F	Rough, Hetero	25.11	0.94	3.04	0	2940	184	3.340	24
13	63 M	Rough, Hetero	266.1	0.19	1.16	0	1360	72	3.868	19
Without diffuse uptake										
14	74 F	Homo	0.033	1.23	3.12	0	147	10	2.492	10
15	68 F	Homo	11.01	1.09	2.45	0	465	8	2.364	39
16	50 M	Homo	5.38	0.96	2.15	0	18	22	1.535	14
17	80 F	Homo	12.27	1.56	0.89	100	18	16	1.337	1
18	74 M	Fine, Homo	11.23	1.11	2.39	0	16	18	1.704	83

F female, *M* male, TSH serum thyroid stimulating hormone, *FT4* serum free T4, *FT3* serum free T3, *L-T4* levothyroxine, *Tg-Ab* anti-thyroglobulin antibody, *TPO-Ab* anti-thyroid peroxidase antibody, *SUVmax* maximum standardized uptake, *FDG* ^{18}F-fluorodeoxyglucose, *PET* positron emission tomography, *F* female, *M* male, *Hetero* heterogenous, *Hypo* hypoechoic, *Homo* homogenous, *n.a.* not assessed

a commercial delivery system (Nihon Medi-Physics Co., Ltd., Tokyo, Japan). All patients were fasted for at least 8 h before the injection of 165.5–352.5 MBq of FDG. Imaging was performed 1 h after injection and 2 h after injection. Three-dimensional scanning data were obtained from the top of the skull through to the pelvis, with a 3-min acquisition time per bed position. The studies were reconstructed using a vendor-supplied iterative reconstruction algorithm.

Laboratory tests

Serum levels of TSH, free T3, and free T4 were measured by using a chemiluminescence enzyme immunoassay (Lumipulse Presto, Fujirebio Co., Tokyo, Japan). Serum Tg, anti-Tg titer, and anti-TPO titer were measured with an electrochemiluminescence immunoassay (Elecsys Tg, Elecsys Anti-TPO, and Elecsys Anti-Tg, respectively; Roche Diagnostics K. K., Tokyo, Japan). The reference ranges for these laboratory tests at our institution were 0.5–5.0 mIU/mL for TSH, 2.3–4.0 pg/mL for free T3, 0.9–1.7 ng/dL for free T4, 0–33.7 ng/mL for serum Tg, 0–27 IU/mL for anti-Tg titer, and 0–15 IU/mL for anti-TPO titer. US examinations were performed with an 8.0-MHz linear phased-array probe (Aplio-XG, Canon Medical Systems Corporation, Tokyo, Japan). FDG uptake was evaluated by two board-certified radiologists (TK and HE).

Statistical analysis

All comparisons between the two groups were analyzed using the nonparametric Mann-Whitney U test. Differences in prevalence between men and women were evaluated by using the χ^2 test. Correlations were assessed by using Spearman's correlation coefficient analysis. All statistical analyses were performed with R version 3.4.1 (The R Foundation for Statistical Computing, Vienna, Austria). Two-tailed p values < 0.05 were considered significant.

Results

Comparison of clinical and laboratory parameters

Table 2 shows comparisons of clinical and laboratory parameters between patients with or without diffuse thyroid uptake of FDG. Anti-Tg titer and anti-TPO titer were significantly higher in group 1 than in group 2. Serum free T4 was also significantly higher in patients with diffuse thyroid uptake, but it was similar in groups 1 and 2 after excluding those undergoing replacement therapy consisting of levothyroxine. No significant differences in other parameters were detected. The patients in group 1 were more likely to exhibit diffusely swollen thyroids with a rough and/or heterogeneous pattern on thyroid US.

Associations between thyroid SUVmax and thyroid autoantibodies

Associations between thyroid SUVmax and thyroid autoantibodies were evaluated in all subjects. Thyroid SUVmax was positively correlated with both anti-TPO titer ($r = 0.856$, $p < 0.01$) and anti-Tg titer ($r = 0.821$, $p < 0.01$). Notably, however, anti-TPO and anti-Tg titers were also strongly correlated with each other ($r = 0.607$, $p < 0.05$). Therefore, univariate analysis of SUVmax was performed for each autoantibody. Anti-TPO titer was a significant

Table 2 Comparisons of clinical and laboratory parameters in the two groups

	Group 1: Patients with diffuse uptake	Group 2: Patients without diffuse uptake	*p*
n (female)	13 (10)	5 (3)	0.583
Serum TSH Median (minimum-maximum)	22.43 (3.24–266.1)	11.01 (0.033–12.27)	0.143
Serum TSH (only patients without replacement therapy) Median (minimum-maximum)	8.45 (3.24–266.1)	8.20 (0.03–11.23)	0.414
Serum free T3 Median (minimum-maximum)	2.20 (1.16–3.21)	2.39 (0.89–3.12)	0.921
Serum free T4 Median (minimum-maximum)	0.93 (0.19–1.32)	1.11 (0.96–1.56)	< 0.05
Serum free T4 (only patients without replacement therapy) Median (minimum-maximum)	0.94 (0.19–1.32)	1.10 (0.96–1.23)	0.247
Serum thyroglobulin Median (minimum-maximum)	1.465 (0.08–175.0)	3.435 (2.94–3.93)	0.533
Tg-Ab titer Median (minimum-maximum)	1360 (122–4000)	18 (16–465)	< 0.01
TPO-Ab titer Median (minimum-maximum)	184 (16–600)	16 (8–22)	< 0.01

TSH thyroid stimulating hormone, *Tg-Ab* anti-thyroglobulin antibody, *TPO-Ab* anti-thyroid peroxidase antibody

predictor of thyroid SUVmax in univariate analysis, but anti-Tg titer was not (Table 3). After transformation into Z-scores, anti-TPO titer yielded a β-coefficient of 0.851 ($p < 0.01$).

Discussion

In this study, we evaluated patients with Hashimoto's thyroiditis, which was diagnosed based on the elevation of either anti-TPO titer or anti-Tg titer; Hashimoto's thyroiditis patients with high titers of anti-thyroid antibodies were likely to exhibit intense diffuse FDG uptake in the thyroid. In contrast, the frequency of hypothyroidism was similar in patients with or without diffuse uptake in the thyroid.

Previous studies suggested that Hashimoto's thyroiditis is the most frequent cause of diffuse FDG uptake in the thyroid. Yasuda et al. [10] reported that, in a sample of 36 patients with diffuse FDG uptake, there were seven with hypothyroidism and 27 who were positive for anti-TPO antibody. In a sample of 45 patients, Kim et al. [11] detected 10 patients with hypothyroidism and six with anti-TPO or anti-Tg antibodies. Karantanis et al. [12] evaluated 133 patients with diffuse uptake in the thyroid, in most of whom the indication for FDG-PET was oncology imaging, and reported that 63 (47.4%) had prior clinical diagnoses of hypothyroidism or autoimmune thyroiditis. This percentage was significantly higher than that of their control group (13/133; 9.8%). In an evaluation of 137 patients with diffuse uptake, Lee et al. [13] found that 76 (55.5%) were positive for anti-microsomal antibody. This frequency was higher than that of patients without diffuse uptake (64/1925; 3.3%).

The mechanisms underlying diffuse FDG uptake in the thyroid have not yet been clarified. Glucose utilization by normal thyrocytes appears to be dependent on TSH. However, in the current study, which evaluated only patients with Hashimoto's thyroiditis, serum TSH and the frequency of hypothyroidism were similar regardless of diffuse FDG uptake. In fact, one patient in the present study required 100 μg levothyroxine despite low FDG uptake in the thyroid. However, Lee et al. [13] evaluated 2062 patients with or without diffuse uptake and found that TSH was significantly higher in patients with diffuse uptake. Therefore, the limited sample size in our study might underpower the results with respect to serum TSH and the frequency of hypothyroidism. Conversely, Yoshida et al. [14] evaluated 70 autopsied cases and reported that positive serum anti-thyroid antibodies in subjects without overt thyroid disease may indicate the existence of lymphocytic infiltration in the thyroid gland. In addition, inflammatory cells were shown to exhibit increased expression of glucose transporter isoforms when activated [15]. This indicates that thyroid FDG uptake may be associated with the degree of lymphocyte infiltration into the thyroid, rather than residual thyroid function, and higher SUVmax and high titers of anti-TPO antibody may indicate a higher degree of lymphocytic infiltration. Furthermore, in the current study, Hashimoto's thyroiditis patients with high titers of anti-TPO antibody were more likely to exhibit diffusely swollen thyroids with a heterogeneous pattern on US. In a previous study, high anti-TPO titer was highly indicative of the degree of hypoechoic pattern in autoimmune thyroiditis [16]. That result is concordant with the results of the current study. Further studies are necessary to clarify the relationships between FDG uptake, the degree of chronic thyroiditis, and the degree of hypothyroidism.

Anti-TPO antibody was predictive of SUVmax in the present study. However, Karantanis et al. [12] studied 21 patients with diffuse uptake and no prior history of thyroid disease and reported no correlation between SUVmax and TSH or anti-TPO titer. The discrepancy between their results and those of the current study may be partially due to differing backgrounds of the subjects in the two studies. The present study only included patients with serologically diagnosed Hashimoto's thyroiditis, while Karantanis et al. [12] included patients with other diseases. Several previous studies have evaluated clinical backgrounds in patients with diffuse uptake in the thyroid [10–13], but the current study is unique in that only patients with Hashimoto's thyroiditis were included. Additionally, in the clinical setting, diffuse FDG uptake may be observed in a patient without thyroid hormone replacement therapy, when his or her anti-TPO antibody titer is high.

The primary limitation of the present study was its small sample size. Notably, the relationship between higher SUVmax and high titers of anti-TPO antibody was observed in this study. However, additional studies with larger sample sizes are required to evaluate the relationship between TSH and diffuse FDG uptake. Another limitation of the present study was the method used for clinical diagnosis of Hashimoto's thyroiditis. We evaluated only clinical symptoms and

Table 3 Anti-TPO antibody titer and anti-Tg antibody titer univariate regression with SUVmax

1. Anti-TPO antibody				
Variate	*B* (S.E.)	β	t	*p*
Intercept	2.312 (0.546)		4.23	< 0.01
TPO-Ab titer	0.010 (0.002)	0.851	6.26	< 0.01
2. Anti-Tg antibody				
Variate	*B* (S.E.)	β	t	*p*
Intercept	2.949 (0.777)		3.80	< 0.01
Tg-Ab titer	0.001 (0.000)	0.390	2.10	0.06

TPO-Ab anti-thyroid peroxidase antibody, *Tg-Ab* anti-thyroglobulin antibody

ultrasonographic findings but did not perform fine needle aspiration, to exclude the possibility of neoplastic diseases (e.g., thyroid lymphoma).

Conclusions

The results of the present study suggest that patients with Hashimoto's thyroiditis and high titers of anti-thyroid antibodies are likely to exhibit intense diffuse FDG uptake in the thyroid. However, the frequency of hypothyroidism was similar in patients with or without diffuse uptake in the thyroid. Therefore, it should be borne in mind that thyroid function may be clearly impaired even in the presence of only mild FDG uptake in the thyroid.

Abbreviations

CT: Computed tomography; FDG: ^{18}F-fluorodeoxyglucose; PET: Positron emission tomography; SUVmax: Maximum standardized uptake value; Tg: Hyroglobulin; TPO: Thyroid peroxidase; TSH: Thyroid stimulating hormone; US: Ultrasonography

Funding

This research did not receive any specific grant from any funding agency in the public, commercial, or not-for-profit sector.

Authors' contributions

NE, KM, and TI were involved in study design, acquisition of data, analysis and interpretation of data and drafting and revising the manuscript. MS, TK, HE, EO, MO, KT and HO were involved in data collection and manuscript drafting. All authors read and approved the final manuscript.

Consent for publication

Not applicable

Competing interests

The authors declare that they have no competing interests.

Author details

Department of Internal Medicine, Teikyo University School of Medicine, 2-11-1, Kaga, Itabashi, Tokyo 173-0003, Japan. [2]Department of Radiology, Teikyo University School of Medicine, 2-11-1, Kaga, Itabashi, Tokyo 173-0003, Japan. [3]Department of Radiology, Toho University Ohashi Medical Center, 2-22-36, Ohashi, Meguro, Tokyo, Japan.

References

1. Strauss LG, Conti PS. The applications of PET in clinical oncology. J Nucl Med. 1991;32:623–48 discussion 649-50.
2. Zhuang H, Alavi A. 18-fluorodeoxyglucose positron emission tomographic imaging in the detection and monitoring of infection and inflammation. Semin Nucl Med. 2002;32:47–59.
3. Nakamoto Y, Tatsumi M, Hammoud D, Cohade C, Osman MM, Wahl RL. Normal FDG distribution patterns in the head and neck: PET/CT evaluation. Radiology. 2005;234:879–85.
4. Tsubaki F, Kurata S, Tani J, Sumi A, Fujimoto K, Abe T. Clinical significance of patterns of increased [18F]-FDG uptake in the thyroid gland: a pictorial review. Jpn J Radiol. 2018;36:181–93.
5. Soelberg KK, Bonnema SJ, Brix TH, Hegedus L. Risk of malignancy in thyroid incidentalomas detected by 18F-fluorodeoxyglucose positron emission tomography: a systematic review. Thyroid. 2012;22:918–25.
6. Nayan S, Ramakrishna J, Gupta MK. The proportion of malignancy in incidental thyroid lesions on 18-FDG PET study: a systematic review and meta-analysis. Otolaryngol Head Neck Surg. 2014;151:190–200.
7. Saif MW, Tzannou I, Makrilia N, Syrigos K. Role and cost effectiveness of PET/CT in management of patients with cancer. Yale J Biol Med. 2010;83:53–65.
8. Kurata S, Ishibashi M, Hiromatsu Y, Kaida H, Miyake I, Uchida M, et al. Diffuse and diffuse-plus-focal uptake in the thyroid gland identified by using FDG-PET: prevalence of thyroid cancer and Hashimoto's thyroiditis. Ann Nucl Med. 2007;21:325–30.
9. Boerner AR, Voth E, Theissen P, Wienhard K, Wagner R, Schicha H. Glucose metabolism of the thyroid in Graves' disease measured by F-18-fluoro-deoxyglucose positron emission tomography. Thyroid. 1998;8:765–72.
10. Yasuda S, Shohtsu A, Ide M, Takagi S, Takahashi W, Suzuki Y, et al. Chronic thyroiditis: diffuse uptake of FDG at PET. Radiology. 1998;207:775–8.
11. Kim TY, Kim WB, Ryu JS, Gong G, Hong SJ, Shong YK. 18F-fluorodeoxyglucose uptake in thyroid from positron emission tomogram (PET) for evaluation in cancer patients: high prevalence of malignancy in thyroid PET incidentaloma. Laryngoscope. 2005;115:1074–8.
12. Karantanis D, Bogsrud TV, Wiseman GA, Mullan BP, Subramaniam RM, Nathan MA, et al. Clinical significance of diffusely increased 18F-FDG uptake in the thyroid gland. J Nucl Med. 2007;48:896–901.
13. Lee JY, Choi JY, Choi Y-H, Hyun SH, Moon SH, Jang SJ, et al. Diffuse thyroid uptake incidentally found on18F-Fluorodeoxyglucose positron emission tomography in subjects without Cancer history. Korean J Radaol. 2013;14: 501–9.
14. Yoshida H, Amino N, Yagawa K, Uemura K, Satoh M, Miyai K, et al. Association of serum antithyroid antibodies with lymphocytic infiltration of the thyroid gland: studies of seventy autopsied cases. J Clin Endocrinol Metab. 1978;46:859–62.
15. Maratou E, Dimitriadis G, Kollias A, Boutati E, Lambadiari V, Mitrou P, et al. Glucose transporter expression on the plasma membrane of resting and activated white blood cells. Eur J Clin Investig. 2007;37:282–90.
16. Raber W, Gessl A, Nowotny P, Vierhapper H. Thyroid ultrasound versus antithyroid peroxidase antibody determination: a cohort study of four hundred fifty-one subjects. Thyroid. 2002;12:725–31.

26

Study of Optimal Replacement of Thyroxine in the Elderly (SORTED)

Salman Razvi[1,2*], Lorna Ingoe[2], Vicky Ryan[3], Simon H. S. Pearce[1] and Scott Wilkes[4]

Abstract

Background: Hypothyroidism is a common condition, particularly in the older population. Thyroid hormone requirements change with age and serum TSH levels also alter, especially in older patients. However, in practice laboratory reference ranges for thyroid function are not age-specific and treatment in older patients aims to achieve a similar target thyroid function level as younger age groups.

Methods: A dual centre, single blind, randomised controlled trial was conducted to determine the feasibility of a future definitive RCT in hypothyroid individuals aged 80 years or older who were treated with levothyroxine. Potential participants were identified from 17 research-active GP practices ($n = 377$), by opportunistic invitations ($n = 9$) or in response to publicity ($n = 4$). Participants were randomly allocated to either usual (0.4–4.0 mU/L) or a higher (4.1–8.0 mU/L) target serum TSH range. Information on participants' willingness to enter the trial, acceptability of study design, length of time to complete recruitment and dose titration strategy was collected.

Results: Fifteen percent (57/390) of potentially eligible hypothyroid individuals consented to participate in this trial and 48 were randomised to trial medication for 24 weeks, giving a recruitment rate of 12 %. Recruitment averaged 5.5 participants per month over approximately 9 months. Eight participants withdrew (3/24 and 5/24 in the usual and higher TSH arms, respectively) with the commonest reason cited (5 patients) being tiredness. Interestingly, 3/5 participants withdrew from the site that required a visit to a Research Facility whereas only 5/43 participants withdrew from the site that offered home visits. In the higher TSH arm, of those participants who completed the study, approximately half of participants (10/19) reached target TSH.

Conclusions: It is feasible to perform a randomised controlled trial of thyroid hormones in hypothyroid patients aged 80 or older. A definitive trial would require collaboration with a large number of General Practices and the provision of home visits to achieve recruitment to time and target. Power calculations should take into account that approximately 12 % of those approached will be randomised and 1 in 6 participants are likely to withdraw from the study. Finally, several dose adjustments may be required to achieve target serum TSH levels in this age group.

Keywords: Hypothyroidism, Older age, Feasibility

* Correspondence: salman.razvi@newcastle.ac.uk
[1]Institute of Genetic Medicine and Queen Elizabeth Hospital, International Centre for Life, Newcastle University, Central Parkway, Newcastle upon Tyne NE1 3BZ, UK
[2]Department of Endocrinology, Queen Elizabeth Hospital, Gateshead NE9 6SX, UK
Full list of author information is available at the end of the article

Background

Thyroid hormones regulate metabolism and impact on several organs in the body. Hypothyroidism (underactive thyroid) is a common endocrine condition in which the thyroid gland produces insufficient thyroid hormones. Hypothyroidism is more prevalent in women and in older individuals with rates of up to 16 % reported in those aged over 80 years [1, 2]. Hypothyroidism is diagnosed based on results of blood tests with low thyroid hormone levels in the presence of high serum Thyroid Stimulating Hormone (TSH) concentrations (usually > 4.0 mU/L). Treatment with the synthetic form of thyroxine (Levothyroxine or LT4) is the treatment of choice in these patients and patients are generally managed in primary care. LT4 is prescribed to 3–4 % of the general population and its use is increasing [3–5]. Thyroid function changes with age and several reports suggest that the upper limit of the TSH reference range increases with age [6–10]. In addition, observational studies have shown that older individuals with a slightly raised serum TSH level have no adverse consequences [11–16]. In fact, one report suggests that a slightly raised TSH may be beneficial for survival in 85-year old individuals followed up for four years [17]. Despite this, all patients are treated uniformly with the aim of achieving a serum TSH target level (usually 0.4–4.0 mU/L) and age-specific ranges are not used. Moreover, evidence obtained from General Practice records suggests LT4 is increasingly being prescribed for older individuals and for minimally raised serum TSH levels [18]. This issue is of increasing importance as the populations in most developed – and many developing – countries are ageing and diagnoses of hypothyroidism are therefore likely to rise. Before a definitive randomised controlled trial (RCT) in the older hypothyroid population can be conducted it would be highly desirable to assess its feasibility. We, therefore, designed a feasibility RCT to investigate lower dose LT4 (aiming for a higher than usual serum TSH) versus usual dose LT4 (aiming for the currently utilised serum TSH range) in hypothyroid individuals aged 80 years or more. We report the feasibility of this trial in this paper.

Methods

The detailed protocol has been published previously [19]. Briefly, a dual-centre single-blind RCT of elderly (≥80 years) individuals with primary hypothyroidism and good biochemical control (as demonstrated by serum TSH levels within the reference range in the preceding 3 months) was organised. After providing written informed consent, participants were randomised in a 1:1 ratio to either usual dose LT4 (aiming to continue to keep serum TSH between 0.4 and 4.0 mU/L) or lower dose LT4 (reduced by 25 mcg daily initially and a further 25 mcg daily, if required at 12 weeks) to aim for a slightly higher serum TSH level of 4.1–8.0 mU/L. After randomisation participants were assessed at 12 and 24 weeks, with a final follow-up phone call at 25 weeks. The inclusion criteria required participants of either gender, aged 80 years or older, living independently in the community, who had been prescribed LT4 (at least 50 mcg daily) for at least 6 months and whose serum TSH was between 0.4 and 4.0 mU/L in the preceding 3 months. Patients were excluded if they were deemed to not have capacity to provide written informed consent, had severe chronic medical conditions that would prevent participation, thyroid cancer, on medications affecting thyroid function, non-English speakers, had participated in another RCT in the previous 3 months or had lactose intolerance.

The primary objectives were to demonstrate that recruitment to such a trial is possible; to gauge participants' acceptability of being part of the study; to assess the length of time required to complete recruitment; to assess the dose titration strategy and the length of time required to achieve desired TSH levels; and to gauge medication compliance.

The design and analysis followed published recommendations for feasibility studies [20, 21]. As such, no formal sample size calculation was performed; a target sample size of 50 randomised participants was deemed sufficient to assess the feasibility of the trial. The data analyses were descriptive, and statistical comparisons between randomised treatment groups were not undertaken.

Results

Screening and recruitment

Participants were screened for their eligibility to participate in the trial via one of three possible routes: from participating GP practices, hospital endocrine clinics or self-referral responding to posters in hospitals and participating GP practices. (See Fig. 1)

Twenty research-active practices agreed to identify potential patients for the trial. These GP practices were identified by the then National Institute for Health Research, Primary Care Research Network. Of these, two practices did not have the capacity to identify patients for the study and a third responded late in the recruitment process. The remaining 17 GP practices facilitated the identification of potential participants and posted letters of invitation (Table 1). The prevalence of treated hypothyroid patients aged ≥ 80 years ranged from 0.5 to 1.4 % of the total number of patients registered in those practices (Table 1). A total of 377 invitation letters (with a reply slip and stamped addressed envelope) were sent by practice staff and 233/377 (62 %) responded, of which 66 (18 % of total invitations) agreed to participate. The protocol allowed the participating GP practices to send reminder letters to patients that had not replied but this

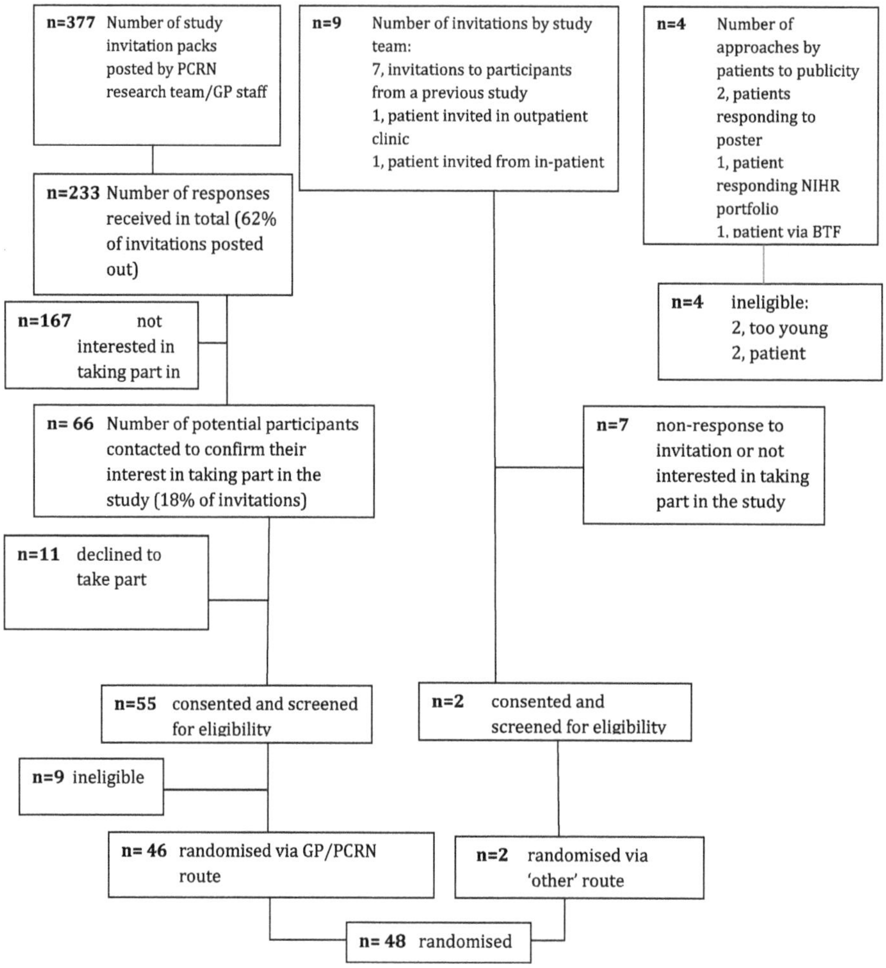

Fig. 1 Recruitment summary

was not followed. Subsequently, 11 individuals changed their mind and declined participation. The reasons given for changing their mind related to either not understanding the study requirements or due to change in circumstances (such as illness). A further 9 patients were deemed ineligible after study-specific screening as either their serum TSH was too low ($n = 6$) or too high ($n = 3$). Therefore, a total of 46 patients (12 % of the 377 potentially eligible participants) were randomised via this route.

Another 13 participants were invited by either the study team or self referred in response to publicity posters in hospitals, the NIHR portfolio or via the patient-led charity the British Thyroid Foundation newsletter. Of these, 2 (15 %) participants were screened and subsequently randomised.

Randomisation process

Participants were randomised in a ratio of 1:1, using random permuted blocks. Randomisation was stratified by usual (pre-study) LT4 dose (50, 75, 100 and 125 mcg daily) and administered by the Newcastle Clinical Trials Unit using a secure password-protected web-based system (Table 2).

Baseline characteristics

The median age of the participants was 83 years (range: 80 to 93 years) and majority (71 %) were women (Table 3).

Primary outcome measures

This feasibility trial had five primary outcome measures.

1. Participants' willingness to enter the trial (as gauged by the ratio of those who consented to participate to those who were potentially eligible and approached): 57 out of 390 (15 %) potentially eligible patients consented to participate but, as stated above, 9 individuals (16 % of the potentially eligible group) were not eligible due to abnormal thyroid function at screening.

Table 1 Number of participants approached and randomised by each GP practice

Practices [a]	Total registered patients (n) (A)	Potentially eligible hypothyroid patients aged ≥ 80 year (% of A)	Invites sent [c] (n) (B)	Replies received (% of B)	Consented to be screened (n) (% of B)	Randomised (n) (% of B)
A	16,340	112 (0.7 %)	112	63 (56 %)	20 (18 %)	13 (12 %)
B	5475	42 (0.8 %)	42	25 (60 %)	6 (14 %)	6 (14 %)
C	8830	75 (0.9 %)	14	14 (100 %)	7 (50 %)	5 (36 %)
D	9230	58 (0.6 %)	39	23 (59 %)	5 (13 %)	3 (8 %)
E	11,019	63 (0.6 %)	20	15 (75 %)	3 (15 %)	3 (15 %)
F	10,141	28 [b]	11	10 (91 %)	4 (36 %)	3 (30 %)
G	5960	82 (1.4 %)	20	14 (70 %)	4 (20 %)	3 (15 %)
H	6875	52 (0.8 %)	10	6 (50 %)	3 (30 %)	3 (30 %)
I	4478	57 (1.3 %)	4	4 (100 %)	2 (50 %)	2 (50 %)
J	7460	36 (0.5 %)	36	20 (50 %)	6 (17 %)	1 (3 %)
K	3728	7 [b]	7	4 (57 %)	1 (14 %)	1 (14 %)
L	11,788	31 [b]	20	14 (70 %)	1 (5 %)	1 (5 %)
M	6893	9 [b]	9	3 (33 %)	1 (11 %)	1 (11 %)
N	19,223	20 [b]	10	7 (70 %)	1 (10 %)	1 (10 %)
O	3274	3 [b]	3	1 (33 %)	1 (33 %)	0 (0 %)
P	3296	12 [b]	5	2 (40 %)	1 (20 %)	0 (0 %)
Q	5565	15 [b]	15	8 (53 %)	0 (0 %)	0 (0 %)
Total	139,575	703	377	233 (62 %)	66 (18 %)	46 (12 %)

[a]The names of the GP practices are not shown to protect identity
[b]For these practices the total number of potentially eligible patients was not provided
[c]Some practices were asked to only send invites to a random selection of patients to be able to obtain a wide spread of responses from GP practices as possible

2. Participants' acceptability of study design (as measured by the completion rate of participants in each randomised group): 21 out of 24 (87.5 %) and 19/24 (79.2 %) randomised participants completed the trial in the usual and higher TSH arms, respectively.
3. Participant recruitment rate (as measured by the number of patients randomised divided by the length of the recruitment period): Participants were recruited between 17th October 2012 and 10th July 2013 with the first participant randomised on 9th November 2012 and the last one on 10th July 2013. The projected recruitment was 5 or 6 participants/month. Over the 267 days that trial recruitment was open 48 participants were recruited (5.5 participants/month) (See Fig. 2).
4. Dose titration strategy and length of time required to achieve desired TSH levels (as calculated by number of participants in each group that reach target TSH range at both 12 and 24 weeks): For the 40 participants who remained in the study until their final study assessment, most participants in the usual dose arm stayed within their target TSH range of 0.4–4.0 mU/L whereas half of the higher target TSH arm achieved their target TSH range (Table 4).
5. Medication compliance (tablet count at each visit): At the end of visits 2 and 3, participants were asked to return any surplus study drug in the original packaging to the study team, who verified and documented compliance. Compliance was deemed to be generally good. In participants who completed the trial, $n = 40$, compliance was 100 and 95 % at

Table 2 Distribution of patients by randomisation strata (pre-study dose of Levothyroxine) and allocated treatment group

Pre-study dose of Levothyroxine	Treatment group		Total randomised
	Target TSH range 0.4–4.0 mU/L	Target TSH range 4.1–8.0 mU/L	
50 µg daily	5	5	10
75 µg daily	9	9	18
100 µg daily	8	7	15
125 or more µg daily	2	3	5
Total	24	24	48

Table 3 Baseline characteristics

	Total *n* =48
Sex	
Female (n,% of females)	34 (71 %)
Male (n, % of males)	14 (29 %)
Age (years) Median (range)	83.0 (80.0 – 93.0)
Blood pressure (mmHg) Median (IQR)	
Systolic	154.5 (141.0 – 168.5)
Diastolic	85.0 (77.0 – 92.5)
Physical examination Mean (sd)	
Height (cm)	158.8 (8.8)
Weight (kg)	68.5 (13.1)
BMI (kg/m^2)	27.1 (4.7)
Pulse (bpm)	67.9 (9.8)
Chronic conditions n (%)	
Type 2 diabetes mellitus	4 (8.3)
Hypertension	24 (50)
Ischaemic heart disease	13 (27.1)
Cerebrovascular disease	7 (14.6)
COPD	6 (12.5)
Blood results Median (IQR)	
TSH (mU/L)	1.43 (0.88 – 2.64)
FT4 (pmol/L)	18.8 (16.7 – 19.7)
FT3 (pmol/L)	3.8 (3.6 – 4.2)
Total Cholesterol (mmol/L)	4.9 (4.4 – 6.2)
HDLc (mmol/L)	1.6 (1.5 – 1.9)
Triglycerides (mmol/L)	1.3 (1.0 – 1.9)
Serum CTX (pg/mL)	0.27 (0.17 – 0.37)
TPO antibodies	
< 35 IU/ml (n, %)	28 (58 %)
≥ 35 IU/ml (n, %)	20 (42 %)

IQR interquartile range, *sd* standard deviation, *bpm* beats per minute, *COPD* chronic obstructive pulmonary disease, *TSH* thyroid stimulating hormone, *FT4* free thyroxine, *FT3* free triiodothyronine, *HDLc* high density lipoprotein cholesterol, *CTX* carboxy-terminal collagen crosslinks, *TPO* thyroid peroxidase

both visits in the usual TSH and higher target TSH arms, respectively (Table 4).

Adverse Events (AEs) and Serious Adverse Events (SAEs): There were 119 AEs reported by 37 patients; 16 patients in the usual TSH arm reporting 49 AEs (mean = 3.1 per patient, sd = 2.1) and 21 patients in the higher TSH arm reporting 70 AEs (mean = 3.3, sd = 2.2). Patients reported between 1 and 10 AEs over the course of the study. The frequency of AEs with regards to the various organ-systems appeared to be broadly similar. For example, the frequency of participants reporting new-onset or worsening tiredness/fatigue was 41.7 % vs 50 % in the usual and higher TSH arms, respectively. Muscle aches and pains (29.2 % vs 16.7 %), dizziness (20.8 % vs 25 %) and constipation (16.7 % vs 29.2 %) were comparable in the two groups.

There were three SAEs, two in the usual TSH arm and one in the higher TSH arm. (See Table 5 for details).

Site of follow-up: At baseline 71 % of patients (34/48) chose to have their first study visit at home and 29 % (14/48) chose to come into hospital out-patients. At visit 2, four patients switched from out-patient visits to home visits with one patient switching in the other direction (this patient had become a hospital inpatient). Of the 40 patients still in the study at visit 3, 80 % (32/40) had their visit at home and 20 % (8/40) had their visit as an out-patient.

Phone contacts: Over the course of the 24 week study period a total of 27 telephone contacts were made by 20 participants and discussed with the research staff. The majority (20/27) were made in the first 12 weeks; of which 15 were in the first 4 weeks. The queries were with regards to new or existing symptoms (20 contacts by 14 participants; $n = 8$ in usual TSH arm and $n = 6$ in higher TSH arm), query relating to study drug (4 phone calls by 3 participants, all in usual TSH arm), and one phone call each for taking study drug in addition to usual dose levothyroxine (usual TSH arm) and problems in swallowing study drug (usual TSH arm).

Withdrawals and reasons: Eight patients withdrew from the study; three from the usual TSH arm and five from the higher TSH arm (Table 6). Five patients withdrew before visit 2 (two usual TSH, three higher TSH), one patient withdrew at visit 2 (higher TSH arm), and two patients withdrew after visit 2 but before visit 3 (one usual TSH and 1 higher TSH arm, respectively). Three of the five participants withdrew (60 %) from the site that required a visit to a Research Facility whereas only 5/43 participants (12 %) withdrew from the site that offered home visits. In seven participants, the reasons cited for withdrawal were AEs (mainly tiredness or constipation in six and infected foot and wrist pain in a seventh). One participant was withdrawn from the study by the research team for safety reasons as she was found to be taking the study drug in addition to her usual levothyroxine medication.

Discussion

It is currently unclear what the best practice for managing hypothyroidism is in older people. There is good evidence that thyroid hormone requirements change with age and that the current practice of treating everyone in a uniform fashion may not be appropriate. This feasibility RCT has demonstrated that reducing the dose of the synthetic thyroid hormone levothyroxine is possible and that patients are willing to participate.

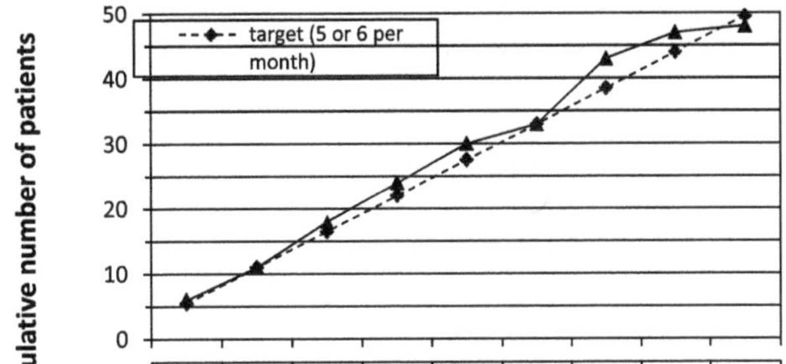

	Nov-12	Dec-12	Jan-13	Feb-13	Mar-13	Apr-13	May-13	Jun-13	Jul-13
target (5 or 6 per month)	5.5	11	16.5	22	27.5	33	38.5	44	49.5
cumulative monthly total	6	11	18	24	30	33	43	47	48
monthly	6	5	7	6	6	3	10	4	1

Fig. 2 Plot of cumulative number of patients randomised, target versus actual

The population of the western world - including the United Kingdom - is ageing. Ageing of the population refers to both the increase in the median age as well as the increase in the absolute number and proportion of older individuals. The number of people aged 75 and over has increased by 89 % over the period 1974 to 2014 and now makes up 8 % of the total population [22]. Between 2015 and 2020, when the general population is expected to increase by 3 %, it is estimated that people aged 65 years or more will rise by 12 % to 1.1 million; those over 85 years by 18 % to 300,000; and the number of centenarians by 40 % (7000) [22]. Similar demographic changes are occurring across much of the Western world. For instance, in the United States it is estimated that there are now about six million persons aged 85 years and older and this number may reach 19 million in 2050 [23]. Data from this feasibility study suggests that the prevalence of treated hypothyroidism in the over 80 age group is between 0.5 and 1.4 % of the entire population. It is also apparent that the majority of hypothyroid patients in this age group are on modest doses of LT4 – which is indicative that treatment was commenced for borderline raised TSH levels. This has significant implications for the management of hundreds of thousands of older hypothyroid individuals in the United Kingdom. Furthermore, as the number of older individuals increases then the absolute number of older people with treated hypothyroidism is also likely to grow.

The result of this feasibility trial has shown that it is possible to recruit participants into an interventional trial to aim for a higher than usual target serum TSH. The randomisation rate was approximately 5.5 participants per month from the 17 GP practices that identified patients and from the other sources of referral. Overall, 12 % of potentially eligible patients consented to participate and were randomised. This feasibility data suggests that a large-scale RCT would have to recruit from hundreds of GP practices. Furthermore, allowance would have to be made for 16 % (possibly even higher in a study of a longer duration) of participants to withdraw from the study. Any subsequent full RCT would have to be of longer duration (probably several years) and designed to be able to answer the important question of the optimum target serum TSH to aim for in older hypothyroid patients. Such a trial would require hard clinical end points including cardiovascular events and fractures as its main outcome measures.

One of the limitations of this trial is that we are unable to assess the characteristics of individuals who refused to participate. This is because study invitations were sent by individual GP practices and the responses were received in an anonymised form by the study team.

Table 4 Dose titration strategy and compliance with study medications

Dose titration strategy: Participants who remained in the study until their final study assessment (i.e. excluding withdrawals), $n = 40$	Usual TSH range (0.4–4.0 mU/L) $n = 21$	Higher TSH range (4. 1–8.0 mU/L) $n = 19$
Percent achieving target TSH range at week 12 (visit 2)	18/21 (85.7 %)	6/19 (31.6 %)
Percent achieving target TSH range at week 24 (visit 3)	18/21 (85.7 %)	10/19 (52.6 %)
Percent compliant at week 12 (visit 2)	21/21 (100 %)	18/19 (94.7 %)
Percent compliant at week 24 (visit 3)	21/21 (100 %)	18/19 (94.7 %)

Table 5 Chronological listing of serious adverse events

Treatment allocation	Randomisation date	Date of initial report	Description	Onset Date	Severity	SAE reason	Outcome
Usual TSH arm	01/03/2013	26/04/2013	Stroke	22/04/2013	mild	Involved patient hospitalisation	Recovered with sequelae
Usual TSH arm	20/03/2013	13/06/2013	Possible overdose on levothyroxine	12/06/2013	mild	Other significant medical event	Completely recovered
Higher TSH arm	21/01/2013	01/07/2013	Cardiac arrest due to acute myocardial infarction	25/06/2013	severe	Life threatening	Death (after study completion: 05/08/2013)

Therefore, it is not possible to assess differences between responders and non-responders.

Adverse events and serious adverse events did appear to be similar in both the usual TSH arm as well as the higher TSH arm in our study. However, this feasibility trial was not powered to detect a significant difference in any effect size. It is therefore possible that there may be a higher incidence of adverse events in a larger trial over a longer follow-up period. This would require support to be available for study participants. In this trial telephone support was made use of by a number of participants and may have contributed to their retention. The telephone contacts were made mostly in the first few weeks after randomisation and related to either symptoms or study drug. It is important to consider providing telephone support in a full large RCT particularly in the first 4 weeks after commencing study drug. In addition, it is also evident that participants in this age group prefer to have home visits rather than to have to come to a hospital research facility. It is unclear how participants would view visits to their local GP practice.

It is important to consider strategies that would help retain participants in the trial and lead to high completion rates. Approximately 4 out of 5 randomised participants completed this trial. This was achieved by offering flexible study dates, times and venue, providing alternative appointments at short notice, being seen by the same member of staff at each visit and availability of telephonic support.

This feasibility trial revealed that of the patients randomised to a higher TSH range, who remained in the study until their final study assessment, only half reach their target. This is not surprising given that up to half the hypothyroid population, irrespective of age does not

Table 6 Chronological listing of withdrawals

Subject ID	Treatment allocation	Randomisation date	Withdrawal date	Days in the study	Reason (severity and relation to study drug)
709	Reduced dose	07/12/2012	09/01/2013	34	Withdrew due to AEs experienced whilst on the study: constipation, tiredness and generally unwell (mild, possibly related)
103	Usual dose	11/01/2013	23/01/2013	13	Withdrew due to "feeling unwell" (mild, possibly related)
104	Reduced dose	11/01/2013	27/03/2013	76	Withdrew due to infected right foot (moderate, not related), loose stools (moderate, unknown relationship to study drug) and sore wrist (mild, unknown relationship to study drug)
509	Reduced dose	26/11/2012	22/04/2013	148	6 weeks after Visit 2 withdrew from the study due to tiredness (moderate, possibly related)
205	Usual dose	01/03/2013	22/04/2013	53	Withdrew due to fatigue which started 2 weeks after commencing the study drug. The patient was hospitalised with a mild stroke on 22/04/13, reported to be linked to ongoing hypertension (severe, not related).
515	Reduced dose	18/02/2013	08/05/2013	80	Withdrew after experiencing several AEs: dry skin, dry hair, feeling cold, weight gain and tiredness (mild, possibly related), and swollen face with itching (mild, not related) - unscheduled home visit: thyroid function normal, weight gain of 0.3kgs.
521	Reduced dose	15/05/2013	12/06/2013	29	Withdrew after experiencing several AEs: nausea and loss of appetite (mild, not related), vertigo (mild, not related) and confusion (mild, not related)
614	Usual dose	20/03/2013	27/06/2013	100	At Visit 2 patient reported that she had been taking her prescribed dose of LT4 as well as the study medication. Patient reported no AEs. Serum thyroid function was normal (TSH 0.60, FT4 20.8). Subsequently the patient changed her mind and withdrew.

AEs adverse events, *LT4* levothyroxine

have good biochemical control as evidenced by their serum TSH level [24, 25]. The implications of this are that more frequent or smaller dose adjustments of levothyroxine may be required in the full trial to be able to achieve a higher proportion of participants in the desired relaxed TSH range.

Conclusion

In conclusion, this feasibility trial has shown that it is possible to recruit and retain patients with levothyroxine treated hypothyroidism aged 80 years or older into a RCT. Several important lessons have been learnt that would help to design a trial that should be able to successfully recruit and retain patients into a longer-term study.

Abbreviations

AEs: Adverse events; BMI: Body mass index; COPD: Chronic obstructive pulmonary disease; CTX: Carboxy-terminal collagen crosslinks; FT3: Free triiodothyronine; FT4: Free thyroxine; GP: General practitioner; IQR: Interquartile range; LT4: Levothyroxine; PCRN: Primary Care Research Network; RCT: Randomised control trial; SAEs: Serious adverse events; sd: Standard deviation; TPO: Thyroid peroxidase; TSH: Thyroid stimulating hormone

Acknowledgments

Primary Care Clinical Research Network Staff, especially Norah Phipps; TSC members: Dr Catherine Watson (trial manager), Mrs Janis Hickey (BTF member) as well as SR, SW, SP, VR and LI); independent DMEC members: Dr Ramzi Ajian (chair), Dr Petros Perros (expert), Dr Barbara Gregson (statistician). This report is independent research arising from a NIHR RfPB award PB-PG-0610 22139 supported by the National Institute for Health Research. The views expressed in this publication are those of the author(s) and not necessarily those of the NHS, the NIHR or the Department of Health.

Funding

This project is funded by the NIHR RfPB (http://www.nihr.ac.uk/funding/fundingdetails.htm?postid=1572, reference PB-PG-0610 22139).

Authors' contributions

The study was designed by SR, SP, VR and SW. LI performed study visits. SR wrote the first draft, and all authors reviewed, commented and approved the final version of the manuscript.

Authors' information

Dr Salman Razvi is Senior Lecturer and Consultant Endocrinologist, Newcastle University, UK.
Ms Lorna Ingoe is a research nurse, Gateshead Health NHS Foundation Trust.
Ms Vicky Ryan is a senior statistician, Institute of Health and Society, Newcastle University, UK.
Prof Simon Pearce is a Professor of Endocrinology, Newcastle University, UK.
Prof Scott Wilkes is a Professor of Primary Care, Sunderland University, UK.

Competing interests

The authors declare that they have no competing interests.

Consent for publication

All authors provide consent for this publication.

Author details

[1]Institute of Genetic Medicine and Queen Elizabeth Hospital, International Centre for Life, Newcastle University, Central Parkway, Newcastle upon Tyne NE1 3BZ, UK. [2]Department of Endocrinology, Queen Elizabeth Hospital, Gateshead NE9 6SX, UK. [3]Institute of Health & Society, Newcastle University, Baddiley Clark Building, Richardson Road, Newcastle upon Tyne NE2 4AX, UK. [4]Department of Pharmacy, Health and Wellbeing, Faculty of Applied Sciences, University of Sunderland, Sunderland SR1 3SD, UK.

References

1. Canaris GJ, Manowitz NR, Mayor G, Ridgway EC. The Colorado thyroid disease prevalence study. Arch Intern Med. 2000;160(4):526–34.
2. Hollowell JG, Staehling NW, Flanders WD, Hannon WH, Gunter EW, Spencer CA. Serum TSH, T(4), and thyroid antibodies in the United States population (1988 to 1994): National Health and Nutrition Examination Survey (NHANES III). J Clin Endocrinol Metab. 2002;87(2):489.
3. Leese GP, Flynn RV, Jung RT, Macdonald TM, Murphy MJ, Morris AD. Increasing prevalence and incidence of thyroid disease in Tayside, Scotland: the Thyroid Epidemiology Audit and Research Study (TEARS). Clin Endocrinol (Oxf). 2008;68(2):311–6.
4. Flynn RW, MacDonald TM, Morris AD, Jung RT, Leese GP. The thyroid epidemiology, audit, and research study: thyroid dysfunction in the general population. J Clin Endocrinol Metab. 2004;89(8):3879–84.
5. Mitchell AL, Hickey B, Hickey JL, Pearce SH. Trends in thyroid hormone prescribing and consumption in the UK. BMC Public Health. 2009;9:132.
6. Surks MI, Hollowell JG. Age-specific distribution of serum thyrotropin and antithyroid antibodies in the US population: implications for the prevalence of subclinical hypothyroidism. J Clin Endocrinol Metab. 2007;92(12):4575–82.
7. Vadiveloo T, Donnan PT, Murphy MJ, Leese GP. Age- and gender-specific TSH reference intervals in people with no obvious thyroid disease in Tayside, Scotland: the Thyroid Epidemiology, Audit, and Research Study (TEARS). J Clin Endocrinol Metab. 2013;98(3):1147–53.
8. Ehrenkranz J, Bach PR, Snow GL, Schneider A, Lee JL, Ilstrup S, Bennett ST, Benvenga S. Circadian and circannual rhythms in thyroid hormones: determining the TSH and free T4 reference intervals based upon time of day, age, and sex. Thyroid. 2015;25(8):954–61.
9. Bremner AP, Feddema P, Leedman PJ, Brown SJ, Beilby JP, Lim EM, Wilson SG, O'Leary PC, Walsh JP. Age-related changes in thyroid function: a longitudinal study of a community-based cohort. J Clin Endocrinol Metab. 2012;97(5):1554–62.
10. Atzmon G, Barzilai N, Hollowell JG, Surks MI, Gabriely I. Extreme longevity is associated with increased serum thyrotropin. J Clin Endocrinol Metab. 2009;94(4):1251–4.
11. Virgini VS, Wijsman LW, Rodondi N, Bauer DC, Kearney PM, Gussekloo J, den Elzen WP, Jukema JW, Westendorp RG, Ford I, Stott DJ, Mooijaart SP, PROSPER Study Group. Subclinical thyroid dysfunction and functional capacity among elderly. Thyroid. 2014;24(2):208–14.
12. Simonsick EM, Newman AB, Ferrucci L, Satterfield S, Harris TB, Rodondi N, Bauer DC, Health ABC Study. Subclinical hypothyroidism and functional mobility in older adults. Arch Intern Med. 2009;169(21):2011–7.
13. Blum MR, Wijsman LW, Virgini VS, Bauer DC, den Elzen WP, Jukema JW, Buckley BM, de Craen AJ, Kearney PM, Stott DJ, Gussekloo J, Westendorp RG, Mooijaart SP, Rodondi N, PROSPER study group. Subclinical thyroid dysfunction and depressive symptoms among the elderly: a prospective cohort study. Neuroendocrinology. 2016;103(3-4):291–9.
14. Hyland KA, Arnold AM, Lee JS, Cappola AR. Persistent subclinical hypothyroidism and cardiovascular risk in the elderly: the cardiovascular health study. J Clin Endocrinol Metab. 2013;98(2):533–40.
15. Waring AC, Arnold AM, Newman AB, Bùzková P, Hirsch C, Cappola AR. Longitudinal changes in thyroid function in the oldest old and survival: the cardiovascular health study all-stars study. J Clin Endocrinol Metab. 2012;97(11):3944–50.
16. Pearce SH, Razvi S, Yadegarfar ME, Martin-Ruiz C, Kingston A, Collerton J, Visser TJ, Kirkwood TB, Jagger C. Serum thyroid function, mortality and disability in advanced old age: The Newcastle 85+ study. J Clin Endocrinol Metab. 2016;23:jc20161935.
17. Gussekloo J, van Exel E, de Craen AJ, Meinders AE, Frolich M, Westendorp RG. Thyroid status, disability and cognitive function, and survival in old age. JAMA. 2004;292(21):2591–9.
18. Taylor PN, Iqbal A, Minassian C, Sayers A, Draman MS, Greenwood R, Hamilton W, Okosieme O, Panicker V, Thomas SL, Dayan C. Falling threshold for treatment of

borderline elevated thyrotropin levels – balancing benefits and risks. Evidence from a large community-based study. JAMA Intern Med. 2014;174(1):32–9.

19. Wilkes S, Pearce S, Ryan V, Rapley T, Ingoe L, Razvi S. Study of Optimal Replacement of Thyroxine in the ElDerly (SORTED): protocol for a mixed methods feasibility study to assess the clinical utility of lower dose thyroxine in elderly hypothyroid patients: study protocol for a randomized controlled trial. Trials. 2013;14:83.
20. Lancaster GA, Dodd S, Williamson PR, et al. Design and analysis of pilot studies: recommendations for good practice. J Eval Clin Pract. 2004;10:307–12.
21. Thabane L, Ma J, Chu R, et al. A tutorial on pilot studies: the what, why and how. BMC Med Res Methodol. 2010;10:1.
22. UK National Statistics. http://www.ons.gov.uk/ons/rel/pop-estimate/population-estimates-for-uk-england-and-wales-scotland-and-northern-ireland/mid-2014/sty-ageing-of-the-uk-population.html. Accessed 17 June 2016.
23. 2014 National Population Projections. 2014; https://www.census.gov/population/projections/data/national/2014/summarytables.html. Accessed 17 June 2016.
24. Parle JV, Franklyn JA, Cross KW, Jones SR, Sheppard MC. Thyroxine prescription in the community: serum thyroid stimulating hormone level assays as an indicator of undertreatment or overtreatment. Br J Gen Pract. 1993;43(368):107–9.
25. Flynn RW, Bonellie SR, Jung RT, MacDonald TM, Morris AD, Leese GP. Serum thyroid-stimulating hormone concentration and morbidity from cardiovascular disease and fractures in patients on long-term thyroxine therapy. J Clin Endocrinol Metab. 2010;95(1):186–93.

27

Embolic suppurative thyroiditis with concurrent carcinoma in pregnancy: lessons in management through a case report

Manish M George*, Jay Goswamy and Susannah E Penney

Abstract

Background: The thyroid undergoes a variety of physiological changes during pregnancy. The relatively low iodine levels seen in pregnancy have been implicated in thyroid growth during this time. Management of thyroid cancer in pregnancy is not immediately apparent. Furthermore, acute suppurative thyroiditis is rare and this is attributed to the glands innate immunity. We thoroughly review the evidence regarding management of thyroid abscess and thyroid malignancy during pregnancy and illustrate it via an extremely rare case of an embolic thyroid abscess highlighting an underlying carcinoma in a pregnant woman.

Case: A 29-year old female was found to have a thyroid mass during an antenatal assessment. Following a wound infection from Caesarian section she developed a rapidly progressive thyroid abscess. Incision and drainage of the abscess, and subsequent histology revealed papillary carcinoma. She subsequently underwent both total thyroidectomy with level 6 dissection and radio-iodine ablation post-natally.

Conclusion: The literature is inconsistent regarding pregnancy as a risk factor for thyroid cancer, but overall it has been suggested as equally or slightly more frequent than in the non-pregnant population. Thyroid mass investigation should be as for the non-pregnant population. In the first trimester any endocrine surgery is associated with miscarriage, whereas these risks are reduced in second trimester. Importantly, there is no survival benefit in undergoing papillary carcinoma surgery in the third trimester versus early post partum and the risks of premature labour may outweigh any benefit gained by operating early. Most importantly, acute suppurative thyroiditis is rare entity and clinicians should have a low threshold for suspicion of underlying malignancy in these patients. This is especially true in the pregnant population who may be especially susceptible whilst undergoing hypertrophic thyroid changes.

Keywords: Abscess, Suppurative, Thyroiditis, Embolic, Pregnancy, Carcinoma

Background

The thyroid undergoes a variety of physiological changes in pregnancy. High circulating levels of human chorionic gonadotrophin crossbind to the thyroid stimulating hormone (TSH) receptor inducing hypertrophy and hyperplasia [1-4]. A raised level of oestrogen promotes higher levels of thyroid binding globulin and this results in both increased bound thyroxine and a reduction in free thyroxine levels [5,6]. Pregnant women have a high overall total body thyroxine level; however even in this population a low free T4 is inversely correlated with TSH [3]. It is therefore biochemically reasonable that the reduction in free T4 may stimulate a compensatory increase in thyroid activity and growth. Low iodine secretion can cause goitre through decreased thyroxine synthesis and compensatory increased TSH. The relatively low iodine levels seen in pregnancy have been implicated in thyroid growth associated with pregnancy, although this has only been studied in low iodine populations [3,7]. The low incidence of acute suppurative thyroiditis is often attributed to the glands innate immunity. The high local concentration of iodine that inhibits bacterial growth, its degree of lymphatic drainage and its encapsulation all contribute to low local infection rates [8,9]. Dysregulation of these processes via hypertrophy or malignancy may change the susceptibility of the thyroid to infection.

* Correspondence: manish.george@nhs.net
Department of Otolaryngology-Head and Neck Surgery, Manchester Royal Infirmary, Oxford Road, Manchester M13 9WL, United Kingdom

We describe a young woman who developed a thyroid mass during her third trimester of pregnancy. A post-caesarean section wound infection was followed by an episode of acute suppurative thyroiditis. At the time of thyroid abscess drainage, a biopsy was taken of the abscess cavity wall. Papillary thyroid carcinoma was diagnosed. This is the first case in the world literature at the time of publication describing a thyroid abscess of embolic origin. This is also the first report of a postnatal suppurative thyroid gland uncovering a papillary thyroid carcinoma in the acute setting.

Case report

A 29-year-old female at 37 weeks of an uneventful pregnancy attended antenatal clinic. During her assessment a large predominantly left sided thyroid mass was noted. She was reviewed during that attendance by the local otolaryngology team. She had no history of thyroid pathology, had no lifetime radiation exposure and no relevant family history. There was no palpable cervical lymphadenopathy. Her vocal cords were mobile and symmetrical. Spirometry revealed no intrinsic pulmonary pathology.

An emergency Caesarian section was performed at term + 2 days for fetal distress without intra-operative complication. The child was healthy. Six days post partum she developed a tender erythematous lower abdominal wound, was diagnosed with a wound site infection. A Caesarean section wound swab grew mixed skin flora with anaerobes and treatment was initiated with 625 mg co-amoxiclav. During this time she underwent an ultrasound examination of the thyroid and neck, which revealed a 35 × 40 mm solid nodule within the left thyroid lobe. The left lobe was noted to be hyper-vascular with a surrounding fluid density collection. An outpatient Otolaryngology appointment was made.

She returned to the emergency department the following day with rapid onset tenderness, oedema and erythema over the thyroid. She became haemodynamically unstable with a white cell count of 14.9×10^9/l and a C-reactive protein of 301 mg/L and was admitted under endocrinology. She was treated with parenterally with 4.5 mg piperacillin/tazobactam three times daily and gentamicin as per trust microbiology advice.

The ultrasound of the thyroid mass was repeated revealing severe expansion of the left lobe with a predominant fluid component. Fine needle aspiration was performed and microbiological assessment again revealed no growth. Cytology however, was suspicious of malignancy. The cytology was repeated and confirmed the likely malignancy.

Due to a lack of response a computed tomographic scan was performed of her neck (Figure 1). A large enhancing soft tissue mass arising from the left lobe of the thyroid with an area of fluid inferolaterally displacing the surrounding structures was reported. The total size of the lesion including the fluid collection was 60 × 43 × 70 mm. Ipsilateral lymphadenopathy was seen in levels II, III and IV. Clinical staging was cT2N1b (according to the International Union Against Cancer staging). During her acute admission the thyroid abscess was incised and drained and a formal biopsy taken of the intra-thyroidal lesion. Systemic improvement was rapid and she completed a further 48 hours of parenteral co-amoxiclav prior to discharge. Histology revealed a papillary thyroid carcinoma (PTC) and a repeat CT for staging was performed (Figure 2). The left common carotid artery and internal jugular vein were displaced and compressed, but there was no evidence of encasement. The mass extended into the sterno-thyroid and sterno-hyoid muscles and appeared inseparable but not invading. Maximal axial dimensions were 29 × 26 mm, with a maximal coronal dimension of 48 mm. The previously enlarged nodes had resolved.

She subsequently underwent a total thyroidectomy and bilateral level VI clearance. As the previous enlarged nodes had resolved, no other neck dissection was performed. Post-operatively she developed hypocalcaemia and received supplementation, which was reduced over the following 2 months. Histology revealed a 40 mm infiltrative unencapsulated classical PTC with extrathyroid invasion. One of 5 lymph nodes contained metastatic PTC. Her pathological staging was pT3N1a. Post operatively she received radioactive iodine ablation and has made a full recovery.

Conclusions

There is no consensus in the literature regarding pregnancy as a risk factor for thyroid cancer, but overall it has been suggested as equally or slightly more frequent than in the non-pregnant population [10-16]. There is also no total agreement on pregnancy as a poor prognostic factor for differentiated thyroid cancer, [17,18,14,19,13] the majority of evidence however proposes it does not have a deleterious effect on natural disease progression.

Thyroid mass investigation should be as for the non-pregnant population, that is, with a combination of biochemical, radiological and cytological investigation [20,21]. Some authors do caution that pregnancy induced hyperplasia may make the interpretation of thyroid cytology difficult [22]. Marley and Oertel however, on their cytological analysis of 57 pregnant and post partum women did not find any distinct or differentiating cytological features [10].

The British Thyroid Association guidelines for the management of thyroid cancer suggest two main options for consideration during pregnancy: the first is to defer thyroidectomy and radioiodine until postpartum and the second to defer thyroidectomy until the second trimester with delay of adjuvant radio-iodine ablation until postpartum [23]. It has also been noted that in extreme cases including highly aggressive cancers, possible termination

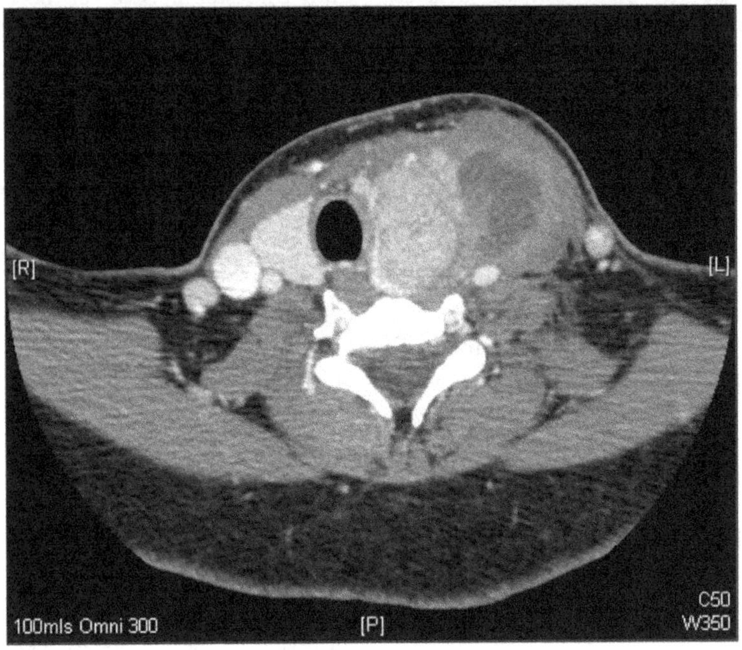

Figure 1 CT with contrast axial slice through neck. CT image demonstrating a large fluid collection arising from left thyroid mass, suggestive of an abscess. Noted compression and deviation of adjacent organs.

of pregnancy followed by surgery and radio-iodine maybe necessary. In the first trimester any endocrine surgery is associated with miscarriage, whereas these risks are reduced in second trimester [24,25]. Importantly, there is no survival benefit in undergoing papillary carcinoma surgery in the third trimester versus early post partum and the risks of premature labour outweigh any possible marginal benefit gained by operating [21,20,24,18]. It is for this reason that most extensive summary of thyroid disorder in pregnancy and post

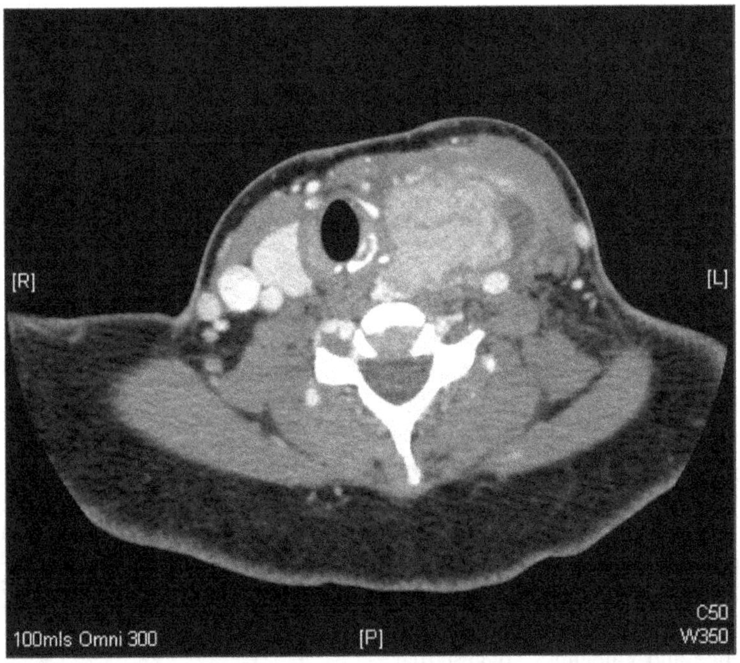

Figure 2 CT with contrast axial slice through neck. A more superior CT neck slice demonstrating a resolving abscess and concurrent left thyroid soft tissue mass, now confirmed as a papillary thyroid carcinoma.

partum recommends that treatment can be delayed unless the nodule has significantly poor prognosis or is rapidly growing [26]. In cases where cancer is suspected during pregnancy, there is no strong evidence for or against administration of exogenous T4 to suppress TSH levels [27,26].

Thyroid abscesses account for less than 1% of thyroid-related diseases and tend to occur in those with underlying pathology [28,8]. This includes immunosuppression, pre-existing thyroid nodules or underlying malignancy, [8,29-31]. Nishihara et al. report seeding of a thyroid abscess from fine needle aspiration in a patient undergoing regular therapeutic drainage of an adenomatous nodule with cystic degeneration [32]. It is however more commonly due to local direct spread with the most frequent source appearing to be pyriform sinus fistulae [33,30]. Pyriform sinus fistulae related to third and fourth branchial pouch anomalies are a known cause but this tends to present initially in childhood [30,31].

Partial or total thyroidectomy maybe necessary in recurrent, progressive or persistent abscesses, especially in cases with suspicion of underlying malignancy [34,8,35]. Due to concurrent inflammation complete surgical margins may be technically difficult. For this reason it has been recommended that drainage of the abscess acutely with delayed elective partial or total thyroidectomy maybe enable adequate resection margins more frequently [8]. If a pyriform sinus fistula is present a procedure to remove or obliterate the tract is advised [8,36,37].

Acute suppurative thyroiditis has been linked to both oesophageal cancer and laryngeal cancer [35,38]. Concurrent cases of thyroid malignancy are rarely described. In a Saudi report from 2002 Haddad et al. discuss a terminal cardiac event secondary to sepsis from a suppurative infarcted papillary carcinoma found at post mortem [39]. Hong et al. in a Korean publication mention Reidel's thyroiditis complicated by suppurative thyroiditis and ultimately, micropapillary carcinoma discovered on histology [40]. In our case the papillary carcinoma was not micropapillary, it was suspected before excision and unusually, the abscess was most probably secondary to haematogenous spread via wound infection to a susceptible gland. Intra-operative thyroid pus samples did not grow positive cultures as prolonged course of antibiotics had been administered prior to aspiration. Given the patient's clear underlying thyroid pathology, once wound infection had been noted, a more cautious approach for monitoring and admission for intravenous antibiotics could have been taken.

Summary

During pregnancy, evidence and guidelines suggest that optimal management of differentiated cancer is dependent on gestation. As in our case, uncomplicated yet suspicious third trimester masses can be investigated during pregnancy with definitive treatment, namely thyroidectomy, delayed in the vast majority of cases until post-partum.

Thyroid malignancy may predispose to embolic infection, due in part to local dysregulation of the immune system, disruption of the capsule and increased vascularity. The distal lymphatic or haematogenous spread as likely happened in this case is not described in the literature.

Although thyroiditis is a commonly encountered condition, acute suppurative inflammation is less common and may represent underlying malignancy. Drainage with antibiotic therapy maybe sufficient in causing resolution acutely but carcinoma needs to be excluded. Appropriate investigations with expeditious follow up should be employed accordingly.

Consent

Written informed consent was obtained from the patient for publication of this case report including the accompanying images. A copy of the written consent is available for review by the Editor-in-Chief of this journal.

Competing interests

The authors declare that they have no competing interests

Authors' contributions

MMG was involved in the care of this patient from diagnosis through to treatment. MMG also led the write up and literature review. JG participated in the surgical management of this patient, gained consent for use of images for publication of this case. JG also made significant contributions to drafting the manuscript. SEP lead the care of this patient, advised on themes to cover for drafting and edited the manuscript on multiple occasions. All authors have read and approved the final manuscript.

References

1. Haddow JE, McClain MR, Lambert-Messerlian G, Palomaki GE, Canick JA, Cleary-Goldman J, et al. First, Second Trimester Evaluation of Risk for Fetal Aneuploidy Research C. Variability in thyroid-stimulating hormone suppression by human chorionic [corrected] gonadotropin during early pregnancy. J Clin Endocrinol Metab. 2008;93(9):3341–7. doi:10.1210/jc.2008-0568.
2. Hershman JM. Physiological and pathological aspects of the effect of human chorionic gonadotropin on the thyroid. Best Pract Res Clin Endocrinol Metab. 2004;18(2):249–65. doi:10.1016/j.beem.2004.03.010.
3. Elahi S, Hussain Z. A Longitudinal Study of Changes in Thyroid Related Hormones among Pregnant Women Residing in an Iodine Deficient Urban Area. ISRN Endocrinol. 2013;2013:234031. doi:10.1155/2013/234031.
4. Yoshimura M, Hershman JM. Thyrotropic action of human chorionic gonadotropin. Thyroid. 1995;5(5):425–34.
5. Chan GW, Mandel SJ. Therapy insight: management of Graves' disease during pregnancy. Nat Clin Pract Endocrinol Metab. 2007;3(6):470–8. doi:10.1038/ncpendmet0508.
6. Lee RH, Spencer CA, Mestman JH, Miller EA, Petrovic I, Braverman LE, Goodwin TM. Free T4 immunoassays are flawed during pregnancy. Am J Obstet Gynecol. 2009;200(3):260 e1-6. doi:10.1016/j.ajog.2008.10.042.
7. Kung AW, Chau MT, Lao TT, Tam SC, Low LC. The effect of pregnancy on thyroid nodule formation. J Clin Endocrinol Metab. 2002;87(3):1010–4. doi:10.1210/jcem.87.3.8285.
8. Paes JE, Burman KD, Cohen J, Franklyn J, McHenry CR, Shoham S, et al. Acute bacterial suppurative thyroiditis: a clinical review and expert opinion. Thyroid. 2010;20(3):247–55. doi:10.1089/thy.2008.0146.
9. Pearce EN, Farwell AP, Braverman LE. Thyroiditis. N Engl J Med. 2003;348 (26):2646–55. doi:10.1056/NEJMra021194.

10. Marley EF, Oertel YC. Fine-needle aspiration of thyroid lesions in 57 pregnant and postpartum women. Diagn Cytopathol. 1997;16(2):122–5.
11. Rosen IB, Walfish PG. Pregnancy as a predisposing factor in thyroid neoplasia. Arch Surg. 1986;121(11):1287–90.
12. Rosen IB, Walfish PG, Nikore V. Pregnancy and surgical thyroid disease. Surgery. 1985;98(6):1135–40.
13. Rosvoll RV, Winship T. Thyroid carcinoma and pregnancy. Surg Gynecol Obstet. 1965;121(5):1039–42.
14. Akslen LA, Nilssen S, Kvale G. Reproductive factors and risk of thyroid cancer. A prospective study of 63,090 women from Norway. Br J Cancer. 1992;65(5):772–4.
15. Kravdal O, Glattre E, Haldorsen T. Positive correlation between parity and incidence of thyroid cancer: new evidence based on complete Norwegian birth cohorts. Int J Cancer. 1991;49(6):831–6.
16. McTiernan AM, Weiss NS, Daling JR. Incidence of thyroid cancer in women in relation to reproductive and hormonal factors. Am J Epidemiol. 1984;120 (3):423–35.
17. Glinoer D, Soto MF, Bourdoux P, Lejeune B, Delange F, Lemone M, et al. Pregnancy in patients with mild thyroid abnormalities: maternal and neonatal repercussions. J Clin Endocrinol Metab. 1991;73(2):421–7. doi:10.1210/jcem-73-2-421.
18. Yasmeen S, Cress R, Romano PS, Xing G, Berger-Chen S, Danielsen B, et al. Thyroid cancer in pregnancy. Int J Gynaecol Obstet. 2005;91(1):15–20. doi:10.1016/j.ijgo.2005.06.022.
19. Hod M, Sharony R, Friedman S, Ovadia J. Pregnancy and thyroid carcinoma: a review of incidence, course, and prognosis. Obstet Gynecol Surv. 1989;44(11):774–9.
20. Moosa M, Mazzaferri EL. Outcome of differentiated thyroid cancer diagnosed in pregnant women. J Clin Endocrinol Metab. 1997;82(9):2862–6. doi:10.1210/jcem.82.9.4247.
21. Cooper DS, Doherty GM, Haugen BR, Kloos RT, Lee SL, Mandel SJ, et al. Revised American Thyroid Association management guidelines for patients with thyroid nodules and differentiated thyroid cancer. Thyroid. 2009;19 (11):1167–214. doi:10.1089/thy.2009.0110.
22. Betsill W. Thyroid fine needle aspiration in pregnant women. Diagn Cytopathol. 1985;1(1):53–4.
23. Perros P, Boelaert K, Colley S, Evans C, Evans RM, Gerrard Ba G, et al. British Thyroid Association: Guidelines for the management of thyroid cancer. Clin Endocrinol (Oxf). 2014;81 Suppl 1:1–122. doi:10.1111/cen.12515.
24. Sam S, Molitch ME. Timing and special concerns regarding endocrine surgery during pregnancy. Endocrinol Metab Clin North Am. 2003;32(2):337–54.
25. Kuy S, Roman SA, Desai R, Sosa JA. Outcomes following thyroid and parathyroid surgery in pregnant women. Arch Surg. 2009;144(5):399–406; discussion doi:10.1001/archsurg.2009.48.
26. De Groot L, Abalovich M, Alexander EK, Amino N, Barbour L, Cobin RH, et al. Management of thyroid dysfunction during pregnancy and postpartum: an Endocrine Society clinical practice guideline. J Clin Endocrinol Metab. 2012;97(8):2543–65. doi:10.1210/jc.2011-2803.
27. Stagnaro-Green A, Abalovich M, Alexander E, Azizi F, Mestman J, Negro R, et al. Postpartum. Guidelines of the American Thyroid Association for the diagnosis and management of thyroid disease during pregnancy and postpartum. Thyroid. 2011;21(10):1081–125. doi:10.1089/thy.2011.0087.
28. Al-Dajani N, Wootton SH. Cervical lymphadenitis, suppurative parotitis, thyroiditis, and infected cysts. Infect Dis Clin North Am. 2007;21(2):523–41. doi:10.1016/j.idc.2007.03.004.
29. Berger SA, Zonszein J, Villamena P, Mittman N. Infectious diseases of the thyroid gland. Rev Infect Dis. 1983;5(1):108–22.
30. Miyauchi A, Matsuzuka F, Takai S, Kuma K, Kosaki G. Piriform sinus fistula A route of infection in acute suppurative thyroiditis. Arch Surg. 1981;116(1):66–9.
31. Yolmo D, Madana J, Kalaiarasi R, Gopalakrishnan S, Kiruba Shankar M, Krishnapriya S. Retrospective case review of pyriform sinus fistulae of third branchial arch origin commonly presenting as acute suppurative thyroiditis in children. J Laryngol Otol. 2012;126(7):737–42. doi:10.1017/S0022215112000898.
32. Nishihara E, Miyauchi A, Matsuzuka F, Sasaki I, Ohye H, Kubota S, et al. Acute suppurative thyroiditis after fine-needle aspiration causing thyrotoxicosis. Thyroid. 2005;15(10):1183–7. doi:10.1089/thy.2005.15.1183.
33. AP F. Sporadic Painless, Painful Subacute and Acute Suppurative Thyroiditis. In: Braverman LE, editor. Werner & Ingbar's the thyroid: a fundamental and clinical text. 10th ed. Philadelphia: Wolters Kluwer/Lippincott Williams & Wilkins Health; 2013. p. xix, 891 p.
34. Mollar-Puchades MA, Camara-Gomez R, Perez-Guillen V, Benavides-Gabernet M, Gomez-Vela J, Pinon-Selles F. Thyroid hematoma and infectious thyroiditis after a neck injury. Thyroid. 2006;16(4):421–2. doi:10.1089/thy.2006.16.421.
35. Premawardhana LD, Vora JP, Scanlon MF. Suppurative thyroiditis with oesophageal carcinoma. Postgrad Med J. 1992;68(801):592–3.
36. Kim KH, Sung MW, Koh TY, Oh SH, Kim IS. Pyriform sinus fistula: management with chemocauterization of the internal opening. Ann Otol Rhinol Laryngol. 2000;109(5):452–6.
37. Nicoucar K, Giger R, Pope Jr HG, Jaecklin T, Dulguerov P. Management of congenital fourth branchial arch anomalies: a review and analysis of published cases. J Pediatr Surg. 2009;44(7):1432–9. doi:10.1016/j.jpedsurg.2008.12.001.
38. Wilson TD, Pickard BH, Whittam DE. Carcinoma of the larynx masquerading as acute suppurative thyroiditis. Br J Surg. 1969;56(12):936.
39. Haddad FH, Malkawi OM, Omari AA, Izzat AS, Khassrof HM, Faiad LM, et al. Diabetes and infarcted papillary thyroid cancer. Saudi Med J. 2002;23(4):467–70.
40. Hong JT, Lee JH, Kim SH, Hong SB, Nam M, Kim YS, et al. Case of concurrent Riedel's thyroiditis, acute suppurative thyroiditis, and micropapillary carcinoma. Korean J Intern Med. 2013;28(2):236–41. doi:10.3904/kjim.2013.28.2.236.

Rapid detection of papillary thyroid carcinoma by fluorescence imaging using a γ-glutamyltranspeptidase-specific probe

Rumi Hino[1,2*], Naoko Inoshita[2], Toyoki Yoshimoto[2], Makiko Ogawa[2], Daishu Miura[3], Ryoko Watanabe[4], Kenta Watanabe[4], Mako Kamiya[5,6] and Yasteru Urano[5,7,8]

Abstract

Background: Nodular lesions of the thyroid gland, including papillary thyroid carcinoma (PTC), may be difficult to diagnose by imaging, such as in ultrasonic echo testing, or by needle biopsy. Definitive diagnosis is made by pathological examination but takes several days. A more rapid and simple method to clarify whether thyroid nodular lesions are benign or malignant is needed. Fluorescence imaging with γ-glutamyl hydroxymethyl rhodamine green (gGlu-HMRG) uses γ-glutamyltranspeptidase (GGT), a cell-surface enzyme, to hydrolyze the γ-glutamyl peptide and transfer the γ-glutamyl group. GGT is overexpressed in several cancers, such as breast, lung, and liver cancers. This imaging method is rapid and useful for detecting such cancers. In this study, we tried to develop a rapid fluorescence detection method for clinical samples of thyroid cancer, especially papillary carcinoma.

Methods: Fluorescence imaging with gGlu-HMRG was performed to detect PTC using 23 surgically resected clinical samples. A portable imaging device conveniently captured white-light images and fluorescence images with blue excitation light. Hematoxylin-eosin (HE) staining was used to evaluate which fluorescent regions coincided with cancer, and immunohistochemical examination was used to detect GGT expression.

Results: All 16 PTC samples exhibited fluorescence after topical application of gGlu-HMRG, whereas the normal sections of each sample showed no fluorescence. HE staining revealed that each fluorescent region corresponded to a region with carcinoma. The PTC samples also exhibited GGT expression, as confirmed by immunohistochemistry.

Conclusions: All PTC samples were detected by fluorescence imaging with gGlu-HMRG. Thus, fluorescence imaging with gGlu-HMRG is a rapid, simple, and powerful detection tool for PTC.

Keywords: Thyroid cancer, Papillary thyroid carcinoma, Fluorescence imaging, γ-glutamyltranspeptidase, γ-glutamyl hydroxymethyl rhodamine green

* Correspondence: rumih0301@ic.daito.ac.jp
[1]Department of Sports and Health Science, Daito Bunka University, 560 Iwadono, Higashimathuyama-shi, Saitama 355-8501, Japan
[2]Department of Pathology, Toranomon Hospital, Tokyo 105-0001, Japan
Full list of author information is available at the end of the article

Background

Papillary thyroid carcinoma (PTC) is the most common thyroid cancer, comprising 70–80% of all thyroid cancers [1]. Although most PTC cases have good prognoses, there is a high-risk group comprising patients with distant metastasis and older patients (> 50 years of age) accompanied with massive extra-thyroidal invasion or large lymph node metastasis (> 3.0 cm), and the case-specific death was reported to be 20% (44/220 cases) [2]. Patients younger than 16 years with PTC, node metastasis > 3.0 cm, and significant extension are reported to have poor prognoses [3]. However, nodular lesions of the thyroid gland, including PTC, may be difficult to diagnose by imaging, such as in ultrasonic echo testing, or by needle biopsy. In differential diagnosis, malignant tumors, benign tumors, and non-neoplastic lesions are predicted. Definitive diagnosis is made by pathological examination, but this takes a long time, i.e., at least 4 days, and requires multiple laboratory technicians because of steps such as processing, fixation, embedding, sectioning, and staining. The more quickly nodular lesions are diagnosed, the earlier the treatment may begin. Furthermore, simplicity of diagnosis is desired, that is, malignant diagnosis should be able to be determined even if there is no laboratory technician or pathologist. These aspects are of particular importance in cases of malignant tumors.

γ-Glutamyltranspeptidase (GGT) is a cell surface enzyme that cleaves glutathione, hydrolyzes the γ-glutamyl peptide, and transfers the γ-glutamyl group. γ-Glutamyl hydroxymethyl rhodamine green (gGlu-HMRG) is a nonfluorescent dye that is converted to highly fluorescent hydroxymethyl rhodamine green (HMRG) upon reaction with GGT [2]. GGT is purportedly overexpressed in several human cancers, such as breast, ovarian, brain, lung, colon, and peritoneum cancers, as well as head and neck squamous cell carcinoma, and methods exploiting gGlu-HMRG and GGT have been applied to detect such cancers [4–11]. When colorless gGlu-HMRG is sprayed on surgically resected breast cancer tissue, the cancer cells exhibit green fluorescence 1–2 min afterwards [12]. The brightness of the fluorescent agent is grossly confirmed, and green fluorescence indicates the presence of cancer [12]. Until the development of this method, there was no technique capable of visualizing cancer during surgery in such a short time; furthermore, this detection method using gGlu-HMRG is reported to be very simple [4, 7, 9]. No study has examined the use of the GGT-gGlu-HMRG detection method on primary human thyroid tumors.

In this study, we examined whether thyroid lesions were distinguishable as benign or malignant by the GGT-gGlu-HMRG method during surgical procedures.

Methods

Fluorescent probe

gGlu-HMRG, a fluorescent probe targeting GGT, was synthesized as previously described[2]. It was resuspended in 10 mM dimethyl sulfoxide (DMSO, Sigma-Aldrich, St. Louis, MO, USA) and restored. The stock solution of gGlu-HMRG was diluted to the final concentration, 100 μM or 1 mM, in phosphate-buffered saline (PBS, Wako Pure Chemical Industries, Tokyo, Japan).

Study of patient specimens

Twenty-three cases of thyroid lesions were examined. All samples were surgically resected by the Department of Breast and Endocrine Surgery or Otorhinolaryngology, Toranomon Hospital, between 2014 and 2017.

The resected specimens were immediately extracted, and approximately 5 mm [5] of the thyroid lesions and normal sites was also excised. Fluorescence imaging was performed using a fluorescence imaging system (Discovery; INDEC Medical Systems, Santa Clara, CA, USA). White-light images of specimens with no fluorescent probe were captured first, and then fluorescence images through yellow emission filter with 450–490 nm blue excitation light were captured after 100 μM gGlu-HMRG was sprayed on both the lesion and normal tissue segments of the specimens. Fluorescence images were captured 0, 0.5, 1, 2, 3, 5, 7, and 10 min after gGlu-HMRG spraying. Subsequently, the specimens were fixed with formalin and subjected to hematoxylin-eosin (HE) staining.

Histopathology by HE and immunohistochemical staining

HE staining was performed to confirm the pathological findings. Specimens were fixed, embedded in paraffin, and cut into 3-μm sections prior to staining with HE. We determined which parts of tissues exhibited green or no fluorescent signals using a fluorescence imaging system with a microscope (Nikon). In the case of tumors, histological type, capsular invasion, and lymph-vascular invasion were evaluated from sections of each sample according to the World Health Organization classification scheme.

Immunohistochemical analysis of GGT1 was performed using an auto-immunostainer, BOND III (Leica, Wetzlar, Germany), with antibodies against GGT1 (mouse.

monoclonal, dilution 1: 600; Abcam, Cambridge, UK). HepG2 cells were used as a positive control. Higher than 10% positivity among tumor cells was considered positive staining.

Cell lines, cell culture, and cell block construction

Two cell lines were prepared with high and low GGT expression. The high GGT expression cell line was

A549, established from human lung adenocarcinoma and reported as a positive control for gGlu-HMRG [9], and the low GGT expression cell lone was SW782, a noncancerous line of human pre-adipocytes.

HepG2 cells were cultured in Dulbecco's modified Eagle's medium (DMEM; Nacalai Tesque, Kyoto, Japan) supplemented with 10% fetal bovine serum (FBS; Life Technologies, Carlsbad, CA, USA), 100 U/mL penicillin, and 100 μg/mL streptomycin (Wako).

Cell blocks were constructed as follows. HepG2 cells were cultured in 100-mm plates (Nacalai Tesque) and harvested using a scraper (Nacalai Tesque). Cells in 200 μL of saline were then centrifuged at 3000 rpm for 5 min, the supernatant was discarded, and the cells were fixed in formaldehyde saline overnight. Fixed cells were embedded in agarose gel. The cell blocks were cut into thin sections for HE and immunohistochemical staining.

Results

Confirmation of the function of the fluorescent probe

To examine the function of the fluorescent probe, two cell lines, aA549 and SW782, were used. A549 cells exhibited bright green fluorescence on detection of gGlu-HMRG, and we determined that they were suitable as a positive control in this study (Fig. 1). SW782, a noncancerous cell line of human pre-adipocytes, showed no fluorescence using the gGlu-HMRG probe method and was suitable as a negative control (Fig. 1).

Imaging of specimens from patients with thyroid cancer

The ability of gGlu-HMRG to detect malignant thyroid cancer was examined using surgically resected thyroid lesion samples from 23 cases. Information related to the 23 cases is documented in Table 1. Representative images of a human thyroid tumor and normal tissue taken using the fluorescence imaging system (Discovery) are shown in Fig. 2. White-light images of the tumor and normal tissue were taken first (Fig. 2a, c), and then fluorescence images were obtained using gGlu-HMRG (Fig. 2b, d). All cases were evaluated by comparison with normal tissue. Thyroid lesions in this study consisted of 16 PTCs, 3 adenomatous goiters, 1 Graves' disease, 1 follicular adenoma, and 1 thyroiditis.

After treatment with gGlu-HMRG, all 16 PTC samples (Figs. 1 and 2; Case 2), including those from recurrence cases (Fig. 3; Case 3), exhibited green fluorescence, whereas normal tissue from the same cases showed no fluorescence. Among the thyroid samples, those from the follicular adenoma, Graves' disease, thyroiditis (Fig. 3; Case 5), and 3 adenomatous goiter cases showed no fluorescence. One of the 3 adenomatous goiter cases was a mediastinal goiter (Fig. 3; Case 4).

Pathological confirmation of thyroid lesions

After fluorescence imaging, all samples were embedded in paraffin blocks, and each tissue was pathologically confirmed by HE staining. Of the 23 cases studied, 19

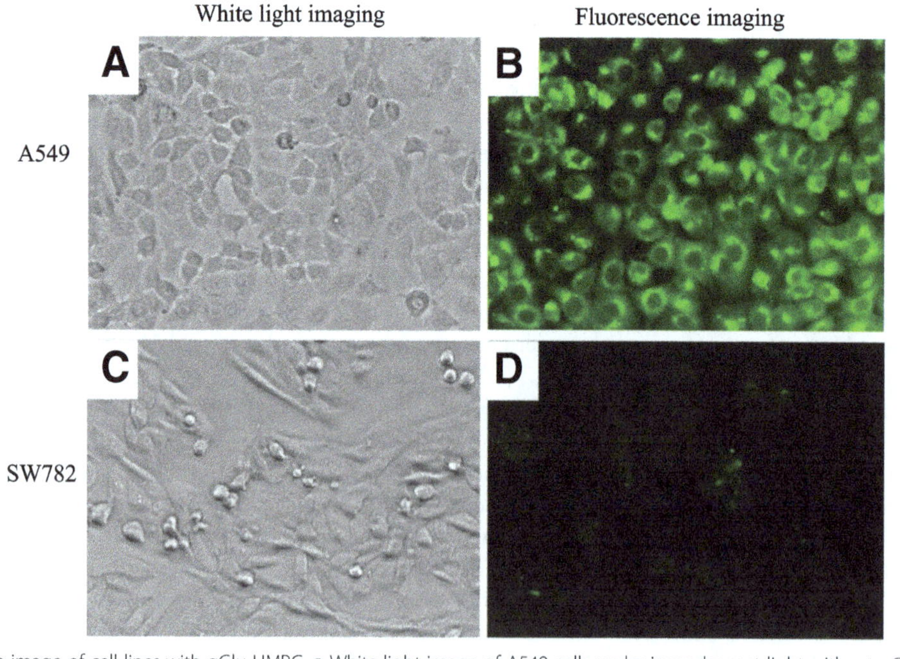

Fig. 1 Fluorescence image of cell lines with gGlu-HMRG. **a** White-light image of A549 cells under incandescent light without gGlu-HMRG. **b** Fluorescence image of A549 cells taken 3 min after spraying with gGlu-HMRG. gGlu-HMRG is converted to highly fluorescent hydroxymethyl rhodamine green (HMRG) upon reaction with γ-glutamyltranspeptidase (GGT). **c** White-light image of SW782 cells under incandescent light without gGlu-HMRG. **d** Fluorescence image of SW782 cells taken 3 min after spraying with gGlu-HMRG

Table 1 Summary of data in patients with thyroid lesion

Patient	Age	Sex	Preoperative clinical diagnosis	Pathological diagnosis	gGlu-HMRG[*a] lesion	normal
1	30	F	PTC[*b]	PTC	positive	negative
2	32	F	PTC	PTC	positive	negative
3	46	F	PTC (recurrence)	PTC(recurrence)	positive	negative
4	55	F	Thyroid malignant tumor	Mediastinal goiter	negative	negative
5	78	M	Lymphoma	Inflammation	negative	negative
6	43	F	PTC	PTC	positive	negative
7	47	F	Thyroid tumor	Follicular adenoma	negative	negative
8	47	F	PTC	PTC	positive	negative
9	44	F	PTC	PTC	positive	negative
10	61	F	PTC	PTC	positive	negative
11	32	F	PTC	PTC	positive	negative
12	48	M	PTC	PTC	positive	negative
13	23	F	Thyroid tumor	Goiter[*c]	negative	negative
14	44	M	PTC	PTC	positive	negative
15	58	F	Thyroid tumor	Goiter	negative	negative
16	72	F	PTC	PTC	positive	negative
17	57	M	PTC	PTC	positive	negative
18	68	F	Thyroid lesion	Graves'[*d]	negative	negative
19	71	F	PTC	PTC	negative	negative
20	55	F	PTC	PTC	positive	negative
21	52	F	PTC	PTC	positive	negative
22	69	M	Goiter	Goiter	negative	negative
23	64	M	PTC	PTC	positive	negative

[*a]gGlu-HMRG: detection results by using γ- glutamyl hydroxymethyl rhodamine green, [*b]PTC: Papillary thyroid carcinoma, [*c]Goiter: Adenomatous goiter, [*d]Graves': Graves' disease or Basedow disease

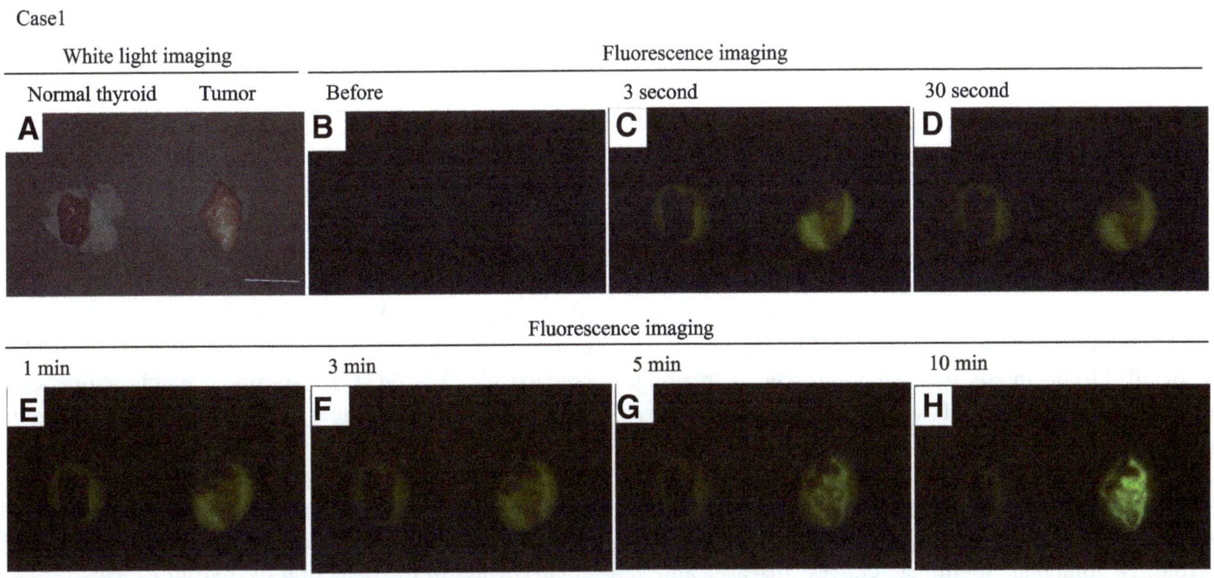

Fig. 2 Representative figure of PTC exhibited green fluorescence of HMRG upon reaction with GGT. **a** White-light image of thyroid tissue, normal (left) and carcinoma (right), taken under incandescent light without gGlu-HMRG. **b-h** Images captured before and 3 s, 30 s, 1, 3, 5 and 10 min after probe application. Green fluorescence signals were observed after 3 s

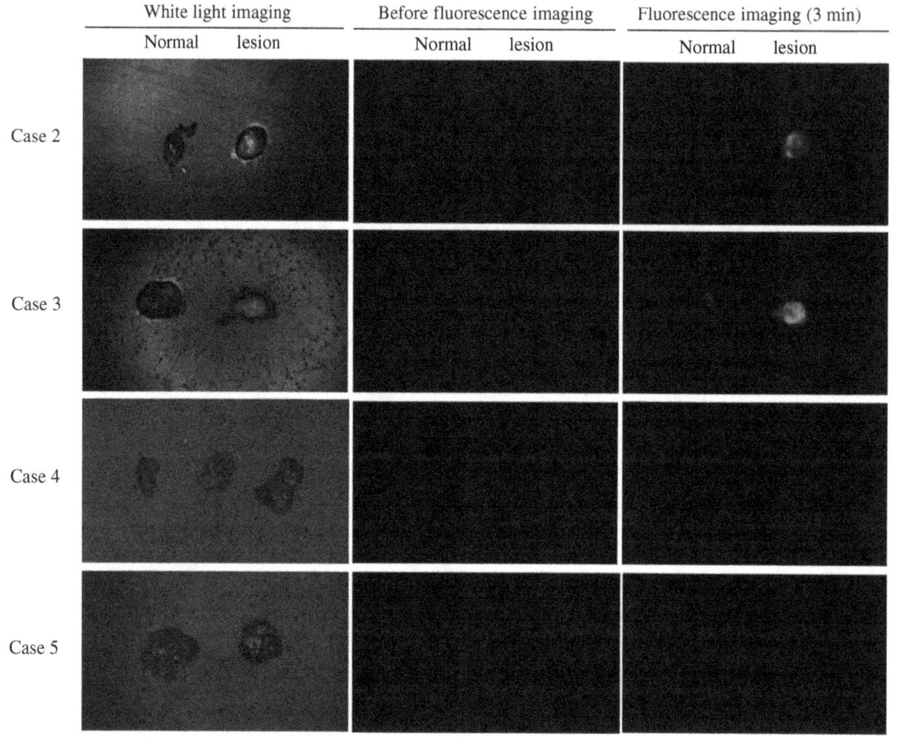

Fig. 3 White-light and fluorescence images of PTC and non-neoplastic cases. In each figure, the left side represents normal tissue and the right side a lesion. Images were captured before and 3 min after gGlu-HMRG application. **Case 2**: PTC case. Green fluorescent light was observed. **Case 3**: PTC recurrence case. Recurrent papillary carcinoma also showed strong green signals from the gGlu-HMRG probe. **Case 4**: Adenomatous goiter case. In this case, almost the entire specimen was goiter tissue, and the three tissues were all goiter. The goiter tissue showed no green signal. **Case 5**: Chronic inflammation case. The lesion was suspected to be PTC but was thyroiditis. The thyroiditis showed no green signal

were papillary carcinoma (Fig. 4; Case 1 and 2), 3 were adenomatous goiter (Fig. 4; Case 4), 1 was follicular adenoma, and 1 was thyroiditis (Fig. 2; Case 5). Two pathologists confirmed the diagnoses. All thyroid lesions were confirmed by HE staining.

Evaluation of GGT expression by immunostaining with anti-GGT1 antibody

To confirm the expression of GGT in all samples, immunohistochemical examination was performed. HepG2 and A549 cells were used as positive controls for GGT immunostaining, whereas SW782 cells were used as a negative control. We conducted GGT1 immunostaining of all 23 specimens used in fluorescence imaging. Representative staining of a thyroid tumor is shown in Fig. 5. Positive staining was seen in thyroid papillary carcinoma tissue (14/16 cases) (Fig. 5a). No GGT1 expression was observed in any normal thyroid tissue (16/16 cases) (Fig. 5c). Samples from the thyroiditis, follicular adenoma, Graves' disease, and 3 adenomatous goiter cases including 1 mediastinal goiter case were judged negative by GGT1 immunohistochemical staining.

Discussion

As GGT is overexpressed on the membranes of various cancer cells, gGlu-HMRG has been reported as a tool to detect breast cancer [12], lung cancer [9], colorectal tumors [10], head and neck squamous cell carcinoma [7], and prostate cancer [13]. The sensitivity and specificity of gGlu-HMRG in lung cancer detection are 43.8 and 84.9%, respectively [9]. gGlu-HMRG also reportedly enabled rapid fluorescence imaging of 54 and 76% of colorectal adenomas and carcinomas, respectively [10]. In a report on 8 head and neck tumor lesions, all samples exhibited fluorescence after application of gGlu-HMRG [7]. The sensitivity and specificity of breast cancer detection by gGlu-HMRG are 92 and 94%, respectively [12]. GGT is reportedly highly expressed in malignant ovarian tumors, breast cancer, carcinoma of the thyroid, and lung cancer [14–16]; however, whether fluorescence imaging using gGlu-HMRG can detect human thyroid cancer remains to be elucidated. This study is the first report demonstrating the efficacy of gGlu-HMRG in the detection of thyroid cancer.

In this study, we evaluated the detection of thyroid cancer, especially PTC, by gGlu-HMRG. All PTCs were detected after spraying with gGlu-HMRG, and

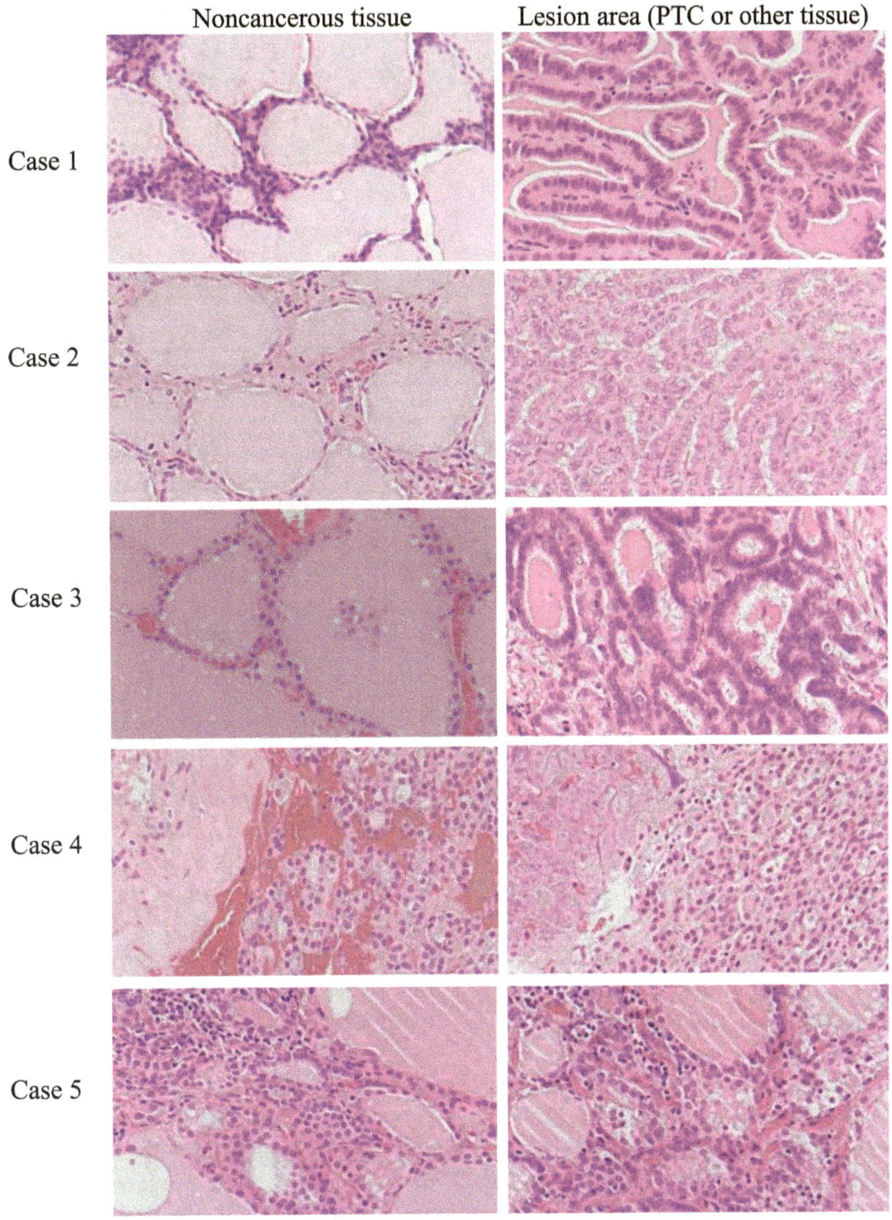

Fig. 4 HE stain images of samples used in fluorescence imaging. Each figure shows noncancerous tissue (left) and lesion area (PTC or other tissue) (right). **Case 1**: This is a representative fluorescence image corresponding to Case 1 in Fig. 2. Papillary carcinoma was well differentiated. Slight inflammation was seen in noncancerous tissue (left). **Case 2**: This PTC was also well differentiated. The noncancerous tissue was accompanied with light inflammation. **Case 3**: This PTC recurrence case was also a well-differentiated papillary carcinoma. **Case 4**: At first, this case was thought to be a malignant tumor because bleeding and necrosis were seen. HE staining established the final diagnosis as mediastinal goiter, an adenomatous goiter in the thymus. **Case 5**: Chronic inflammation case

fluorescence images were obtained (16/16 cases, 100%); in contrast, normal tissue counterparts from the same cases exhibited no fluorescent signals (0/16 cases, 0%). As only 16 cases were studied, evaluation of sensitivity and specificity is difficult, but both are expected to be higher than 95%. Future clinical trials studying larger numbers of PTC cases would help to clarify these concerns. Additionally, the cases of adenomatous goiter, thyroiditis, Graves' disease, and follicular adenoma showed no fluorescent signals after gGlu-HMRG application. These results indicate that the gGlu-HMRG method is useful for the specific detection of PTC and that the method is easy and fast when used on surgically resected specimens.

Frozen-section diagnosis is performed during surgical operation. The process involves preparation of frozen

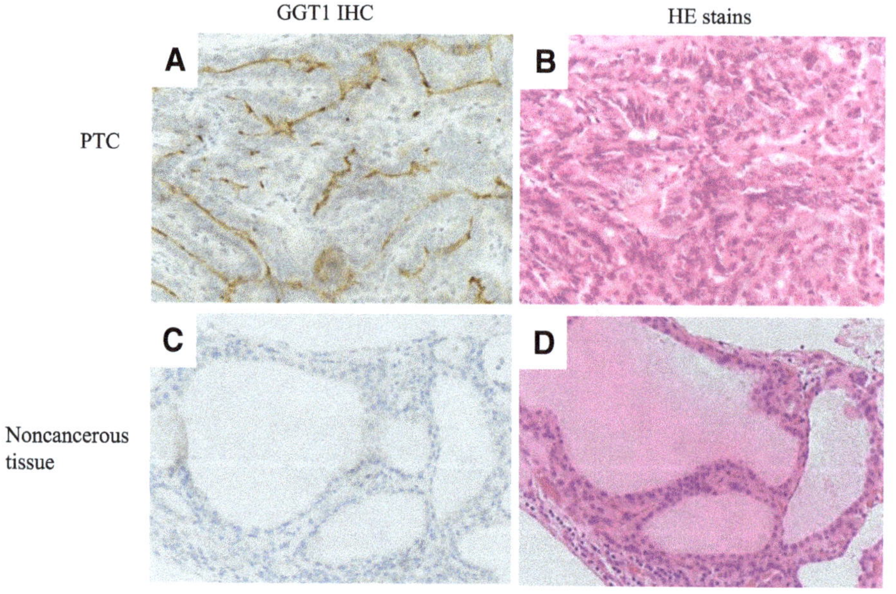

Fig. 5 Immunohistochemical investigation for GGT1. **a** Immunohistochemical detection of anti-GT1 antibody. PTC cases were positive for GGT expression, especially at the cell membranes. **b** HE staining of a PTC case in concordance with A. **c** Immunohistochemical detection of anti-GT1 antibody. Noncancerous tissue of thyroid tumor cases was negative for GGT expression. **d** HE staining of a noncancerous tissue in concordance with C

sections, HE staining, and diagnosis by a pathologist and takes 15–20 min. It has been a useful method for judging whether tissue is malignant during an operation. However, the gGlu-HMRG detection method requires much less time than frozen-section diagnosis, taking only 2–3 min. Tumor lesions become fluorescent within a few minutes of gGlu-HMRG application. The judgment is very simple; green fluorescence indicates the presence of a malignant tumor, whereas benign or non-neoplastic lesions show no fluorescence. Frozen-section diagnosis requires several years of pathological training, whereas recognition of green fluorescence requires no training. Therefore, gGlu-HMRG detection of malignant tumors is simpler than frozen-section diagnosis, and it could be applied in hospitals without laboratory technicians or pathologists.

There were 2 interesting cases in this experiment. The first was a mediastinal goiter case. When the specimen was carried to the pathology laboratory from the operating room, a malignancy was strongly suspected because the tissue exhibited massive bleeding and necrosis. Spraying with gGlu-HMRG resulted in no fluorescent green signal, suggesting no malignancy. The final pathological diagnosis made by HE staining was mediastinal goiter, which is neither a tumor nor malignant, but rather an enlarged thyroid gland. The second case was thyroiditis. The lesion was preoperatively expected to be PTC. Applying gGlu-HMRG to the sample resulted in no green signal. HE staining revealed that the lesion was not PTC, but thyroiditis. Both cases demonstrated that the gGlu-HMRG method was capable of correctly judging malignancy. In both cases, PTC was suspected, but the fluorescent probe showed that the lesions were not PTC before pathological diagnosis.

Immunohistochemical examination of cancer and normal tissue was used to validate GGT expression. GGT1 is reportedly expressed in the cell membrane, and GGT is a membrane-bound enzyme involved in the metabolism of glutathione (γ-glutamyl-cysteinyl-glycine; GSH) [17]. Studies have suggested that GGT plays an important role in tumor development, progression, invasion, drug resistance, and prognosis [17–22]. Small tumors are reportedly rapidly detectable by fluorescence imaging in vivo [23–28]. Several studies have reported that GGT is highly expressed in cancer cell membranes, as determined by immunohistochemical methods [7, 9]. In this study, 14 thyroid cancer samples among 16 cases were positive for GGT in the cell membranes; in contrast, cases involving non-cancerous or inflammatory lesions were negative. The negativity of the two cancer cases for GGT1 antibody might be attributable to the low specificity of the GGT antibody to the GGT1 antigen. However, all the cancer tissues were confirmed pathologically according to the parts exhibiting fluorescence. The results of immunostaining also supported the pathological diagnosis. These results showed that GGT is expressed in PTC and that the gGlu-HMRG method depends on GGT.

In this study, we showed that the GGT fluorescent probe could be applied to thyroid cancer detection, especially PTC. This is the first time that thyroid cancer detection by the fluorescent probe has been demonstrated. We began the examination using PTC because we had access to more papillary carcinoma than other thyroid cancer samples. As a next step, we plan to perform a similar experiment for other thyroid carcinomas, such as follicular carcinoma.

Conclusions

In this study, all PTC samples exhibited green fluorescence after application of gGlu-HMRG, whereas normal tissue showed none. Furthermore, samples from cases of other diseases, including thyroiditis, adenomatous goiters, Graves' disease, and follicular adenoma, exhibited no fluorescence. These results were supported by immunohistochemistry using an antibody against GGT1. The main characteristic of this gGlu-HMRG fluorescence detection method is its specific detection of PTC. Thus, the gGlu-HMRG method is expected to be a very effective method for pathologically and clinically identifying PTC. A large clinical study of thyroid cancer to confirm the utility of this fluorescent probe method is warranted.

Abbreviations

DMEM: Dulbecco's modified Eagle's medium; DMSO: Dimethyl sulfoxide; FBS: Fetal bovine serum; gGlu-HMRG: γ-glutamyl hydroxymethyl rhodamine green; GGT: γ-glutamyltranspeptidase; GSH: Glutathione; HE: Hematoxylin-eosin; HMRG: Hydroxymethyl rhodamine green; PBS: Phosphate-buffered saline; PTC: Papillary thyroid carcinoma

Acknowledgments

We thank Mamoru Iijima and Sayaka Ogikubo (Toranomon Hospital, Tokyo, Japan) for supporting pathological staining. This work was in part supported by Okinaka Memorial Institute for Medical Research.

Funding

Grant support: Grant-in aid for Scientific Research on Priority Areas from the Ministry of Education, Science, Sports, and Culture of Japan (17 K01824).

Authors' contributions

All authors read and approved the final manuscript.

Consent for publication

Written informed consent was obtained from the patients' guardian/parent/next of kin for the publication of this report and any accompanying images.

Competing interests

The authors declare that they have no competing interests.

Author details

[1]Department of Sports and Health Science, Daito Bunka University, 560 Iwadono, Higashimathuyama-shi, Saitama 355-8501, Japan. [2]Department of Pathology, Toranomon Hospital, Tokyo 105-0001, Japan. [3]Akasaka Miura Clinic, Tokyo 107-0052, Japan. [4]Department of Otolaryngology, Toranomon Hospital, Tokyo 105-0001, Japan. [5]Graduate School of Medicine, The University of Tokyo, Tokyo 113-0033, Japan. [6]PRESTO, Japan Science and Technology Agency (JST), Saitama 332-0012, Japan. [7]Graduate School of Pharmaceutical Sciences, The University of Tokyo, Tokyo 113-0033, Japan. [8]AMED CREST, Japan Agency for Medical Research and Development, Tokyo 100-0004, Japan.

References

1. Gonzalez-Gonzalez R, Bologna-Molina R, Carreon-Burciaga RG, Gomezpalacio-Gastelum M, Molina-Frechero N, Salazar-Rodriguez S. Papillary thyroid carcinoma: differential diagnosis and prognostic values of its different variants: review of the literature. ISRN Oncol. 2011;2011:915925.
2. Urano Y, Sakabe M, Kosaka N, Ogawa M, Mitsunaga M, Asanuma D, et al. Rapid cancer detection by topically spraying a gamma-glutamyltranspeptidase-activated fluorescent probe. Sci Transl Med. 2011;3:110–9.
3. Ito Y, Kihara M, Takamura Y, Kobayashi K, Miya A, Hirokawa M, et al. Prognosis and prognostic factors of papillary thyroid carcinoma in patients under 20 years. Endocrine. 2012;59:539–45.
4. Shinden Y, Ueo H, Tobo T, Gamachi A, Utou M, Komatsu H, et al. Rapid diagnosis of lymph node metastasis in breast cancer using a new fluorescent method with gamma-glutamyl hydroxymethyl rhodamine green. Sci Rep. 2016;6:2752–5.
5. Hanigan MH, Frierson HF Jr, Brown JE, Lovell MA, Taylor PT. Human ovarian tumors express gamma-glutamyl transpeptidase. Cancer Res. 1994;54:286–90.
6. Harada T, Nakamura Y, Sato K, Nagaya T, Choyke PL, Seto Y, et al. Surgical tissue handling methods to optimize ex vivo fluorescence with the activatable optical probe gamma-glutamyl hydroxymethyl rhodamine green. Contrast Media Mol Imaging. 2016;11:572–8.
7. Mizushima T, Ohnishi S, Shimizu Y, Kato M, Sakamoto N, Urano Y. Fluorescent imaging of superficial head and neck squamous cell carcinoma using a gamma-glutamyltranspeptidase-activated targeting agent: a pilot study. BMC Cancer. 2016;16:411.
8. Schafer C, Fels C, Brucke M, Holzhausen HJ, Bahn H, Wellman M, et al. Gamma-glutamyl transferase expression in higher-grade astrocytic glioma. Acta Oncol. 2001;40:529–35.
9. Hino H, Kamiya M, Kitano K, Mizuno K, Tanaka S, Nishiyama N, et al. Rapid cancer fluorescence imaging using a gamma-glutamyltranspeptidase-specific probe for primary lung cancer. Transl Oncol. 2016;9:203–10.
10. Sato C, Abe S, Saito Y, So Tsuruki E, Takamaru H, Makazu M, et al. A pilot study of fluorescent imaging of colorectal tumors using a gamma-glutamyl-transpeptidase-activatable fluorescent probe. Digestion. 2015;91:70–6.
11. Nakamura Y, Harada T, Nagaya T, Sato K, Okuyama S, Choyke PL, et al. Dynamic fluorescent imaging with the activatable probe, gamma-glutamyl hydroxymethyl rhodamine green in the detection of peritoneal cancer metastases: overcoming the problem of dilution when using a sprayable optical probe. Oncotarget. 2016;7:51124–37.
12. Ueo H, Shinden Y, Kobayashi H, Ueo H, Urano Y, Mimori K. Rapid intraoperative visualization of breast lesions with gamma-glutamyl hydroxymethyl rhodamine green. Sci Rep. 2015;5:12080.
13. Yogo T, Umezawa K, Kamiya M, Hino R, Urano Y. Development of an activatable fluorescent probe for prostate cancer imaging. Bioconjug Chem. 2017;28:2069–76.
14. Pompella A, De Tata V, Paolicchi A, Zunino F. Expression of gamma-glutamyltransferase in cancer cells and its significance in drug resistance. Biochem Pharmacol. 2006;71:231–8.
15. Hanigan MH, Frierson HF Jr, Swanson PE, De Young BR. Altered expression of gamma-glutamyl transpeptidase in human tumors. Hum Pathol. 1999;30:300–5.
16. Hanigan MH, Gallagher BC, Taylor PT Jr, Large MK. Inhibition of gamma-glutamyl transpeptidase activity by acivicin in vivo protects the kidney from cisplatin-induced toxicity. Cancer Res. 1994;54:5925–9.

17. Corti A, Franzini M, Paolicchi A, Pompella A. Gamma-glutamyltransferase of cancer cells at the crossroads of tumor progression, drug resistance and drug targeting. Anticancer Res. 2010;30:1169–81.
18. Wen YF, Yang XZ, Zeng LS, Peng HH, Huang WJ, Cai LM, et al. Prognostic impact of pretherapeutic gamma-glutamyltransferase on patients with nasopharyngeal carcinoma. PLoS One. 2017;12:e0172345.
19. Hanigan MH, Gallagher BC, Townsend DM, Gabarra V. Gamma-glutamyl transpeptidase accelerates tumor growth and increases the resistance of tumors to cisplatin in vivo. Carcinogenesis. 1999;20:553–9.
20. Pompella A, Corti A, Paolicchi A, Giommarelli C, Zunino F. Gamma-glutamyltransferase, redox regulation and cancer drug resistance. Curr Opin Pharmacol. 2007;7:360–6.
21. Van Hemelrijck M, Jassem W, Walldius G, Fentiman IS, Hammar N, Lambe M, et al. Gamma-glutamyltransferase and risk of cancer in a cohort of 545,460 persons - the Swedish AMORIS study. Eur J Cancer. 2011;47:2033–41.
22. Matsuzaki H, Kamiya M, Iwatate RJ, Asanuma D, Watanabe T, Urano Y. Novel hexosaminidase-targeting fluorescence probe for visualizing human colorectal cancer. Bioconjug Chem. 2016;27:973–81.
23. Kamiya M, Urano Y. Rapid and sensitive fluorescent imaging of tiny tumors in vivo and in clinical specimens. Curr Opin Chem Biol. 2016;33:9–15.
24. Shimane T, Aizawa H, Koike T, Kamiya M, Urano Y, Kurita H. Oral cancer intraoperative detection by topically spraying a γ-glutamyl transpeptidase-activated fluorescent probe. Oral Oncol. 2016;54:e16–8.
25. Mori K, Ishizawa T, Yamashita S, Kamiya M, Urano Y, Kokudo N. Intraoperative visualization of pancreatic juice leaking from the pancreatic stump in a swine model. Gastroenterology. 2015;149:1334–6.
26. Asanuma D, Sakabe M, Kamiya M, Yamamoto K, Hiratake J, Ogawa M, et al. Sensitive β-galactosidase-targeting fluorescence probe for visualizing small peritoneal metastatic tumours in vivo. Nat Commun. 2015;6:6463.
27. Miyata A, Ishizawa T, Kamiya M, Shimizu A, Kaneko J, Ijichi H, et al. Photoacoustic tomography of human hepatic malignancies using intraoperative indocyanine green fluorescence imaging. PLoS One. 2014;9:e112667.
28. Fujii T, Kamiya M, Urano Y. In vivo imaging of intraperitoneally disseminated tumors in model mice by using activatable fluorescent small-molecular probes for activity of cathepsins. Bioconjug Chem. 2014;25:1838–46.

29

Concordance between the TIRADS ultrasound criteria and the BETHESDA cytology criteria on the nontoxic thyroid nodule

Hernando Vargas-Uricoechea[1], Ivonne Meza-Cabrera[2] and Jorge Herrera-Chaparro[3*]

Abstract

Background: Thyroid nodule is a common disorder of the thyroid. Despite their benign nature, they can be associated with multiple pathologic conditions, including thyroid cancer.

Methods: This cross-sectional study determined the concordance of Ultrasound (TIRADS criteria) and Fine Needle Aspiration Biopsy (FNA-BETHESDA system) in the assessment of the nontoxic thyroid nodule. A total of 180 subjects 18 years old or older underwent the two diagnostic tests and their results were compared using kappa index.

Results: Participants were mostly women, with average age of 57 years. The frequency of BETHESDA II was 65/180 versus 45/180 in TIRADS 2. In contrast, the highest frequency in category 4-IV was 62/180 for TIRADS 4 versus 41/180 for BETHESDA IV. The highest concordance was found among the category 2-II classification. The observed agreement was 87.2% with a linear weighted kappa of 0.69 (95% CI: 0.59-0.79). The heterogeneity analysis showed a trend towards a higher weighted kappa value in nodules ≥4 cm in males and individuals aged ≥50 years, with accelerated nodular growth, binding to adjacent structures, vocal folds paralysis, urban origin, and a history of head and neck radiation therapy.

Conclusions: The TIRADS criteria has a good concordance with the Bethesda system. The ultrasound findings of benign pathology are aligned with the cytology results. The correct interpretation of the two findings helps the clinician to reduce the risk of unnecessary invasive procedures in patients with a low probability of presenting thyroid cancer, while facilitating the identification of patients at higher risk of cancer.

Keywords: Thyroid, Nodule, TIRADS, Bethesda, Concordance

Background

A steady increase in the incidence rate of thyroid cancer has been noted in recent decades all over the world, and the causes of this increase are still controversial. Thyroid cancer is the most common endocrine malignancy (1.0–1.5% of all newly diagnosed cancers in the United States of America every year are originally thyroid). The increased frequency in thyroid cancer is almost exclusively due to the rise in the number of papillary cancers, with no significant changes in other histologic subtypes [1, 2]. The typical presentation is as small tumors, though there is a growing incidence of large tumors; it has been hypothesized that the rise in the incidence of thyroid cancer is mostly due to improved detection rather than to a real increase in frequency [3]. Thyroid nodule can be defined as a discrete lesion within the thyroid gland that is radiologically distinct from the surrounding thyroid parenchyma. It may be solitary, multiple, solid, or cystic, and may or not be functional. Thyroid nodules are frequent among the general population and thyroid Ultrasound (US) has considerably increased the number of cases identified. Thyroid nodules may be palpated in about 4–8% of the general population (however, neck palpation is

* Correspondence: hernandovargasuricoechea@gmail.com
[3]Department of surgery, Universidad del Cauca, Carrera 6 No 41 N-135 apto 202B terrazas del campestre, Popayán, Cauca, Colombia
Full list of author information is available at the end of the article

very imprecise in terms of determining the size and morphology). US identifies the presence of nodules in 19-67% of the cases, and is an accurate method for the detection of thyroid nodules; however, US has a low accuracy in differentiating between benign from malignant thyroid nodules [4]. The sonographic characteristics of a thyroid nodule associated with a higher likelihood of malignancy include hypoechogenicity, increased intranodular vascularity, irregular margins, microcalcifications, absent halo, and a taller-than-wide shape measured in the transverse dimension. Thus, several benign and malignant ultrasound gray scale and Doppler features have emerged over the last ten years that may be used in different ways to assign probabilities, together with a method based on the Breast Imaging Reporting and Data System (BIRADS). Likewise, several US Thyroid Imaging Reporting and Data Systems (TIRADS) have been proposed for risk stratification of thyroid nodules [5].

The nodules are usually divided into different categories based on TIRADS and are then referred for Fine-Needle Aspiration (FNA) Biopsy or follow-up, according to the variable risk of malignancy. The terminology of TIRADS was first used by Horvath et al. [6]. They described 10 US patterns of thyroid nodules and related the rate of malignancy based on the pattern. The initial purpose of TIRADS was to improve patient management and cost-effectiveness by avoiding unnecessary FNA Biopsies in patients with thyroid nodules (Table 1), with a sensitivity, specificity, positive predictive value, negative predictive value, and accuracy of 88, 49, 49, 88, and 94%, respectively. However, its clinical use is still very limited and its practical application in clinical practice is questioned. Moreover, FNA Biopsy is the most accurate method for determining malignancy, and is a fundamental part of current thyroid nodule evaluation. The Bethesda System for Reporting Thyroid Cytopathology is a standardized reporting system for classifying thyroid FNA Biopsy results that comprises six diagnostic categories with unique risks of malignancy and recommendations for clinical management. Since its inception, the Bethesda System has been widely adopted, each category conveys a risk of malignancy and recommended next steps, though it is unclear if each category also predicts the type and extent of malignancy (Table 1). Nevertheless, the implementation of this reporting system has shown significant diagnostic variability, both inter and intra pathologists, particularly when read as "atypical cells of undetermined significance, follicular lesion of undetermined significance, or follicular neoplasm" (also termed as Bethesda Category III, comprising a heterogeneous population of low-risk lesions that contain follicular cells exhibiting either architectural abnormalities or nuclear atypia that do not fit into other definitive cytological categories). A recent meta-analysis evaluated the validity of the Bethesda reporting system and found 97% sensitivity, 50.7% specificity and 68.8% diagnostic accuracy; the negative and positive predictive values were 96.3 and 55.9%, respectively [7, 8]. Notwithstanding the fact that both US and FNA biopsy are widely recommended procedures to study patients with thyroid nodules, the value of the existing concordance between the two methods has not been established. Consequently, the purpose of this study was to assess the existing concordance between the two diagnostic methods used in the initial evaluation of individuals with non-toxic thyroid nodule (TIRADS and Bethesda systems).

Methods

The overall objective of the study was to determine the level of concordance between the ultrasound criteria established under TIRADS (The Thyroid Imaging Reporting and Data System for US of the thyroid); and the cytology criteria according to The Bethesda System for Reporting Thyroid Cytopathology [9, 10]. Additionally, the study population was characterized from the socio-demographic point of view, the concordance of the classification systems was estimated, and the heterogeneity of the factors influencing the consistency of the various classification systems was analyzed.

Ethics approval and consent to participate

All personal data were confidential and managed exclusively by the principal investigator, according to the legal standards on the confidentiality of the medical record and adhering to the rules of the Institutional Review Committee of Human Ethics (reference number: 221–011). Universidad del Valle, Valle del Cauca-Colombia.

Design of the study

This was a cross-sectional study to evaluate the concordance between two diagnostic systems (TIRADS and Bethesda), administered simultaneously to the same individual. The population consisted of consecutive patients consulting the outpatient endocrinology, internal medicine, or general surgery departments at a high complexity referral center, with a diagnosis of nodular or non-nodular "thyroid dysfunction". The inclusion criteria were as follows: male and females aged 18 years and older, with a non-toxic thyroid nodule (ranges for normal thyroid tests were Thyrotrophin (TSH): 0.4 to 4 mIU/L; Free thyroxine: 0.8 to 1.8 ng/dL, according to the National Academy of Clinical Biochemistry) identified either clinically or through imaging [11]. The exclusion criteria were: TIRADS 1 and Bethesda I (Table 1); Graves-Basedow–associated hyperthyroidism, patients with toxic thyroid nodular disease, chronic hypothyroidism (with

Table 1 Thyroid imaging reporting and data system (TIRADS) and the Bethesda System for Reporting Cytopathology (ref. 6, 8, 9)

TIRADS		BETHESDA	
Categories	Features	Diagnostic Categories	Risk of malignancy
TIRADS 1	Normal thyroid gland.	I. Nondiagnostic or unsatisfactory.	-
TIRADS 2	Benign conditions (0% malignancy).	Cyst fluid only.	
TIRADS 3	Probably benign nodules (5% malignancy).	Virtually acellular specimen.	
TIRADS 4	Suspicious nodules (5–80% malignancy rate). A subdivision into 4a (malignancy between 5 and 10%) and 4b (malignancy between 10 and 80%) was optional.	Other (obscuring blood, clotting artifact, etc.).	
TIRADS 5	Probably malignant nodules (malignancy >80%).	II. Benign.	0-3
TIRADS 6	Category included biopsy proven malignant nodules.	Consistent with a benign follicular nodule (includes adenomatoid nodule, colloid nodule, etc.).	
		Consistent with lymphocytic (Hashimoto) thyroiditis in the proper clinical context.	
		Consistent with granulomatous (subacute) thyroiditis.	
		III. Atypia of undetermined significance/follicular lesion of undetermined significance.	5-15
		IV. Follicular neoplasm/"suspicious" for follicular neoplasm. Specify if Hürthle cell type.	15-30
		V. Suspicious for malignancy.	60-75
		Suspicious for papillary carcinoma.	
		Suspicious for medullary carcinoma.	
		Suspicious for metastatic carcinoma.	
		Suspicious for lymphoma.	
		VI. Malignant.	97-99
		Papillary thyroid carcinoma.	
		Poorly differentiated carcinoma.	
		Medullary thyroid carcinoma.	
		Undifferentiated (anaplastic) carcinoma.	
		Squamous cell carcinoma.	
		Carcinoma with mixed features.	
		Metastatic.	

a minimum of six-months on treatment with levothyroxine sodium), iatrogenic hyperthyroidism resulting from high-dose sodium levothyroxine therapy regardless of the indication; a history of surgically resected thyroid cancer, and patients with a history of partial thyroidectomy (lobectomy) or subtotal/near total thyroidectomy under levothyroxine sodium therapy (the latter criterion is based on the fact that a constant high stimulus of thyroid hormones and the concomitant TSH suppression in patients with endogenous hyperthyroidism and levothyroxine management may impact the size of the thyroid nodules) [12, 13].

This study was supported by the Internal Medicine Department from The Faculty of medicina of the Universidad del Cauca (Popayán-Colombia), who provided funding to conduct the analysis and prepare the manuscript.

Sample size estimate and sampling

To estimate the sample size, matched categories in both reporting systems were considered. Based on the data from a pilot study with 32 subjects that met the above selection criteria, and using the formula below, the N value was established at 128 subjects:

$$n = \frac{P_e}{ee^2(1-P_e)}$$

Where:

P_e: Expected percentage of random concordance

Ee: Kappa index standard error [14–16].

A consecutive non-probabilistic sampling was used based on an initial review of 217 medical records; however the final analysis was limited to 180 patients and 37 patients were excluded due to:

1. Incomplete family history and missing socio-demographic information in 26 records.
2. The echography was not reported according to TIRADS criteria in 4 records.
3. The cytology results were not reported according to the Bethesda criteria in 5 cases.
4. The ultrasound examination had been done at a different institution or by a different radiologist in 2 cases.

The source of the information in this study is a registry of consecutive data from an outpatient center for patients with a diagnosis of thyroid dysfunction. A standard form collected socio-demographic information, family and personal history of diseases, in addition to the data available from the medical record. Patients undergoing thyroid ultrasound imaging and FNA Biopsy due to non-toxic nodular thyroid disease were analyzed in accordance with the medical opinion of the institution's study group on thyroid disease (endocrinology, pathology, radiology and surgery). All patients were informed about the procedure and after signing the informed consent, the thyroid ultrasound was performed, and the node(s) were sampled according to Crockett's FNA Biopsy protocol [17].

The same radiologist read all the tests. One out of every 20 patients was randomly selected to repeat the ultrasound examination. The principal researcher interpreted the results in accordance with the TIRADS criteria and if the second reading was inconsistent with the first, a second radiologist was asked for an opinion to arrive at a consensus between the two radiologists and establish a TIRADS-based ultrasonographic diagnosis. 9 of the 180 participants were randomly selected to assess the radiologists' agreement. One of the nine US results showed disagreement because the first radiologist reported TIRADS 3, while the second one reported TIRADS 2, based on the original classification. Upon further analysis the conclusion was TIRADS 3. The material obtained via the FNA Biopsy was placed on a glass slide previously impregnated with 96% alcohol and then a second glass slide was placed on top. The smear was again immersed in 96% alcohol and then stained using the Papanicolaou technique. To ensure the quality of the cytology specimens, the same experienced pathologist read the slides and reported a diagnosis based on the Bethesda criteria. One out every ten specimens was randomly selected to be analyzed by a second pathologist. In case of disagreement between the two pathologists, a pathologist meeting was convened (five pathologist). The second pathologist disagreed with two of the 18 specimens subject to a second evaluation; in both cases, the first pathologist classified the cytology specimen as Bethesda V, while the second pathologist classified the specimens as Bethesda VI. Both specimens were further evaluated at a pathologist meeting, and the final classification was Bethesda VI. The radiologists and the pathologists were blinded to the patients' medical record data for both the ultrasound examination and the FNA biopsy.

Statistical analysis

The weighted Kappa statistical method with a 95% confidence interval and the statistical Z-test were used to estimate the level of concordance between the two systems. In order to pursue the Kappa analysis, categories 5 and 6 of both the TIRADS and the Bethesda classification were combined since the highest risk for malignancy is usually described in these two categories. Category 1 in both classifications was excluded from the selection process because a TIRADS 1 ultrasound examination is considered normal, and Bethesda I is considered an unsatisfactory specimen. The purpose of excluding category 1 was to avoid invalidating further comparisons since category 1 is inconclusive, particularly Bethesda I. Consequently, the analysis categories are as follows:

- TIRADS 2: "BENIGN"
- TIRADS 3: "PROBABLY BENIGN"
- TIRADS 4: "SUSPICIOUS"
- TIRADS 5: "PROBABLY MALIGNANT"
- Bethesda II: "BENIGN".
- Bethesda III: "PROBABLY BENIGN".
- Bethesda IV: "SUSPICIOUS".
- Bethesda V: "PROBABLY MALIGNANT"

Weighted Kappa statistic with linear weight was used to estimate the level of agreement between the two systems; Kappa with quadratic weighting was used for comparative purposes. A descriptive analysis was used to indicate the distribution of the quantitative variables. Based on that distribution, the average represented the central trend and the scatter represented the standard deviation. The qualitative variables were defined in terms of percentages by category. A stratified analysis was performed to explore heterogeneity factors, resulting in a linear weighted Kappa for the following categories: Gender, age, nodule size, urban/non-urban origin, accelerated nodule growth, vocal folds paralysis, hard nodule, attached to underlying structures, history of head and neck radiation therapy, and family history of thyroid cancer. All the analyses used STATA 10.1

Results

The average age was 57 years old. Over 75% of the participants were females and 68.9% came from the urban area; however, there was a remarkable high frequency of risk factors for thyroid cancer. (Table 2) The frequency

Table 2 Socio-demographic characteristics and risk factors for thyroid cancer

Characteristic	Frequency
Mean age	57 y (SD:±14y)
Sex	Fem: 141 (78.3%)
	Male: 39 (21.7%)
Origin	Urban: 124 (68.9%).
	Non-Urban: 56 (31.1%).
Thyroid cancer family backgrounds	N (%)
No	119 (66.1%)
Yes	61 (33.9%)
Accelerated Growth of the Thyroid Nodules	
No	121 (67.2%)
Yes	59 (32.8%)
Head Radiation	
No	163 (90.6%)
Yes	17 (9.4%)
Firm Nodule	
No	94 (51.7%)
Yes	86 (47.8%)
Adjacent structure Attachment	
No	130 (72.2%)
Yes	50 (27.8%)
Vocal Chord Paralysis	
No	130 (72.2%)
Yes	50 (27.8%)
≥4 cm nodule	
No	109 (60.6%)
Yes	71 (39.4%)

distribution according to the scales was strikingly different for categories 2-II and 4-IV. The frequency of category II in Bethesda was 65/180 versus 45/180 in TIRADS 2. In contrast, the highest frequency in category 4-IV was 62/180 for TIRADS 4 versus 41/180 for Bethesda IV. (Table 3) The highest concordance was found for categories TIRADS 2-Bethesda II (23.33%). None of the patients classified as TIRADS 2 were rated as Bethesda IV or V. In contrast, 4 subjects classified as Bethesda II were classified as TIRADS 4 ($n = 2$) or V ($n = 2$). Of the 35 patients classified as Bethesda V none were classified as TIRADS 2 or 3, but 3 of the 32 subjects with TIRADS 5 were classified as Bethesda II ($n = 2$) or III ($n = 1$). The weighted Kappa value according to the linear weights was 0.69 (95% CI: 0.59–0.79). The overall Kappa and the Kappa with quadratic weighting were also estimated for comparative purposes. (Table 4) The heterogeneity analysis showed a trend towards a higher weighted kappa

Table 3 Joint distribution of BETHESDA & TIRADS categories

Diagnostic categories		TIRADS				Total
		2	3	4	5	
BETHESDA	II	42	19	2	2	65
		23.33%	10.56%	1.11%	1.11%	
	III	3	21	14	1	39
		1.67%	11.67%	7.78%	0.56%	
	IV	0	1	33	7	41
		0%	0.56%	18.33%	3.89%	
	V	0	0	13	22	35
		0%	0%	7,22%	12,22%	
	Total	45	41	62	32	180

value in nodules ≥4 cm in males and individuals aged ≥50 years, with accelerated nodular growth, binding to adjacent structures, vocal folds paralysis, urban origin, and a history of head and neck radiation therapy (Tables 5 and 6).

Discussion

This study evaluated the concordance between the TIRADS and the Bethesda reporting systems on the non-toxic thyroid nodule. The result showed a "good or substantial" concordance and the most frequent consistency was found for categories II and IV. The kappa index measures the level of inter-observer concordance, or as in this particular case, the concordance between two diagnostic methods rather than the "quality" of the observation, so it is not possible to establish the validity of the resulting classifications. This study addresses the level of discrepancy, the report categories, and which categories tend to exhibit a higher frequency of discrepancies between the two methods. When particular types of disagreements are more frequent, this information shall be kept in mind when developing the kappa index [18, 19]. For this reason, the weighted kappa analysis was used, without neglecting the fact that although using weights is logical and attractive, it introduces a component of subjectivity since assigning weights is subjective and may impact the interpretation of the data when used for a different population –the weights assigned may vary based on the frequency of the disease-. This is evidenced through the variation in the kappa estimates when weighing is used, and depends on the weighing method used. The weighted kappa estimate with linear weights assigned to the categories shows a value of 0.69. The weighted kappa value based on quadratic weights was higher than the overall kappa or the linear weighted kappa (the quadratic weighted kappa value was 0.80). The difference is based on the fact that the linear and quadratic methods are based on the relative separation among the classification categories but

Table 4 Kappa comparison according to the estimation method

Kappa	Observed Agreement	Expected agreement	Kappa	Standard error	IC 95%	Z	Value p
Global	65.56%	25.27%	0.5391	0.0425	0.46–0.62	12.68	<0.001
Weighted (linear weights)	87.22%	58.76%	0.6901	0.0528	0.59–0.79	13.07	<0.001
Estimated (quadratic weights	94.63%	72.86%	0.8021	0.0731	0.66–0.94	10.97	<0.001

the quadratic approach uses square differences, while the linear approach uses absolute values [20, 21]. Consequently, quadratic weights tend to assign a higher weight to disagreements that were relatively few in this study; when the kappa interpretation is based on quadratic weights, the level of concordance remains unchanged versus the interpretation of the linear weighted kappa; but if analyzed as an absolute value, it is evidently overestimated. Since the kappa value is affected by the prevalence of the characteristic studied, caution is of the essence when generalizing the results of inter-observer comparisons in the presence of varying prevalence. The prevalence of malignancy based on cytology findings (Bethesda V in the matched scale) was reported at 19.4% (35/180); however, using the TIRADS scale (maximum value of 5 in the matched scale), the prevalence of malignancy was 17% (32/180), showing a non-significant difference between the two methods. This is extremely relevant when considering that a prevalence of close to 50% results in a higher kappa value for the same proportion of agreements observed [22, 23]. Thus, the interpretation of the kappa index requires identifying the value of the marginal frequencies on the table (prevalence observed per observer). Since the difference between the prevalence estimated by both methods is not significant, the conclusion is than that the prevalence of the event did not affect the kappa value reported. When evaluating heterogeneity based on characteristics such as gender, age, size of the nodule, place of origin, accelerated nodular growth, vocal folds paralysis, hard nodule, binding to adjacent structures, a history of head and neck radiation therapy, a family history of thyroid cancer, the trend indicates a stronger concordance (expressed as a weighted kappa value). This is also the case for variables such as nodule size ≥4 cm, male gender, and age ≥50 years. Despite this trend, the study failed to show statistically significant differences. The TIRADS classification attempts to improve the interpretation of the findings of a thyroid nodule by defining categories that in the end are exclusive, although the original classification indicates a risk of malignancy between 5-80% for TIRADS 4, and this fact makes it difficult to clinically define a follow-up and management strategy. Notwithstanding this consideration, from the clinical perspective, in a subject with low probability of having thyroid cancer (and a TIRADS 2 or 3) the US negative predictive value will be greatly enhanced. The best US diagnostic performance is probably with extreme results of the classification (TIRADS 2–3 and TIRADS 5–6 of the original classification). Depending on the clinical probability of malignancy, the US findings may be more or less useful and applicable [24].

Table 5 Stratification according to nodule size, sex, and age in order to assess heterogeneity

Strata	Observed Agreement	Expected Agreement	Kappa	Standard Error	IC 95%
Nodule Size					
<4 cm	85.63%	65.15%	0.5876	0.067	0.46-0.72
≥4 cm	89.67%	66.26%	0.6938	0.083	0.53-0.86
Sex					
Men	89.74%	58.32%	0.7539	0.117	0.53-0.98
Women	86.52%	59.30%	0.6689	0.059	0.55-0.78
Age					
<50 years old	82.49%	59.91%	0.5632	0.092	0.38-0.74
≥50 years old	89.53%	59.18%	0.7435	0.064	0.62-0.87

Previous studies have evaluated the diagnostic performance of both US and FNA Biopsy in the initial study of thyroid nodules. A recent study was aimed at developing a diagnostic algorithm using the data reported in the US (in accordance with a scoring system evaluating the risk of malignancy based on several US patterns) and the results of the FNA Biopsy (according to Bethesda). This study showed that classifying an individual in accordance with the presence of different US patterns as low, intermediate or high risk, together with the results of the FNA Biopsy, enables optimal clinical decision-making with regards to treatment strategies [25]. Along the same lines, other studies classify the risk of malignancy in accordance with the US characteristics and based on such risk, establish the need to perform a FNA Biopsy. The higher the risk of malignancy (according to the US) the greater the need to do the FNA Biopsy, and vice-versa –the lower the risk of malignancy based on the US, the lower the indication for a FNA Biopsy– [26–28].

Our study showed that the highest concordance was found among both the lowest risk (TIRADS 2 and Bethesda II) and the higher risk categories (TIRADS 4 and Bethesda IV), which is consistent with the previously described trials. This indicates that the US characteristics suggesting a higher or lower risk of malignancy, will be associated with higher

Table 6 Heterogeneity assessment by stratifying the variables according to: thyroid cancer family history, accelerated growth of the nodules, firm nodule, underlying structure, vocal chords paralysis, origins, and history of radiation

Strata	Observed Agreement	Expected Agreement	Kappa	Standard Error	95% CI
Thyroid Cancer Family history					
Yes	87.98%	60.71%	0.694	0.086	0.53–0.86
No	86.83%	58.81%	0.680	0.066	0.55–0.81
Accelerated Growth of the nodule					
Yes	90.40%	60.12%	0.759	0.090	0.58–0.94
No	85.67%	59.89%	0.643	0.065	0.52–0.77
Firm Nodule					
Yes	86.82%	58.55%	0.682	0.076	0.53–0.83
No	87.59%	60.10%	0.689	0.073	0.55–0.83
Adjacent Structure Attachment					
Yes	94.00%	65.52%	0.826	0.096	0.64–1.01
No	84.62%	59.42%	0.621	0.062	0.50–0.74
Vocal Chords Paralysis					
Yes	94.67%	66.11%	0.843	0.096	0.65–1.03
No	84.36%	58.52%	0.623	0.062	0.50–0.74
Origin					
Urban (exclusive)	88.70%	58.99%	0.7245	0.065	0.60–0.85
Urban or Rural	84.41%	58.26%	0.6265	0.0881	0.45–0.8
Head and neck radiation therapy					
Yes	96.08%	61.48%	0.8982	0.1689	0.57–1.23
No	86.30%	58.55%	0.6695	0.0557	0.56–0.78

or lower probability of malignancy according to the FNA Biopsy report (Bethesda), respectively.

Finally, the interpretation of the results in this study requires acknowledging that over two thirds of the subjects were women. Probably this trend is due to the fact that autoimmune thyroid disease is significantly more frequent in females than in males, so these patients with autoimmune thyroid disease visit the physician more often increasing the probability of detecting the nodules either through palpation or ultrasound; clinically this situation may be defined as a "medical surveillance bias" [29, 30]. The geographical distribution indicates that most of the patients were from urban areas and those from the rural areas were mostly from municipalities with accessible specialized care. The participants in the study had information about exposure/disease since they had been referred for a study of the thyroid nodule with a probable diagnosis of malignancy. In cross-section studies the participants may be more prone to participate based on their knowledge about exposure and disease and the convenience of their geographical location leading to a higher "selection bias" that in turn could overestimate the frequency of malignancies [31, 32]. This study highlights the high frequency of factors that have been historically associated with thyroid cancer. Those factors were evaluated with the survey administered to the study subjects that had been previously referred for tests to rule out malignancies, so these participants were more likely to recall past exposures (accurate or vague) potentially leading to a "recall bias" [30, 33]. Furthermore, since the data collection from the participants was not masked (they had been previously identified as nodular thyroid disease patients screened for malignancies), the interviewer's interest in evaluating the exposure factors could have resulted in an "interviewer bias" [34, 35].

Conclusions

The thyroid ultrasound report using the TIRADS criteria has a good concordance with the Bethesda cytology findings using FNA Biopsy. The ultrasound findings of benign pathology are aligned with the cytology results and vice-versa; ultrasound findings of malignancy shall be consistent with cytology-identified malignant disease. The correct interpretation of the two findings helps the clinician to reduce the risk of unnecessary invasive procedures in patients with a low probability of presenting thyroid cancer, while facilitating the identification of patients at higher risk of cancer. There is a need to develop study and monitoring protocols for cases classified as "discordant", particularly when extreme categories are identified (TIRADS 5-Bethesda II, TIRADS 2-Bethesda V).

Abbreviations
BIRADS: Breast Imaging Reporting and Data System; FNA: Fine-Needle Aspiration; TIRADS: The Thyroid Imaging Reporting and Data System for US of the thyroid; TSH: Thyrotrophin; US: Ultrasound

Acknowledgements
None.

Funding
This study was supported by the Internal Medicine Department from The Faculty of medicina of the Universidad del Cauca (Popayán-Colombia), who provided funding to conduct the analysis and prepare the manuscript.

Authors' contributions
H V-U, I M-C and J H-Ch were involved in study design, acquisition of data, analysis and interpretation of data and drafting and revising the manuscript. H V-U, and I M-C were involved in data collection and analysis and manuscript drafting. All authors read and approved the final manuscript.

Competing interests
All authors declare no financial competing interests, nor any other type of conflicts of interest.

Consent for publication
All authors gave their approval for the final version to be published and agree to be accountable for this work.

Author details
[1]Department of Internal Medicine, Division of Endocrinology and Metabolism, Universidad del Cauca, Popayán, Colombia. [2]Laboratory of Pathology, Hospital Universitario San José, Popayán, Cauca, Colombia. [3]Department of surgery, Universidad del Cauca, Carrera 6 No 41 N-135 apto 202B terrazas del campestre, Popayán, Cauca, Colombia.

References
1. Ferlay J, Soerjomataram I, Dikshit R, Eser S, Mathers C, Rebelo M, Parkin DM, Forman D, Bray F. Cancer incidence and mortality worldwide: sources, methods and major patterns in GLOBOCAN 2012. Int J Cancer. 2015;136(5): 359-86.
2. Torre LA, Bray F, Siegel RL, Ferlay J, Lortet-Tieulent J, Jemal A. Global cancer statistics, 2012. CA Cancer J Clin. 2015;65(2):87–108.
3. Wiltshire JJ, Drake TM, Uttley L, Balasubramanian SP. Systematic review of trends in the incidence rates of thyroid cancer. Thyroid. 2016;26(11):1541–52.
4. Gharib H, Papini E, Garber JR, Duick DS, Harrell RM, Hegedüs L, Paschke R, Valcavi R, Vitti P, AACE/ACE/AME Task Force on Thyroid Nodules. American Association Of Clinical Endocrinologists, American College Of Endocrinology, And Associazione Medici Endocrinologi Medical Guidelines For Clinical Practice For The Diagnosis And Management Of Thyroid Nodules–2016 Update. Endocr Pract. 2016;22(5):622–39.
5. Yoon JH, Lee HS, Kim EK, Moon HJ, Kwak JY. Malignancy risk stratification of thyroid nodules: comparison between the thyroid imaging reporting and data system and the 2014 American thyroid association management guidelines. Radiology. 2016;278(3):917–24.
6. Horvath E, Majlis S, Rossi R, Franco C, Niedmann JP, Castro A, Dominguez M. An ultrasonogram reporting system for thyroid nodules stratifying cancer risk for clinical management. J Clin Endocrinol Metab. 2009;94(5):1748–51.
7. Pusztaszeri M, Rossi ED, Auger M, Baloch Z, Bishop J, Bongiovanni M, Chandra A, Cochand-Priollet B, Fadda G, Hirokawa M, Hong S, Kakudo K, Krane JF, Nayar R, Parangi S, Schmitt F, Faquin WC. The Bethesda system for reporting thyroid cytopathology: proposed modifications and updates for the second edition from an international panel. Acta Cytol. 2016;60(5):399–405.
8. Garg S, Desai NJ, Mehta D, Vaishnav M. To establish bethesda system for diagnosis of thyroid nodules on the basis of fnac with histopathological correlation. J Clin Diagn Res. 2015;9(12):EC17–21.
9. Russ G, Bigorgne C, Royer B, Rouxel A, Bienvenu-Perrard M. The Thyroid Imaging Reporting and Data System (TIRADS) for ultrasound of the thyroid. J Radiol. 2011;92(7–8):701–13.
10. Cibas ES, Ali SZ. NCI Thyroid FNA State of the Science Conference. The Bethesda System for reporting thyroid cytopathology. Am J Clin Pathol. 2009;132:658–65.
11. Baloch Z, Carayon P, Conte-Devolx B, Demers LM, Feldt-Rasmussen U, Henry JF, LiVosli VA, Niccoli-Sire P, John R, Ruf J, Smyth PP, Spencer CA, Stockigt JR, Guidelines Committee, National Academy of Clinical Biochemistry. Laboratory medicine practice guidelines. Laboratory support for the diagnosis and monitoring of thyroid disease. Thyroid. 2003;13(1):3–126.
12. Zelmanovitz F, Genro S, Gross JL. Suppressive therapy with levothyroxine for solitary thyroid nodules: a double-blind controlled clinical study and cumulative meta-analyses. J Clin Endocrinol Metab. 1998;83:3881–5.
13. Grussendorf M, Reiners C, Paschke R, Wegscheider K. Reduction of thyroid nodule volume by levothyroxine and iodine alone and in combination: a randomized, placebo-controlled trial. J Clin Endocrinol Metab. 2012;96:2786–95.
14. Kramer M, Feinstein AR. Clinical Biostatistics. The biostatistics of concordance. Clin Pharmacol Ther. 1981;29:111–23.
15. Cantor AB. Sample-size calculation for Cohen's kappa. Psychol Methods. 1996;1:150–3.
16. Sim J, Wrigth CC. The Kappa statistic in reliability studies: Use, interpretation, and sample size requirements. Phys Ther. 2005;85:257–68.
17. Crockett JC. The thyroid nodule fine-needle aspiration biopsy technique. J Ultrasound Med. 2011;30:685–94.
18. Landis JR, Koch GG. The measurement of observer agreement for categorical data. Biometrics. 1977;33:159–74.
19. Barnhart HX, Williamson JM. Weighted least-squares approach for comparing correlated kappa. Biometrics. 2002;58(4):1012–109.
20. McHugh ML. Interrater reliability: the kappa statistic. Biochem Med (Zagreb). 2012;22(3):276–82.
21. Cyr L, Francis K. Measures of clinical agreement for nominal and categorical data: the kappa coefficient. Comput Biol Med. 1992;22(4):239–46.
22. Brenner H, Kliebsch U. Dependence of weighted kappa coefficients on the number of categories. Epidemiology. 1996;7(2):199–202.
23. Guggenmoos-Holzmann I, Vonk R. Kappa-like indices of observer agreement viewed from a latent class perspective. Stat Med. 1998;17(8):797–812.
24. Rosario PW. Thyroid Nodules with Atypia or Follicular Lesions of Undetermined Significance (Bethesda Category III): Importance of Ultrasonography and Cytological Subcategory. Thyroid. 2014;24:1115–20.
25. Adamczewski Z, Lewiński A. Proposed algorithm for management of patients with thyroid nodules/focal lesions, based on ultrasound (US) and fine-needle aspiration biopsy (FNAB); our own experience. Thyroid Res. 2013;6:6. doi:10.1186/1756-6614-6-6.
26. Cavaliere A, Colella R, Puxeddu E, Gambelunghe G, Falorni A, Stracci F, d'Ajello M, Avenia N, De Feo P. A useful ultrasound score to select thyroid nodules requiring fine needle aspiration in an iodine-deficient area. J Endocrinol Invest. 2009;32(5):440–4.
27. Petrone L, Mannucci E, De Feo ML, Parenti G, Biagini C, Panconesi R, Vezzosi V, Bianchi S, Boddi V, Di Medio L, Pupilli C, Forti G. A simple ultrasound score for the identification of candidates for fine needle aspiration of thyroid nodules. J Endocrinol Invest. 2012;35(8):720–4.
28. Remonti LR, Kramer CK, Leitão CB, Pinto LC, Gross JL. Thyroid ultrasound features and risk of carcinoma: a systematic review and meta-analysis of observational studies. Thyroid. 2015;25(5):538–50.
29. Haut ER, Pronovost PJ. Surveillance bias in outcomes reporting. JAMA. 2011;305(23):2462–3.
30. Hoppin JA, Tolbert PE, Taylor JA, Schroeder JC, Holly EA. Potential for selection bias with tumor tissue retrieval in molecular epidemiology studies. Ann Epidemiol. 2002;12(1):1–6.

31. Holford TR, Stack C. (1995) Study design for epidemiologic studies with measurement error. Stat Methods in Med Res. 1995;4(4):339–58.
32. Flanders WD, Eldridge RC. Summary of relationships between exchangeability, biasing paths and bias. Eur J Epidemiol. 2015;30(10):1089–99.
33. Sanderson S, Tatt ID, Higgins JP. Tools for assessing quality and susceptibility to bias in observational studies in epidemiology: a systematic review and annotated bibliography. Int J Epidemiol. 2007;36(3):666–76.
34. Wynder EL. Investigator bias and interviewer bias: the problem of reporting systematic error in epidemiology. J Clin Epidemiol. 1994;47(8):825–7.
35. Davis RE, Couper MP, Janz NK, Caldwell CH, Resnicow K. Interviewer effects in public health surveys. Health Educ Res. 2010;25(1):14–26.

30

The ratio of serum free triiodothyronine to free thyroxine in children: a retrospective database survey of healthy short individuals and patients with severe thyroid hypoplasia or central hypothyroidism

Yuji Oto, Koji Muroya, Junko Hanakawa, Yumi Asakura and Masanori Adachi*

Abstract

Background: The ratio of serum free triiodothyronine (FT3) to free thyroxine (FT4) has been shown to be constant in healthy adults. However, this ratio has been found to be decreased in athyreotic adult patients on levothyroxine (L-T4) supplementation. In order to better evaluate thyroid-related pathologies in children as well as to establish a reference range, we investigated the FT3/FT4 ratio in a pediatric population. Furthermore, we evaluated this ratio in children with congenital hypothyroidism as well as those with central hypothyroidism.

Methods: A reference range for the FT3/FT4 ratio was obtained from 129 Japanese children (3–17 y) with idiopathic short stature who were designated as the 'Control' group. Patients with congenital hypothyroidism due to athyreosis or severe thyroid hypoplasia (designated as 'A/Hypoplasia'), as well as patients with central hypothyroidism ('Central'), were recruited from the institutional database. For each group, the mean FT3/FT4 ratio was obtained.

Results: In the Control group, the FT3/FT4 ratio was $3.03 \pm 0.38\ 10^{-2}$ pg/ng (mean ± standard deviation) with no age or gender differences. A/Hypoplasia patients showed a significantly decreased mean FT3/FT4 ratio (2.17 ± 0.33, $P < 0.001$) compared to Control patients, with decreased FT3 and elevated FT4 levels. The Central group also showed a significantly decreased FT3/FT4 ratio (2.55 ± 0.45, $P < 0.001$) compared to the Control group, with decreased FT3 and equivalent FT4 levels.

Conclusions: The FT3/FT4 ratio appears to be constant between the ages of 3–17 y. Children on L-T4 due to congenital thyroid a/hypoplasia or central hypothyroidism have a decreased FT3/FT4 ratio compared to short normal children.

Keywords: Congenital hypothyroidism, Deiodinase, L-thyroxine therapy, Hypopituitarism, Triiodothyronine, Thyroxine

Background

Triiodothyronine (T3) is the most active form of thyroid hormone. While one fifth of net T3 production is performed by the thyroid gland, the remaining 80 % is derived from the extrathyroidal conversion of thyroxine (T4) to T3, which is mediated by either iodothyronine deiodinase 1 or 2 (DIO 1 or DIO 2, respectively). In contrast, T4 is produced exclusively in the thyroid gland [1, 2].

The ratio of serum free T3 (FT3) over free T4 (FT4) (FT3/FT4 ratio) may reflect the degree of extrathyroidal T4 to T3 conversion activity. Whereas FT3/FT4 ratio has been reported to be constant in healthy adult individuals [3], the consistency of this ratio has not yet been clearly determined in the pediatric population.

Abnormally high or low FT3/FT4 ratios are seen in several congenital disorders that may affect peripheral thyroid hormone economy, such as Allan-Herndon-Dudley syndrome (MCT8 deficiency) [4], selenocysteine insertion sequence binding protein 2 deficiency [5], and thyroid hormone resistance [6, 7]. Therefore, investigating the

* Correspondence: madachi@mars.sannet.ne.jp
Department of Endocrinology and Metabolism, Kanagawa Children's Medical Center, Mutsukawa 2-138-4 Minami-ku, Yokohama 232-8555, Japan

consistency of the FT3/FT4 ratio in the pediatric population, as well as the establishment of a reference range, is of vital importance.

Decreased FT3/FT4 ratios has been observed in postoperative athyreotic adult patients under oral levothyroxine (L-T4) supplementation [3, 8]. This presents the therapeutic problem of setting a target thyroid-stimulating hormone (TSH) range when treating athyreotic populations with L-T4. It also indicates the potential benefit of combination therapy with L-T4 and liothyronine (L-T3). It is therefore probable that these same challenges may apply to children with congenital hypothyroidism, especially those with athyreosis. Additionally, we anticipated that the FT3/FT4 ratio may be unbalanced in children with central hypothyroidism, owing to diminished TSH stimulation on thyroidal T3 production.

The purpose of this study was twofold: First, to investigate any age-dependent variations in the FT3/FT4 ratio in the pediatric population without thyroidal morbidity; and second, to evaluate this ratio in children with congenital hypothyroidism owing to athyreosis or severe thyroid hypoplasia, and in those with central hypothyroidism of any etiology.

Methods

This study was conducted as a retrospective database survey of the patients who attended the endocrine unit in Kanagawa Children's Medical Center, the regional children's hospital near metropolitan Tokyo between April 2004 and March 2010. The Ethics Committee of Kanagawa Children's Medical Center reviewed and approved the study protocol. Informed consent from the patients and/or their caregivers was not required.

To obtain a reference range for the FT3/FT4 ratio, 129 patients who were diagnosed with idiopathic short stature without any underlying morbidities were selected. Hereafter, this category is referred to as the 'Control'. They were divided into 5 groups according to their chronological ages: 3–5 y, 6–8 y, 9–11 y, 12–14 y, and 15–18 y. For each interval, mean and standard deviation (SD) of the FT3/FT4 ratio, expressed as 10^{-2} pg/ng, was obtained.

Next, we searched for patients with congenital hypothyroidism due to athyreosis or severe thyroid hypoplasia (designated as 'A/Hypoplasia'). Thyroid morphology was evaluated by ultrasound imaging and/or scintigraphy with ^{123}I or $^{99m}TcO_4^-$. Among all candidate patients, only those who presented with a TSH value greater than 100 μIU/mL during the neonatal period were selected. For each patient, the FT3/FT4 ratio obtained at various ages throughout childhood was extracted from the database only when the concurrently determined TSH level was adequate (0.30–5.0 μIU/mL). If a patient had measured FT3 and FT4 more than once during a chronological year, the mean FT3/FT4 ratio for that age was used.

Finally, patients with central hypothyroidism, whether congenital or acquired, were enrolled; these were designated as 'Central'. As for patients with growth hormone (GH) deficiency, only GH-replaced patients were included. In each patient, the FT3/FT4 ratio was selected only when the FT4 level was adequate (0.80–1.80 ng/dL). As with congenital hypothyroidism patients, the mean FT3/FT4 ratio at each age was obtained.

During the study period, serum FT3 and FT4 levels were determined by electrochemiluminescence immunoassay (ECLIA) kits: FT3 by Elecsys® FT3II and FT4 by Elecsys® FT4 (Roche Diagnostics, Tokyo, Japan). Antibodies used for FT3 and FT4 determination were ovine monoclonal and polyclonal antibodies, respectively. Serum TSH levels were determined via the ECLIA kit Elecsys® TSH (Roche Diagnostics).

Statistical analysis

Statistical analysis was performed using the SPSS software (Version 16.0; SPSS, IL, Chicago, USA). Data were compared using paired *t*-tests with normal distributions. Differences between groups were evaluated by the covariance analysis test. FT3/FT4 ratios lower than –2 SD or higher than +2 SD were regarded as outliers. A *P* value less than 0.05 was considered significant.

Results

The profiles of the 129 children with idiopathic short stature (the Control group) are shown in Table 1. Table 2 shows the reference ranges for the FT3/FT4 ratio in each age group, together with individual FT3 and FT4 values, obtained from the Control group. The FT3/FT4 ratio was constant across each age interval, although a significant decrease of FT3 was observed in the 12–14 y age group compared to the 6–8 y age group ($P = 0.037$). There was no significant difference between males and females in the Control group (Table 3).

There were 22 patients with congenital hypothyroidism due to A/Hypoplasia with neonatal TSH levels greater than 100 μIU/mL (Table 1). A total of 101 sets of FT3 and FT4 values obtained with adequate TSH levels (0.30–5.0 μIU/mL) from these patients were utilized for FT3/FT4 ratio calculation.

Results of FT3/FT4 ratio analysis in A/Hypoplasia patients, with their respective FT3 and FT4 values, are presented in Table 2 and Fig. 1. For all age intervals, the FT3/FT4 ratio was significantly lower than that of the respective Control, whereas the FT4 levels in A/Hypoplasia were significantly higher than that of the Control. Although there was no difference in FT3 levels between A/Hypoplasia and Control when comparing within each age interval, the

Table 1 Profiles of the three categories of patients enrolled in this study

Category[a]	n (male)	Age range at study in years	Median latest L-T4[b] dose (range)	Total number of FT3 and FT4 measurements[c]	Mean TSH[d] level (range)
Control	129 (81)	3.1–17.1	Not applicable	129	2.16 ± 1.03 (0.56–4.96)
A/Hypoplasia	22 (11)	3.0–18.4	125 (25–200)	156	1.81 ± 1.19 (0.30–4.96)
Central	27 (13)	3.0–18.9	100 (50–200)	366	Not applicable

[a]See text for the definition of each category
[b]L-T4: L-thyroxine, in μg per day
[c]These numbers represent all the individual FT3 and FT4 measurements taken before averages were calculated. In A/Hypoplasia and Central, the values exceed the number of patients owing to repetitive measurements
[d]Values are μIU/mL; mean ± standard deviation

difference was significant when compared as a whole group ($P = 0.004$, Table 2).

There were 27 patients in the Central group who were GH sufficient or replete (Table 1). Of these, 11 patients had congenital hypopituitarism (including 5 with septo-optic dysplasia) and 16 had acquired hypopituitarism (11 with craniopharyngioma, 4 with germinoma, and 1 with ROHHADNET syndrome). A total of 145 sets of values for FT3 and FT4 (where FT4 levels were 0.80–1.80 ng/dL) were utilized for FT3/FT4 ratio calculation.

In Table 2 and Fig. 1, the FT3 and FT4 values, as well as the FT3/FT4 ratio, in the Central group are also presented. The total FT3/FT4 ratio was significantly lower than that of the Control group, as was the case in all individual age groups except for the youngest. The FT4 value in the Central group was not different than that of the Control group, whereas the total FT3 value of the Central group was significantly lower than that of the Control group ($P = 0.02$).

Table 4 depicts a schematic summary of the FT3/FT4 ratio, as well as the levels of FT3 and FT4, in the A/Hypoplasia and Central groups compared to the Control group.

Discussion

We observed a marked consistency in the FT3/FT4 ratio (mean, 3.03 ± 0.38) among healthy short Japanese children between 3–17 years of age, with no differences owing to gender. This finding is in line with a previous study conducted in an adult population by Gullo et al. [3], which reported a consistent FT3/FT4 ratio with a median molar ratio of 0.32 (corresponding to 2.71 10^{-2} pg/ng), in 3,875 euthyroid subjects (with minor age and gender variability). The difference in the absolute value of the ratio between Gullo et al.'s data [3] and ours may be multifactorial, owing to both the methodological differences in hormone detection (particularly the types of the antibodies used) and ethnic differences that influence iodine sufficiency.

Our report is the first to specifically investigate the FT3/FT4 ratio in the pediatric population. While reference values for FT3 and FT4 in children have been reported [9–13], these reports did not refer to the FT3/FT4 ratio. Additionally, most studies provided only the ranges or centile values of FT3 and FT4, and calculation of the FT3/FT4 ratio was therefore impractical. More research is needed to evaluate the distribution of the FT3/FT4 ratio

Table 2 FT3 and FT4 levels, as well as their ratios, in patient groups according to age

		3–5 y	6–8 y	9–11 y	12–14 y	15–18 y	Total
Control ($n = 129$)	n	24	19	31	36	19	129
	FT3	4.11 ± 0.56	4.29 ± 0.43[α]	4.14 ± 0.38	3.89 ± 0.50[α]	3.93 ± 0.56	4.06 ± 0.50
	FT4	1.36 ± 0.14	1.38 ± 0.11	1.36 ± 0.14	1.33 ± 0.16	1.31 ± 0.10	1.35 ± 0.14
	FT3/FT4	3.02 ± 0.38	3.12 ± 0.31	3.07 ± 0.38	2.95 ± 0.35	3.01 ± 0.50	3.03 ± 0.38
A/Hypoplasia ($n = 22$)	n[b]	14	20	22	21	24	101
	FT3	4.15 ± 0.51	3.86 ± 0.42	3.91 ± 0.45	3.84 ± 0.60	3.52 ± 0.60	3.82 ± 0.55*
	FT4	1.95 ± 0.20**	1.81 ± 0.31**	1.76 ± 0.26**	1.85 ± 0.59**	1.90 ± 0.69**	1.85 ± 0.47**
	FT3/FT4	2.15 ± 0.25**	2.18 ± 0.30**	2.25 ± 0.39**	2.23 ± 0.34**	2.03 ± 0.30**	2.17 ± 0.33**
Central ($n = 27$)	n[b]	11	31	46	31	26	145
	FT3	3.50 ± 0.48	3.49 ± 0.53**	3.51 ± 0.64**	3.63 ± 0.64	3.46 ± 0.54	3.52 ± 0.58**
	FT4	1.24 ± 0.23	1.31 ± 0.17	1.43 ± 0.29	1.45 ± 0.30	1.49 ± 0.25	1.41 ± 0.27
	FT3/FT4	2.94 ± 0.58	2.68 ± 0.51*	2.49 ± 0.37**	2.52 ± 0.37*	2.37 ± 0.40**	2.55 ± 0.45**

Values are pg/mL (FT3) and ng/dL (FT4); mean ± standard deviation
[α]$P < 0.05$, *$P < 0.05$; **$P < 0.01$, compared to control, respectively
[b]In A/Hypoplasia and Central, patients underwent repetitive measurements of FT3 and FT4. All the values are averaged according to the chronological age of the patients. The same patients may have average independent measurement values in more than one age category if they were evaluated over multiple years

Table 3 Gender difference of FT3/FT4 ratio in Control

		3–5 y	6–8 y	9–11 y	12–14 y	15–18 y	Total
Male	n	10	11	19	29	12	81
	FT3/FT4	3.03 ± 0.27	3.23 ± 0.32	3.06 ± 0.30	3.02 ± 0.34	3.09 ± 0.37	3.06 ± 0.32
Female	n	14	8	12	7	7	48
	FT3/FT4	3.02 ± 0.0.46	2.97 ± 0.25	3.08 ± 0.50	2.83 ± 0.16	3.11 ± 0.23	3.02 ± 0.40

Values are mean ± standard deviation

in both the longitudinal and cross-sectional aspects. The influence of pubertal development on this ratio also ought to be investigated, because FT3 levels in the 12–14 y groups were found to be lower than in the younger age groups.

The consistency of the FT3/FT4 ratio during childhood is useful for the screening of several genetic disorders related to peripheral thyroid hormone metabolism, including Allan-Herndon-Dudley syndrome (MCT8 deficiency) [4], selenocysteine insertion sequence binding protein 2 deficiency [5], thyroid hormone resistance [6, 7], and others.

Furthermore, evaluating the FT3/FT4 ratio in patients on L-T4 supplementation due to various thyroidal disorders may be a method of assessing the sufficiency of the L-T4 therapy. Observing differences of FT3/FT4 ratios in pathological situations was the main feature of this study, which is the first to evaluate this ratio in pediatric patients with congenital hypothyroidism and central hypothyroidism.

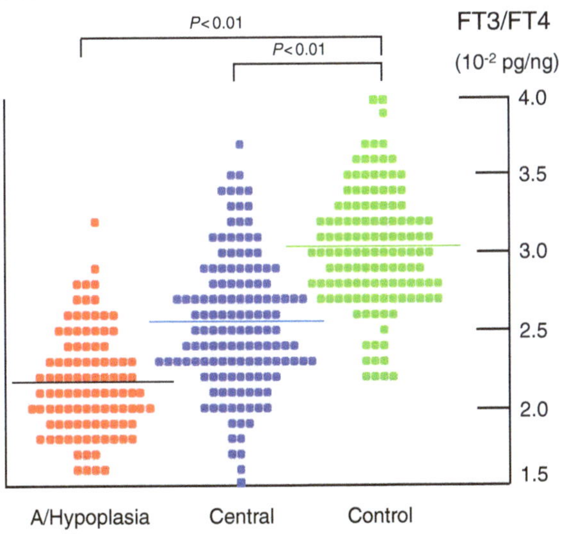

Fig. 1 Serum free triiodothyronine (FT3) to free thyroxine (FT4) ratio distribution in the Control, A/Hypoplasia, and Central groups. In the A/Hypoplasia and Central groups, the number of dots exceeds the patients' number because all the individual FT3/FT4 measurements with averaging per chronological age groups are included. Note the significantly decreased FT3/FT4 ratio in both the A/Hypoplasia and Central groups compared to the Control group

The FT3/FT4 ratio in patients with A/Hypoplasia, which is defined by extremely high neonatal TSH levels (>100 μIU/mL), was significantly lower than that in the Control group (Table 2 and Fig. 1). As depicted in Table 4, this decrease is mainly due to the elevation of the denominator (FT4 level), although a slightly decreased numerator (FT3 level) also contributed. This finding is consistent with recent studies conducted in adult populations. For example, Ito et al. found that athyreotic adult patients ($n = 51$) who underwent total thyroidectomy for papillary thyroid carcinoma and who are on L-T4 therapy with normal TSH level (0.3–5 μIU/mL) had increased FT4 and slightly decreased FT3, resulting in a decreased FT3/FT4 ratio [8]. Additionally, Gullo et al. reported that 29.6 % of 1,811 patients who were thyroidectomised because of thyroid cancer and were on L-T4 therapy with TSH levels of 0.4–4.0 μIU/mL, had FT3/FT4 ratios below the lower limit of euthyroid controls [3].

Elevated FT4 levels in our A/Hypoplasia group and athyreotic adult patients is expected because, in athyreotic patients, thyroid hormone is solely derived from exogenous L-T4 whereas thyroidal T3 production is almost absent. Thus, normalization of TSH is achieved at the expense of higher FT4 levels. This is the inverse situation of the increased FT3/FT4 ratio in untreated or refractory Graves' disease, where thyroidal T3 production is predominant [14].

Ito et al. explained the pathophysiology of decreased FT3 levels in their athyreotic adult patients as follows [8]: First, TSH secreting cells have T3 in their cytoplasm transported directly from the circulation. Second, these cells also have T3, which is generated from T4 by intracellular deiodinase. Third, referring to a classical study [15], it was shown that the proportion of the latter T3 is increased in hypothyroid patients on L-T4. Thus, when target TSH levels are set to approximate the physiologically

Table 4 Summary of FT3/FT4 ratio and individual levels in congenital hypoplasia and central hypothyroidism

	Congenital thyroid hypoplasia[a]	Central hypothyroidism[a]
FT3/FT4 ratio	↓↓	↓
FT3	↓	↓↓
FT4	↑↑	→

[a]Compared to the control group

normal range, circulating FT3 will be maintained at lower level. As Gullo et al. pointed out, the reason for this phenomenon is the inadequacy of peripheral T3 production, which cannot compensate for the absent thyroidal T3 production [3]. This same scenario likely applies to our A/Hypoplasia patients.

The Central group was also found to have a significantly decreased FT3/FT4 ratio compared to the Control group. This decrease is mainly due to grossly decreased FT3 levels with maintained FT4 levels, resulting in a less prominent decrease of the ratio than that found in the A/Hypoplasia group (Table 2 and Fig. 1). There does not appear to be a precedent study investigating the FT3/FT4 ratio in subjects with central hypothyroidism in either adult or pediatric populations.

The explanation for decreased FT3/FT4 values in the Central group is straightforward: As TSH level cannot be used as a therapeutic guide in patients with central hypothyroidism [16], they instead undergo L-T4 therapy to achieve normal FT4 levels. Thus, FT3 levels must be lower because T3 is generated mainly from the peripheral conversion of exogenous L-T4 to T3, and thyroidal T3 production is diminished under attenuated TSH stimulation.

The clinical significance of the decreased FT3/FT4 ratio in the A/Hypoplasia and Central groups is unclear. It has been reported that 5–10 % of hypothyroid patients treated with L-T4 therapy suffered from symptoms indicative of persistent hypothyroidism such as impaired well-being, diminished cognitive functions, anxiety, and depression despite adequate TSH suppression [17–19]. Whether these symptoms are related to abnormal FT3/FT4 ratios is unknown. In clinical trials, L-T4 and L-T3 combination therapy was found to be beneficial in terms of quality-of-life and the severity of depression, and was also found to ameliorate tissue hypothyroidism [20, 21]. Alternatively, Ito et al. suggested that TSH-suppressive doses of L-T4 are required to achieve preoperative native serum FT3 levels in patients who have undergone total thyroidectomy [8]. Further studies are required to determine the significance of decreased FT3/FT4 ratios and their effects of therapeutic interventions [17].

The main drawback of this study is that the Control group constituted children with normal short stature. Although it is clearly more ideal to compare our subjects to the general population, we could not evaluate thyroid function in such subjects because of ethical limitations. In the pediatric field, however, other studies have utilized data obtained from normal short children as references [22, 23]. Additionally, all patients in the Control group underwent thorough evaluation for possible underlying diseases, including hypothalamic-thyroid axis. Therefore, we anticipate that the data from the Control group can be utilized as an alternative to currently used references.

Conclusions

The FT3/FT4 ratio appears to be constant between 3–17 y. Pediatric populations with congenital hypothyroidism due to severe thyroidal hypoplasia and with central hypothyroidism with exogenous L-T4 supplementation were found to have decreased FT3/FT4 ratios compared to short normal children. The clinical significance of this finding should be further investigated.

Abbreviations

TSH: Thyroid stimulating hormone; T3: Triiodothyronine; FT3: Free triiodothyronine; T4: Thyroxine; FT4: Free thyroxine; L-T3: Liothyronine; L-T4: Levothyroxine; SD: Standard deviation.

Competing interests

The authors declare that they have no competing interests.

Authors' contributions

MA conceptualized and designed the study. MA and YO contributed to the data collection, analysis, and writing the manuscript. JH, KM, and YA contributed to preparation of the manuscript by critically analyzing it. All authors read and approved the final manuscript.

References

1. Brent GA. Mechanisms of thyroid hormone action. J Clin Invest. 2012;122:3035–43.
2. Pilo A, Iervasi G, Vitek F, Ferdeghini M, Cazzuola F, Bianchi R. Thyroidal and peripheral production of 3,5,3'-triiodothyronine in humans by multicompartmental analysis. Am J Physiol. 1990;258:E715–26.
3. Gullo D, Latina A, Frasca F, Le Moli R, Pellegriti G, Vigneri R. Levothyroxine monotherapy cannot guarantee euthyroidism in all athyreotic patients. PLoS One. 2011;6, e22552.
4. Schwartz CE, May MM, Carpenter NJ, Rogers RC, Martin J, Bialer MG, et al. Allan-Herndon-Dudley syndrome and the monocarboxtylate transporter gene. Am J Hum Genet. 2005;77:41–53.
5. Di Cosmo C, McLellan N, Liao XH, Khanna KK, Weiss RE, Papp L, et al. Clinical and molecular characterization of a novel selenocysteine insertion sequence-binding protein 2 (SBP2) gene mutation (R128X). J Clin Endocrinol Metab. 2009;94:4003–9.
6. Ferrara AM, Onigata K, Ercan O, Woodhead H, Weiss RE, Refetoff S. Homozygous thyroid hormone receptor β-gene mutations in resistance to thyroid hormone: three new cases and review of the literature. J Clin Endocrinol Metab. 2012;97:1328–36.
7. Bochukova E, Schoenmakers N, Agostini M, Schoenmakers E, Rajanayagam O, Keogh JM, et al. A mutation in the thyroid hormone receptor alpha gene. N Engl J Med. 2012;366:243–9.
8. Ito M, Miyauchi A, Morita S, Kudo T, Nishihara E, Kihara M, et al. TSH-suppressive doses of levothyroxine are required to achieve preoperative native serum triiodothyronine levels in patients who have undergone total thyroidectomy. Eur J Endocrinol. 2012;167:373–8.
9. Djemli A, Van Vliet G, Belgoudi J, Lambert M, Delvin EE. Reference intervals for free thyroxine, total triiodothyronine, thyrotropin and thyroglobulin for Quebec newborns, children and teenagers. Clin Biochem. 2004;37:328–30.
10. Kapelari K, Kirchlechner C, Högler W, Schweitzer K, Virgolini I, Moncayo R. Pediatric reference intervals for thyroid hormone levels from birth to adulthood: a retrospective study. BMC Endocr Disord. 2008;8:15.
11. Soldin OP, Jang M, Guo T, Soldin SJ. Pediatric reference intervals for free thyroxine and free triiodothyronine. Thyroid. 2009;19:699–702.
12. Verburg FA, Kirchgässner C, Hebestreit H, Steigerwald U, Lentjes EG, Ergezinger K, et al. Reference ranges for analytes of thyroid function in children. Horm Metab Res. 2011;43:422–6.
13. Iwaku K, Noh JY, Minagawa A, Kosuga Y, Suzuki M, Sekiya K, et al. Determination of pediatric reference levels of FT3, FT4 and TSH measured with ECLusys kits. Endocr J. 2013;60:799–804.

14. Yoshimura Noh J, Momotani N, Fukada S, Ito K, Miyauchi A, Amino N. Ratio of serum free triiodothyronine to free thyroxine in Graves' hyperthyroidism and thyrotoxicosis caused by painless thyroiditis. Endocr J. 2005;52:537–42.
15. Silva JE, Larsen PR. Contributions of plasma triiodothyronine and local thyroxine monodeiodination to triiodothyronine to nuclear triiodothyronine receptor saturation in pituitary, liver, and kidney of hypothyroid rats. Further evidence relating saturation of pituitary nuclear triiodothyronine receptors and the acute inhibition of thyroid-stimulating hormone release. J Clin Invest. 1978;61:1247–59.
16. Persani L. Clinical review: Central hypothyroidism: pathogenic, diagnostic, and therapeutic challenges. J Clin Endocrinol Metab. 2012;97:3068–78.
17. Wiersinga WM. Paradigm shifts in thyroid hormone replacement therapies for hypothyroidism. Nat Rev Endocrinol. 2014;10:164–74.
18. Saravanan P, Chau WF, Roberts N, Vedhara K, Greenwood R, Dayan CM. Psychological well-being in patients on 'adequate' doses of l-thyroxine: results of a large, controlled community-based questionnaire study. Clin Endocrinol (Oxf). 2002;57:577–85.
19. Wekking EM, Appelhof BC, Fliers E, Schene AH, Huyser J, Tijssen JG, et al. Cognitive functioning and well-being in euthyroid patients on thyroxine replacement therapy for primary hypothyroidism. Eur J Endocrinol. 2005;153:747–53.
20. Grozinsky-Glasberg S, Fraser A, Nahshoni E, Weizman A, Leibovici L. Thyroxine-triiodothyronine combination therapy versus thyroxine monotherapy for clinical hypothyroidism: meta-analysis of randomized controlled trials. J Clin Endocrinol Metab. 2006;91:2592–9.
21. Nygaard B, Jensen EW, Kvetny J, Jarløv A, Faber J. Effect of combination therapy with thyroxine (T4) and 3,5,3'-triiodothyronine versus T4 monotherapy in patients with hypothyroidism, a double-blind, randomised cross-over study. Eur J Endocrinol. 2009;161:895–902.
22. Tanaka T, Hibi I, Shimizu N, Imura H, Tanaka K, Fukata J, et al. Evaluation of hypothalamo-pituitary-adrenocortical function in children by human corticotropin-releasing hormone (MCI-028) test. Endocr J. 1993;40:581–9.
23. Tanaka N, Miyamoto J, Hasegawa Y. A response to human chorionic gonadotropin test in boys with normal gonadal function and with hypogonadism. Clin Pediatr Endocrinol. 2001;10:147–50.

Characteristics and natural course of hypoechoic thyroid lesions diagnosed as possible thyroid lymphomas by fine needle aspiration cytology

Tomoe Nakao[1*], Mitsushige Nishikawa[1], Mako Hisakado[1], Toshihiko Kasahara[1], Takumi Kudo[1], Eijun Nishihara[1], Mitsuru Ito[1], Shuji Fukata[1], Hirotoshi Nakamura[1], Mitsuyoshi Hirokawa[2] and Akira Miyauchi[3]

Abstract

Background: There is little information regarding the natural course of hypoechoic thyroid lesions that are probable or possible thyroid lymphoma based on fine needle aspiration cytology (FNAC) results.

Methods: Sixty-five patients who were diagnosed as probable or possible thyroid lymphoma by ultrasonography (US) and FNAC were investigated. Forty-three patients with strong suspicion underwent thyroid surgery for the diagnosis at our hospital, and 22 patients were followed up with periodic US examination. Thyroid lymphoma was definitely diagnosed in 41 out of 43 patients who underwent thyroid surgery, and such patients were defined as Group A. The outcomes of 22 patients who were followed up without an immediate therapy were analyzed. Their hypoechoic lesions decreased in size ($n = 10$) or disappeared ($n = 2$) in 12 of 22 patients, and such patients were defined as Group B. Patients in Group A and B were compared using the Kuma Hospital-US classification (USC), the diagnostic categories of the Bethesda System for Reporting Thyroid Cytopathology, and the κ/λ deviation of the immunoglobulin light chain in the FNAC specimens. Mann-Whitney *U*-test and chi-squared test (with Yate's continuity correction) were used to compare the two groups.

Results: The USC of < 3.5 [9/12 (75.0%) in Group B; 10/41 patients (24.4%) in Group A] and the κ/λ deviation ratio of < 3.40 [11/12 (91.7%) in Group B; 17/41 patients (41.5%) in Group A] were significantly more frequent ($p < 0.01$), and the FNAC of 'benign' or 'atypia of undetermined significance or follicular lesion of undetermined significance (AUS)' with a comment of possible lymphoma [9/12 (75.0%) in Group B; 12/41 patients (29.3%) in Group A] was significantly more frequent ($p < 0.05$) in Group B than Group A.

Conclusions: Our study suggests that some hypoechoic thyroid lesions that are possible thyroid lymphoma based on US and FNAC might decrease in size or disappear during the careful observation.

Keywords: Thyroid lymphoma, Hypoechoic thyroid lesion, Regression, Fine needle aspiration cytology, κ/λ deviation

* Correspondence: tomoenakao@gmail.com
[1]Department of Internal Medicine, Kuma Hospital, Centre for Excellence in Thyroid Cares, 8-2-35 Shimoyamate-dori, Chuo-ku, Kobe 650-0011, Japan
Full list of author information is available at the end of the article

Background

Primary thyroid lymphoma is a rare cause of malignancy, accounting for 2–5% of all thyroid malignancies [1] and < 2% of extranodal lymphomas [2, 3]. A rapidly enlarging mass was the most common clinical manifestations in earlier series, but recently small lesions are found at the early stage [4]. It is a potentially lethal disease, but often responds well to appropriate treatments [5]. Thyroid lymphoma is not always diagnosed easily, especially in its early phase, because most of the cases are associated with Hashimoto's thyroiditis.

Ultrasonography (US) of the thyroid is initially used for the diagnosis of thyroid lymphoma. On US, lymphoma is shown as hypoechoic lesions, but subacute thyroiditis, focal chronic thyroiditis, some thyroid cancers, and metastatic thyroid cancer is also shown as hypoechoic lesions mimicking thyroid lymphoma. Based on US findings of internal echo levels, borders, and posterior echoes, thyroid lymphoma can be classified as the nodular, diffuse, or mixed type [6]. Although the nodular type often resembles follicular tumor or adenomatous nodule and the mixed type often resembles adenomatous goiter on US, these lesions can be often distinguished by an enhancement of posterior echoes. The diffuse type shows homogeneous and hypoechoic internal echoes, but these findings are also typical for severe chronic thyroiditis [6, 7].

Fine needle aspiration cytology (FNAC) is the next diagnostic strategy for thyroid lymphoma, but is challenging, particularly due to its histological similarities with mucosa-associated lymphoid tissue (MALT) lymphoma and chronic thyroiditis [8, 9]. The flow cytometry with CD45 gating on the FNAC specimen can be used to analyze the proportions of lymphocytic cells with κ and λ immunoglobulin light chains. The κ/λ deviation ratio of the light chain assessment is an important criterion for discriminating between polyclonal reactive processes such as chronic thyroiditis and monoclonal lymphomas. Strong deviation in the κ/λ ratio is regarded as suggestive monoclonal growth of lymphocytes, thus indicating thyroid lymphoma [10].

Even with these modalities, a definite diagnosis is not established easily. A surgical interventions is often needed for the histopathological diagnosis, but it might be unnecessary for the benign lesions. This is especially true for the small or moderate-size lesions. Needle biopsy is usually useful for the diagnosis of diffuse large B-cell type lymphoma, but is often insufficient in the case of MALT lymphoma.

We have observed some hypoechoic lesions that were diagnosed as possible thyroid lymphoma based on the FNAC decrease in size or disappear during their clinical courses without definitive treatment. However, there is little information regarding the natural course of such hypoechoic lesions that were possible thyroid lymphoma based on FNAC findings. We conducted the present study to (*1*) clarify the natural course of hypoechoic thyroid lesions that were possible thyroid lymphoma, and (*2*) identify clinical features that might be used to discriminate benign non-progressive lesions from those with progressive character.

Methods

Between April 2012 and July 2016, 136 patients were suspected of having thyroid lymphoma on US examination at Kuma Hospital, where approximately 15,000 new patients with thyroid diseases are evaluated annually. US examinations were routinely performed by our well-experienced operators. US was performed using an APLIO 500 TUS-A500 system (Toshiba Medical Systems Co., Ltd., Otawara, Japan) with a PLT-805AT (Toshiba) or PLT-1005BT probe (Toshiba). Patients with systemic lymphoma or previously diagnosed lymphoma were excluded. Of these 136 patients, 122 were diagnosed as having probable or possible thyroid lymphoma by FNAC (Fig. 1). The remaining 14 patients were excluded from the study, because they had other diagnoses based on FNAC findings (eight specimens were normal or benign, one anaplastic carcinoma of the thyroid, one subacute thyroiditis or thyroid papillary carcinoma, and one metastatic renal cell carcinoma; the remaining three specimens were inadequate for diagnosis). Among the 122 patients, 57 were excluded from the study, because 56 were referred to other hospitals for the definitive diagnosis and chemo radiotherapy, and one patient dropped out from the follow-up study. Thus, the remaining 65 patients were investigated in this study. Forty-three patients strongly suspected of having thyroid lymphoma underwent thyroid surgery at our hospital for the definite diagnosis and 22 patients with comments of possible lymphoma on cytology were followed up with periodic US examination for 1–41 (median 11.5) months. Whether surgery or follow-up examination was determined by each doctor in charge based on clinical and radiological findings, including the rapidity of the enlargement of the thyroid mass, and the US and FNAC findings. Of 43 patients who underwent thyroid surgery at our hospital, 41 (95.3%) were diagnosed as definite thyroid lymphoma, and the other two (4.7%) were diagnosed as chronic thyroiditis (Fig. 1). Among the 41 patients who were diagnosed as definite thyroid lymphoma, 34 were diagnosed as MALT lymphoma and seven were diagnosed as diffuse large B-cell lymphoma. Whether the lesions of all 41 patients were limited to the thyroid was not known because all were referred to other hospitals to undergo further diagnostic examinations, including the determination of the disease stage, and treatment.

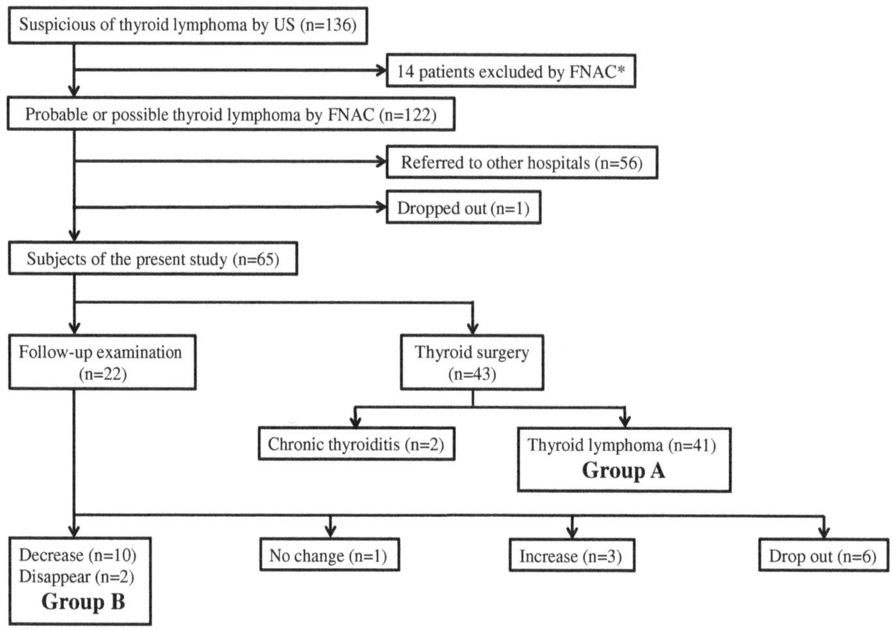

*described in text. Group A: patients with definite thyroid lymphoma diagnosed pathologically. Group B: patients with hypoechoic lesions which decreased in diameter or disappeared.

Fig. 1 Clinical flow and outcomes of patients with possible thyroid lymphoma based on US and FNAC

Hypoechoic lesions of the periodically followed-up 22 patients were analyzed. The US examination was repeated 1–3 month-interval at first and then 6 month-interval when no deterioration was observed. None of 22 patients were treated with steroids or immunosuppressive drugs during the follow-up examination. Other medications or supplementations, or dietary habit including iodine intake were not known in detail. When the maximum diameter of a hypoechoic lesion increased by ≥3 mm, we defined the case as an "increase" of the hypoechoic lesion. When

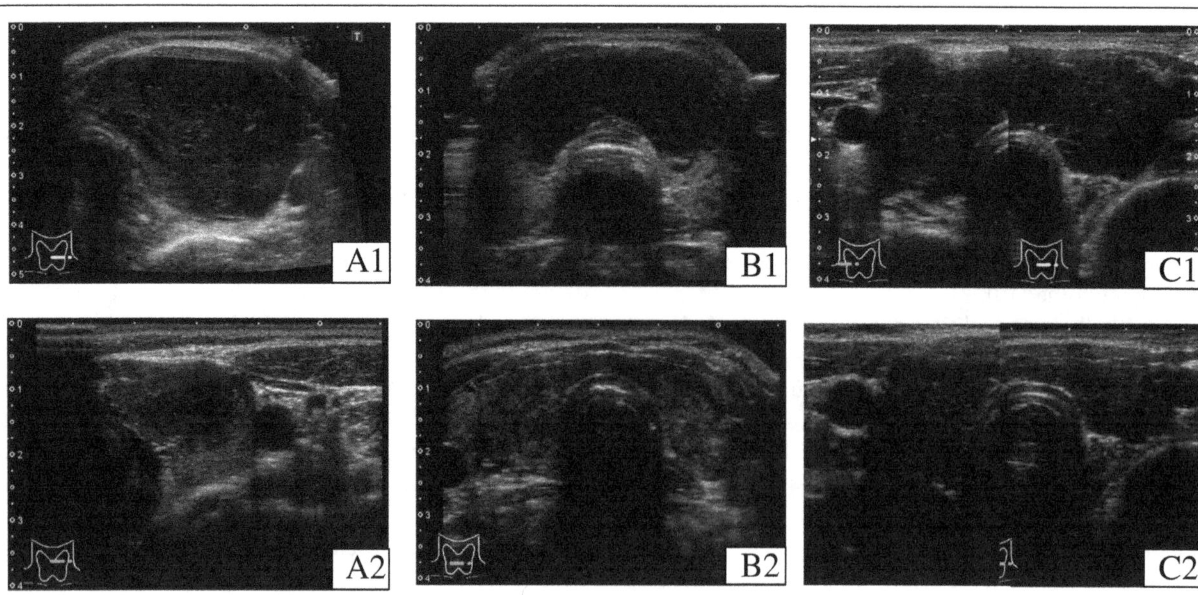

Fig. 2 Echograms of three representative patients whose hypoechoic lesions decreased or disappeared on careful follow-up examination. **a** A 74-year-old woman with a nodular hypoechoic lesion at presentation (A1) that had markedly decreased in size one month later (A2) (case No. 9 in Table 2). **b** A 69-year-old woman with a severely hypoechoic lesion involving the both thyroid lobes (B1) that had almost disappeared 10 months later (B2), although the irregularity remained possibly due to underlying chronic thyroiditis (case No. 4 in Table 2). **c** A 53-year-old woman with a diffuse severely hypoechoic lesion involving the whole thyroid (C1) that had markedly decreased in size 27 months later (C2) (case No. 1 in Table 2)

the maximum diameter of a hypoechoic lesion reduced by ≥3 mm, we defined the case as a "decrease." When the hypoechoic lesions were not detected clearly at follow-up examination, it was defined as "disappeared." We established this parameter because, in our previous study, plus or minus 2 mm was recognized as an observation variation [11]. In the present study, in some cases in which the entire thyroid volume was observed to have decreased, the maximum diameter of the hypoechoic lesions was measured and analyzed.

Representative US images showing "decrease" and "disappearance" are shown in Fig. 2. Our hospital uses its own ultrasound classification system for the diagnosis of thyroid nodules, which consists of five US classes (USC) based on the characteristics of thyroid nodules, such as a regular or irregular shape, solid or cystic content, the presence or absence of microcalcifications, extraglandal invasion, and other factors. The classification consists of five classes from 1 to 5. Intermediate classes from class 2 to class 4 (designated as classes 2.5 and 3.5) are also used (Table 1) [12]. Some cases of lymphoma with diffuse or mixed lesion are hardly classified according to USC, because this classification is mainly scored to thyroid nodules. However, in the present study, the US classification was applied to the hypoechoic lesions. The present study was approved by the Institutional Review Board of Kuma Hospital and the Ethics Committee in Kuma Hospital.

The hypoechoic lesions in 22 patients who were followed up with periodic US examination decreased in size ($n = 10$), disappeared ($n = 2$), showed no change ($n = 1$) or increased in size ($n = 3$). The remaining six patients dropped out from the follow-up examination. Of the three patients whose hypoechoic lesions increased in size, one patient was referred to another hospital and diagnosed as diffuse large B-cell lymphoma; the other two patients were carefully followed up without further progression (Fig. 1).

Forty-one patients with histopathologically diagnosed thyroid lymphoma were defined as Group A, and 12 patients whose hypoechoic lesions decreased in diameter or disappeared as defined Group B (Fig. 1). Their clinical features, the diameter of hypoechoic lesions, US features at the first presentation, and the diagnostic categories of the Bethesda System for Reporting Thyroid Cytopathology (BethSys categories) were compared between Group A and B. Mann-Whitney *U*-test and chi-squared test (with Yate's continuity correction) were used to compare the two groups.

Results

Table 2 summarizes the clinical features of 16 patients who underwent follow-up US examinations of hypoechoic lesions that were diagnosed as possible thyroid lymphoma. Thyroid function tests at presentation showed hypothyroid ($n = 1$), subclinical hypothyroid ($n = 4$) and euthyroid ($n = 11$). Some patients were taking levothyroxine (LT4) before and during the follow-up examination. However, whether LT4 supplementation was involved in the decrease or disappearance of the hypoechoic lesions is unclear, because of the small number of the cases. All Group B patients were thyroglobulin antibody (TgAb)- and/or thyroid peroxidase antibody (TPOAb)-positive. As a result of FNAC, 'atypia of undetermined significance or follicular lesion of undetermined significance (AUS)' was diagnosed in eight, 'suspicious for 'malignancy' in two, 'malignancy' in one, and 'benign' in one patient. The pathological report of case 2 in Table 2 said that it was probably benign; however, lymphoma could not be completely excluded. On flow cytometry of the fine needle aspirations, the κ/λ ratio varied from 0.31 to 4.61. When κ/λ ratio was lower than 1.00, we converted κ/λ ratio to λ/κ ratio (deviation ratio) to discriminate between the polyclonal reactive process and the monoclonal reactive process that is characteristic to lymphomas.

There were no significant differences in age, sex, thyroid function, TgAb, TPOAb, echo pattern of hypoechoic lesions, USC, BethSys, the diameter of hypoechoic lesions, κ/λ deviation ratio, LT4 supplementation or TSH between the patients whose hypoechoic lesions decreased in size or disappeared and patients whose lesions were unchanged or increased in size.

There were no significant differences in patient age, sex, or the diameter of the hypoechoic lesions between Groups A and B (Mann-Whitney *U*-test) (Table 3). The USC and the κ/λ deviation ratio were significantly lower in Group B than Group A ($p < 0.001$ and $p < 0.02$, respectively). The USC of < 3.5 [9/12 (75.0%) in Group B; 10/41 patients (24.4%) in Group A] was significantly more frequent ($p < 0.01$), and the FNAC finding of 'benign' or 'AUS' [9/12 (75.0%) in Group B; 12/41 patients

Table 1 Ultrasonographic classification for thyroid nodule at Kuma Hospital

Class	Description
1	Round or anechoic lesion.
2	Regular-shaped nodule with cystic change. The echo level of solid lesion is similar to that of normal thyroid.
3	Solid and regular-shaped nodule. Internal echo is homogeneous, or may have strong echoes internally or at the capsule.
4	Solid and irregular-shaped nodule. Internal echo is usually low and may have fine strong echogenic spots.
5	Solid and irregular-shaped nodule with extrathyroid extension.

Intermediate classes from class 2 to class 5 (designated as classes 2.5,3.5 and 4.5) are also used

Table 2 Clinical features of 16 patients who underwent follow-up US examinations of hypoechoic lesions that were diagnosed as possible thyroid lymphoma

Case	Age	Sex	Thyroid function[a]	TgAb (IU/mL)	TPOAb (IU/mL)	Echo pattern of hypoechoic lesions	US class	BethSys[b]	Duration of follow-up (months)	Before (mm)	After (mm)	κ/λ deviation ratio[c]	LT4 supplementation (μg/day)	TSH during follow-up	Outcome
1	53	F	subclinical hypothyroid (with LT4 50 μg/day)	4000≦	535	diffuse	3	AUS[d]	27	61	47	1.21	75	normal	decrease
2	62	F	hypothyroid	4000≦	600≦	diffuse	3.5	benign[e]	30	120	80	1.50	112.5	suppressed	decrease
3	66	F	euthyroid	28	89	nodular	3.5	AUS	12	25	11	4.61	50	normal	decrease
4	69	F	euthyroid	120.7	600≦	nodular	3	AUS	10	37	disappearance	3.14	–	normal	disappearance
5	70	M	euthyroid	54	118	nodular	3	AUS	37	15	12	1.84	–	normal	decrease
6	71	M	subclinical hypothyroid	1171	–	nodular	3	malignancy	6	37	23	3.20	50	normal	decrease
7	72	F	euthyroid	906	–	nodular	2.5	Suspicious for malignancy	3	27	14	2.90	50	normal	decrease
8	74	F	euthyroid	512.9	151	nodular	3	AUS	41	12	disappearance	2.75	–	normal	disappearance
9	74	F	euthyroid	688.8	16	nodular	3	Suspicious for malignancy	1	105	25	1.72	–	normal	decrease
10	74	F	euthyroid	121.8	–	nodular	3	AUS	7	16	9	2.06	75	suppressed	decrease
11	77	F	subclinical hypothyroid	1402	–	diffuse	3	AUS	25	46	40	1.53	50	normal	decrease
12	83	F	euthyroid	89.9	–	nodular	3.5	AUS	6	23	19	3.21	–	normal	decrease
13	66	F	euthyroid	235.5	–	nodular	4	AUS	22	22	22	0.86	75	suppressed	no change
14	46	F	euthyroid	609.6	–	nodular	3	Suspicious for malignancy	7	22	30	–	–	normal	increase
15	87	M	euthyroid	750.4	≦16	nodular	3	Suspicious for malignancy	6	19	23	4.09	–	normal	increase
16	94	F	subclinical hypothyroid	586.3	26.5	diffuse	3	Suspicious for malignancy	11	65	160	1.81	62.5	normal	increase

The normal range of TgAb is ≤39.9 U/mL; TPOAb: ≤27.9 U/mL. –: TPOAb not done or no levothyroxine (LT4) supplementation
Intermediate US classes from class 2 to class 4 (designated as classes 2.5 and 3.5) are also used
[a]Thyroid function at the first examination and diagnosis as possible thyroid lymphoma by FNAC
[b]The Bethesda System for Reporting Thyroid Cytopathology
[c]The κ/λ deviation ratio was calculated by λ/κ ratio when the κ/λ ratio was < 1.00
[d]Atypia of undetermined significance or follicular lesion of undetermined significance
[e]Lymphoma cannot be denied

Table 3 Comparison of clinical features of Group A and B

	Group A ($n = 41$)	Group B ($n = 12$)	p-value
Age (year)	67 (48–91)	72 (53–83)	0.35
Sex (Male, number)	11	2	0.48
Diameter of hypoechoic lesions (mm)	35 (16–75)	38 (12–120)	0.51

Group A is the patients with thyroid lymphoma diagnosed histopathologically following thyroid surgery. Group B is the patients whose hypoechoic lesions decreased or disappeared. Data are median and (ranges). The p-values were calculated by Mann-Whitney U-test

(29.3%) in Group A] was significantly more frequent ($p < 0.05$) in Group B than Group A (Tables 4 and 5). Lastly, the κ/λ deviation ratio of the immunoglobulin (Ig) light chain in the FNAC specimens of < 3.40 [11/12 (91.7%) in Group B; 17/41 patients (41.5%) in Group A] was significantly more frequent in Group B than Group A ($p < 0.01$) (Table 6).

Discussion

The characteristics and natural course of hypoechoic lesions that were diagnosed as possible thyroid lymphoma based on the FNAC findings were investigated. Careful US examinations were repeatedly performed in 22 of 65 patients, and hypoechoic lesions decreased in diameter in 10 patients (10 of the 22; 45.5% or 10 of 65 patients; 15.4%), and disappeared in two patients (two of 22; 9.1% or two of 65 patients; 3.1%).

The USC and the κ/λ deviation ratio were significantly lower in Group B than Group A, and the FNAC finding of 'benign' or 'AUS' was significantly more frequent in Group B than Group A. Although thyroid lymphoma typically presents with a rapidly enlarging neck mass leading to compressive symptoms [4], some hypoechoic lesions diagnosed as possible thyroid lymphoma might regress in their natural courses in the present study.

Several studies have demonstrated that *Helicobacter pylori* infection is associated with low-grade gastric MALT lymphoma, and that the eradication of *Helicobacter pylori* can cause histological regression of the lymphoma [13, 14]. Uohashi et al. reported that a hypoechoic lesion in the right lobe disappeared spontaneously after being diagnosed pathologically as non-Hodgkin's lymphoma following a contralateral lobe resection, and suggested spontaneous regression of acute inflammation [15]. Okamoto et al. reported a patient whose primary thyroid lymphoma of cytotoxic T-cell origin regressed spontaneously [16]. Although its cause remains unknown, it may be attributable to an association of acute inflammation [17, 18], and immune mechanisms such as those involving T-helper cells or natural killer cells of the peripheral blood [19].

However, to our best knowledge, there has been no report that the natural course of hypoechoic lesions suspected of being possible thyroid lymphoma was studied extensively. With the combination of US, FNAC, and CD gating analysis for κ/λ deviation, candidate for the surgery could be accurately selected in 41 out of 43 patients (95%) as demonstrated in Group A. However, the management of not strongly suggestive of lymphoma may be controversial. In the present study, the hypoechoic lesion decreased in size in 10, and disappeared in two out of 22 patients, suggesting the careful observation for such lesions.

The limitation of the present study concerns the retrospective analysis that may eliminate the ability to obtain the strong conclusions. Selection of open surgery or careful observation depends on various factors including the results of FNAC and patients' previous courses. Therefore, the proper diagnostic rate of Group A was higher than in that of Group B, and the selection bias might cause the difference of the course of the two groups. The nature of the hypoechoic lesions that regressed during the follow-up examination is unclear in the present study, because open biopsies were not performed in these patients. Some could be actually low-grade thyroid lymphoma, but others could be focal or regional lymphocytic thyroiditis, atypical subacute thyroiditis, or other etiology-unknown lesion(s). Further prospective studies including histopathology and factor(s) involved in the regression or progression of the

Table 4 Comparisons of US classification between the Group A ($n = 41$) and Group B ($n = 12$)

US class	Group A	Group B
2.5	1	1
3	9	8
3.5	9	3
4	21	0

$P < 0.01$

Classes 2.5 and 3.5 designate intermediate classes between 2 &3 and 3 & 4, respectively

Table 5 Comparisons of the diagnostic categories of the Bethesda System for Reporting Thyroid Cytopathology between the Group A (n = 41) and Group B (n = 12)

Diagnostic categories	Group A	Group B
Benign	1	1
AUS	11	8
Suspicious for malignancy	22	2
Malignant	7	1

$P < 0.02$

US: ultrasound. *AUS*: atypia of undetermined significance or follicular lesion of undetermined significance

Benign: benign, but with the comment that lymphoma cannot be denied

Table 6 Comparisons of Groups A and B regarding the κ/λ deviation ratio of Ig light chain

κ/λ deviation ratio	Group A	Group B	Total
≥3.40	24	1	25
< 3.40	17	11	28
Total	41	12	53

The κ/λ deviation ratio of < 3.40 was significantly more frequent in Group B compared to Group A ($p < 0.01$, chi-square test (with Yate's continuity correction)). When the κ/λ deviation ratio was lower than 1.00, we converted it to the λ/κ ratio (deviation ratio)

lesions are needed to investigate the true nature of such lesions, and to clarify the best method of managing such patients.

Hypoechoic lesions suspected of having possible lymphoma decreased in size or disappeared in 12 out of 22 patients (55%), and such a regression should be emphasized in the present study. Because most of these lesions cannot be diagnosed definitely by core needle biopsy, open surgery might be considered. But unnecessary surgeries for benign lesions might be avoided.

Conclusion

Our study suggests that some hypoechoic thyroid lesions that are possible thyroid lymphoma based on US and FNAC might decrease in size or disappear during the careful observation. A careful observation before surgery is suggested for those lesions such as USC < 3.5, a κ/λ deviation ratio < 3.4, and the FNAC classification of 'benign' or 'atypia of determined significance or follicular lesions of undetermined significance'. However, an open biopsy or thyroid surgery should be considered in case of the increasing lesion in diameter on follow-up US examination.

Abbreviations

AUS: Atypia of undetermined significance or follicular lesion of undetermined significance; BethSys categories: Bethesda System for Reporting Thyroid Cytopathology; FNAC: Fine needle aspiration cytology; Ig: Immunoglobulin; MALT: Mucosa-associated lymphoid tissue; TgAb: Thyroglobulin antibody; TPOAb: Thyroid peroxidase antibody; US: Ultrasonography; USC: US classification

Authors' contributions

TN and MN were involved in study design, acquisition of data, analysis and interpretation of data and drafting and revising the manuscript. TN, MN, MH, TK, TK, EN, MI, SF, HN, MH and AM were involved in data collection and manuscript drafting. All authors read and approved the final manuscript.

Consent for publication

The patient has provided their consent for the contents of this report to be published.

Competing interests

The authors declare that they have no competing interests.

Author details

[1]Department of Internal Medicine, Kuma Hospital, Centre for Excellence in Thyroid Cares, 8-2-35 Shimoyamate-dori, Chuo-ku, Kobe 650-0011, Japan. [2]Department of Diagnostic Pathology and Cytology, Kuma Hospital, Centre for Excellence in Thyroid Cares, 8-2-35 Shimoyamate-dori, Chuo-ku, Kobe 650-0011, Japan. [3]Department of Surgery, Kuma Hospital, Centre for Excellence in Thyroid Care, 8-2-35 Shimoyamate-dori, Chuo-ku, Kobe 650-0011, Japan.

References

1. Klopper JP, Kane MA, Haugen BR. Anaplastic thyroid cancer and miscellaneous tumors of the thyroid. In: Braverman LE, Cooper DS, editors. Werner & Ingbar's The Thyroid. 10th ed; 2013. p. 765–74.
2. Freeman C, Berg JW, Occurrence CSJ. Prognosis of extranodal lymphomas. Cancer. 1972;29:252–60.
3. Thieblemont C, Mayer A, Dumontet C, Barbier Y, Callet-Bauchu E, et al. Primary thyroid lymphoma is a heterogeneous disease. J Clin Endocrinol Metab. 2002;87:105–11.
4. Matsuzuka F, Miyauchi A, Katayama S, Narabayashi I, Ikeda H, et al. Clinical aspects of primary thyroid lymphoma: diagnosis and treatment based on our experience of 119 cases. Thyroid. 1993;3:93–9.
5. Watanabe N, Noh JY, Narimatsu H, Takeuchi K, Yamaguchi T, et al. Clinicopathological features of 171 cases of primary thyroid lymphoma: a long-term study involving 24553 patients with Hashimoto's disease. Brit J Hematol. 2011;153:236–43.
6. Ota H, Ito Y, Matsuzuka F, Kuma S, Fukata S, et al. Usefulness of ultrasonography for diagnosis of malignant lymphoma of the thyroid. Thyroid. 2006;16:983–7.
7. Mizokami T, Hamada K, Maruta T, Higashi K, Yamashita H, et al. Development of primary thyroid lymphoma during an ultrasonographic follow-up of Hashimoto's thyroiditis: a report of 9 cases. Intern Med. 2016;55:943–8.
8. Sangalli G, Serio G, Zampatti C, Lomuscio G, Colombo L. Fine needle aspiration cytology of primary lymphoma of the thyroid: a report of 17 cases. Cytopathology. 2001;12:257–63.
9. Aleskow S, Wartofsky L. Primary thyroid lymphoma: a clinical review. J Clin Endocrnol Metab. 2013;98:3131–8.
10. Zeppa P, Cozzolino I, Peluso AL, Troncone G, Lucariello A, et al. Cytologic, flow cytometry, and molecular assessment of lymphoid infiltrate in fine-needle cytology samples of Hashimoto thyroiditis. Cancer Cytopathology. 2009;117:174–84.
11. Ito Y, Miyauchi A, Inoue H, Fukushima M, Kihara M, et al. An observational trial for papillary thyroid microcarcinoma in Japanese patients. World J Surg. 2010;34:28–35.
12. Ito Y, Amino N, Yokozawa T, Ota H, Ohshita M, et al. Ultrasonographic evaluation of thyroid nodules in 900 patients: comparison among ultrasonographic, cytological, and histological findings. Thyroid. 2007;17:1269–76.
13. Montalban C, Manzanal A, Boixeda D, Redondo C, Alvarez I. Helicobacter pylori eradication for the treatment of low-grade gastric MALT lymphoma: follow-up together with sequential molecular studies. Ann Oncol. 1997;2:37–9.
14. Grgov S, Katić V, Krstić M, Nagorni A, Radovanović-Dinić B. Treatment of low-grade gastric MALT lymphoma using Helicobactert pylori eradicateon. Vojnosanit Pregl. 2015;72:431–6.
15. Uohashi A, Imoto S, Matsui T, Murayama T, Okimura Y, et al. Spontaneous regression of diffuse large-cell lymphoma associated with Hashimoto's thyroiditis. Am J Hematol. 1996;53:201–11.
16. Okamoto A, Namura K, Uchiyama H, Kajita Y, Inaba T, et al. Cytotoxic T-cell non-Hodgkin's lymphoma of the thyroid gland. Am J Hematol. 2005;80:77–8.
17. Drobyski WR, Qazi R. Spontaneous regression in non-Hodgkin's lymphoma. Clinical and pathologic considerations. Am J Hematol. 1989;31:138–41.
18. Seachrist L. Spontaneous cancer remissions spark questions. J Natl Cancer Inst. 1993;85:1892–5.

32

Apoptosis induction by combination of drugs or a conjugated molecule associating non-steroidal anti-inflammatory and nitric oxide donor effects in medullary thyroid cancer models: implication of the tumor suppressor p73

Thierry Ragot[1,2,3], Claire Provost[4], Aurélie Prignon[4], Régis Cohen[5], Michel Lepoivre[6] and Sylvie Lausson[4*]

Abstract

Background: Medullary thyroid cancer (MTC) is a C-cell neoplasm. Surgery remains its main treatment. Promising therapies based on tyrosine kinase inhibitors demand careful patient selection. We previously observed that two non-steroidal anti-inflammatory drugs (NSAID), indomethacin, celecoxib, and nitric oxide (NO) prevented tumor growth in a model of human MTC cell line (TT) in *nude* mice.

Methods: In the present study, we tested the NO donor: glyceryl trinitrate (GTN), at pharmacological dose, alone and in combination with each of the two NSAIDs on TT cells. We also assessed the anti-proliferative potential of NO-indomethacin, an indomethacin molecule chemically conjugated with a NO moiety (NCX 530, Nicox SA) on TT cells and indomethacin/GTN association in rMTC 6–23 cells. The anti-tumoral action of the combined sc. injections of GTN with oral delivery of indomethacin was also studied on subcutaneous TT tumors in *nude* mice. Apoptosis mechanisms were assessed by expression of caspase-3, TAp73α, TAp73α inhibition by siRNA or Annexin V externalisation.

Results: The two NSAIDs and GTN reduced mitotic activity in TT cells versus control (cell number and PCNA protein expression). The combined treatments amplified the anti-tumor effect of single agents in the two tested cell lines and promoted cell death. Moreover, indomethacin/GTN association stopped the growth of established TT tumors in *nude* mice. We observed a significant cleavage of full length PARP, a caspase-3 substrate. The cell death appearance was correlated with a two-fold increase in TAp73α expression, with inhibition of apoptosis after TAp73α siRNA addition, demonstrating its crucial role in apoptosis.

Conclusion: Association of NO with NSAID exhibited amplified anti-tumoral effects on *in vitro* and *in vivo* MTC models by inducing p73-dependent apoptotic cell death.

Keywords: Medullary thyroid carcinoma, Non-steroidal anti-inflammatory drugs, NO-donors, Apoptosis, TT cells, rMTC 6–23 cells

* Correspondence: sylvielausson@aol.com
[4]Sorbonne Universités, UPMC University Paris 06, plateforme LIMP, Laboratoire d'Imagerie Médicale Positonique, Hôpital Tenon, Paris 75020, France
Full list of author information is available at the end of the article

Introduction

Medullary thyroid carcinoma (MTC) is a neuroendocrine neoplasm of C cells (for reviews see [1, 2]). This cancer releases large amounts of calcitonin (CT) correlated to tumor size [3]. MTC is sporadic in about 75 % of cases, and patients with sporadic carcinoma are usually diagnosed at late stage. Nowadays, surgical removal of the thyroid with lymph node dissection is the gold standard curative treatment of MTC. Prognostic remains poor since 40 to 60 % of patients are not cured. Current chemo- and radiotherapies are still ineffective. Hereditary germ-line mutations or somatic mutations of the RET proto-oncogene are involved in the carcinogenesis of familial and sporadic MTCs respectively. Several tyrosine kinase inhibitors (TKIs) that are notably RET receptor inhibitors are used and under evaluation for patients with advanced MTC with promising results [2, 4]. Thus TKIs vandetanib or cabozantinib can be used as single agent for first line systemic therapy in selected patients with advanced progressive MTC. But TKIs give only a significant increase of progression-free survival with no effect on death rate [5]. Thus, other or combined curative approaches are necessary to improve MTC treatments in the future.

The anti-tumor potential of non-steroidal anti-inflammatory drugs (NSAIDs) was recognized a few years ago [6–8]. The anti-proliferative effects of NSAIDs can result from the decrease of prostaglandin (PG) synthesis by inhibition of cyclooxygenase (COX) activity but also from anti-tumoral actions independent of PGs and COXs. We have previously demonstrated that the classical NSAID, indomethacin, reduced the development of xenografted TT tumors induced by injection of human MTC TT cells in *nude* mice [9]; indomethacin lowered PGE_2 secretion by TT cells. We also reported that a low dose of the selective COX-2 inhibitor, celecoxib (with less gastro-intestinal side effects than conventional drugs) significantly diminished the growth of TT tumors. This anti-tumor action was independent of PGE_2 and COX-2 [10].

Otherwise, we observed a very strong anti-tumor potential of nitric oxide (NO) on MTCs for two rat cell lines and TT cells [11]. More recently, authors reported that the chemical association of NO donors with a NSAID not only prevented side effects of the NSAID but also was able to amplify its anti-tumor action [12–14]. Elevation of the NO concentration can cause DNA damage, mutation and apoptosis [15]. The tumor suppressor protein p53 is a key player in the DNA damage response and the onset of apoptosis. NO has been shown to activate p53 which promotes pro-apoptotic effects [16]. Two *p53* related genes, *p63* and *p73*, have also been identified more than 15 years after the discovery of *p53* [17, 18]. The human *p*73 gene generates two groups of isoforms, some with a complete transactivation (TA) domain (TAp73) and others exhibiting a truncated TA domain (ΔNp73). Growth suppression or induction of apoptosis can be accomplished by the TAp73 isoforms. Studies have shown that p73 is required for apoptosis induction in response to DNA damage by chemotherapeutic drugs such as cis-platin [19]. Thus, p53 and p73 could be interesting targets to study in MTC chemotherapies: *p53* is not mutated in this cancer; in contrast, p73 was never studied in C cell but mutations in the *p*73 gene are rare in cancer patients. p73 is not only involved in tumor suppression but has important functions in neural cells and it also could be well expressed in neuroendocrine C cells.

In the present study, we compared the anti-proliferative actions of a pharmacological dose of the NO-donor, glyceryl trinitrate (GTN) or Trinitrine, a drug used in cardiology, of two NSAID, indomethacin and celecoxib, of the combinations of one NSAID with GTN, and finally, of a chemically conjugated molecule, NO-indomethacin (NCX 530) from Nicox SA, an indomethacin molecule conjugated with a NO donor group. We also studied the implications of cell death mediators p53 and p73 in TT cells. The NSAID doses used in these cultures were those reproducing the anti-tumoral benefits with low side effects we have previously described *in vivo*. Moreover, we assessed the anti-proliferative effect of the indomethecin/GTN association in another MTC cell line, rMTC 6–23 and studied the anti-tumoral action of a combined administration of GTN in sc. injections with oral delivery of indomethacin on xenografted TT tumors.

Materials and methods

Materials

Celecoxib was a generous gift from Pfizer (USA). Indomethacin was purchased from Cayman Chemical (Ann Arbor, MI). The NO-donor glyceryl trinitrate (GTN) was obtained from Merck (Lyon, France). The conjugated molecule NO-indomethacin (NCX 530) was a gift from Nicox SA (Sophia Antipolis, France). The TT and rMTC 6–23 cell lines were from the American Type Culture Collection (Rockville, MD). Primary antibodies to p73 (IMG 313A, Imgenex, A300-126A, Bethyl Laboratories), p53 (sc 6243, Santa Cruz Biotechnology), PCNA (Santa Cruz Biotechnology), PARP-1 (c-2-10, Calbiochem) and α-tubulin (T9026, Sigma) were used for western blots. Detections were performed with fluorescent Alexa Fluor 680-conjugated anti-mouse (A 21057, Invitrogen/Molecular Probes) or IRDye 800CW-anti-rabbit (926–32211, LI-COR Biosciences) IgG. Rabbit anti-caspase-3 antibody (ab52293, Abcam), Starr Trek Universal detection kit (Biocare Medical/Eurobio) and AEC Peroxidase Substrate kit (Vector Laboratories/Eurobio) were used for the immunohistochemitry of TT tumor slides.

Cell culture

TT cells were cultured in RPMI 1640 medium (Invitrogen, Cergy-Pontoise, France) supplemented with 2 mM L-glutamine, 25 mM HEPES, 10 % heat-inactivated fetal calf serum (FCS), 100 U/mL penicillin and 100 μg/mL streptomycin (Invitrogen). RMTC 6–23 cells were cultured in Dulbecco's Modified Eagle's medium (DMEM) GlutaMAX™ (Life Technologies, Cergy-Pontoise, France) supplemented with 1 % of Non-Essential Amino Acids (Life Technologies) and ~5 % heat-inactivated FCS. To determine the anti-proliferative effects of the NSAID/GTN combinations or NCX 530, TT or rMTC 6–23 cells were seeded out in 6-well-plates at a density of 2 to 3 × 10^5 cells per well, respectively. Three days later, NSAIDs and/or GTN were added (or not, or vehicles only, for the controls) to cell culture medium. Medium was changed every two days (TT cells) or every 36 h (rMTC 6–23 cells). After various periods of treatment, cells were dissociated 5 min with trypsin-EDTA or TrypLE™ Express (Life Technologies) for TT or rMTC 6–23 cells, respectively. Cells were counted with an hemocytometer (Trypan Blue exclusion) and/or using counting slides with an automated cell counter (TC20™ Bio-Rad, Marnes-la-Coquette, France). NSAIDs were dissolved in DMSO and GTN in ethanol. The following doses were used: celecoxib 25 μM, indomethacin 100 or 200 μM, GTN 100 μM, and NCX 530, 100 and 200 μM for short term experiments, and 150 μM for long term experiments. Controls were performed in the presence of drug vehicules (DMSO and ethanol) at the same concentrations as in experimental wells (DMSO ≤ 0.4 % and ethanol = 0.2 %). For western blot analyses, cells were seeded out in 6-well plates at a density of 10^6 cells per well. Treatments began 3 days later. In proliferation and apoptosis detection experiments, triplicates were performed for each category; in experiments for immunoblotting analyses, duplicates were used.

Apoptosis detection

After cell counts, the cell suspensions were adjusted to 10^6 cells/ml in microfuge tubes. An Annexin V-FITC Apoptosis Detection kit (Calbiochem, Merck Millipore, Darmstadt, Germany), was used to quantify apoptosis/necrosis. The "Rapid Annexin V binding" protocol provided by the suppliers was followed. After incubation with Annexin V-FITC and addition of Propidium Iodide, fluorescence was immediately analyzed by flow cytometry (BD Accuri™ C6 Flow Cytometer, BD Biosciences) using 530/30 and 670 LP emission filters preventing spillover. Unlabeled samples were used to adjust the gates.

Immunoblotting analyses

Immunoblots were performed as described in Tebbi et al. [20]. After harvest, cells were washed twice in ice-cold phosphate buffered saline (PBS). Crude cell extracts were prepared in a 50 mM Tris–HCl lysis buffer, pH 7.4, supplemented with 150 mM NaCl, 1 % Triton X-100, 0.5 % sodium deoxycholate, 1 mM EDTA, 1 mM DTT and protease inhibitors including 1 mM Pefablock (Merck/Calbiochem). Soluble proteins (30 μg per lane) were separated by SDS-PAGE using a 10 %-acrylamide gel and transferred onto nitrocellulose membranes. These ones were blocked in 3 % skimmed milk. After overnight incubation at 4 °C with primary antibodies and four washes in PBS/Tween, membranes were incubated for 1 h with fluorescent dye-conjugated secondary antibodies. After washing, the infrared fluorescent signals at 680 and 800 nm were quantified with an Odyssey scanner (LI-COR Biosciences). Protein contents were standardized using α-tubulin band density.

Transfections with TAp73 siRNA

SiRNA sequences were reported and validated in Guittet et al. [21]. Cells were transfected with TAp73 Select siRNA (Ambion) or control siRNA (MWG) using Interferin transfection reagent (Polyplus Transfection). TT cells were plated in 6-well plates and grown to approximately 30-50 % confluency. Before transfection, culture medium was replaced by the same medium without antibiotics (4 mL per well). Interferin (corresponding to 15 μL per well) was incubated with siRNA for 10 min in antibiotic-free medium. Then, the mixture was added dropwise to wells, resulting in a siRNA concentration of 30 nM. We have previously verified that this method led to 80 % reduction of TAp73α expression, 3 days after mixture addition. Cells were maintained in the transfection medium for 16 h. They were then cultured in usual medium with GTN (100 μM) and celecoxib (25 μM) treatment or with DMSO and ethanol (control wells) during 2 days and 8 h.

In vivo experiment

5 × 10^6 TT cells were inoculated subcutaneously (sc) on the back of each *nude* mouse. When tumors became palpable, their diameters were regularly measured with a caliper and tumor volume (mm^3) was calculated using the following formula: (the shortest diameter)^2 × (the longest diameter) × 0.5. When the mean volume of tumors reached about 70 mm^3, animals were randomly divided into three groups: one control group (5) and two treated groups, one receiving sc injections of Nitronal each two days, (0.1 mg GTN/20 g of body weight during 6 days, then 0.15 mg, $n = 5$), the other group receiving the same doses of Nitronal with indomethacin (2 mg/day/kg of body weight in drinking water, $n = 4$). Animal manipulations were performed according to the recommendations of the French Ethical Committee and under the supervision of authorized investigators.

Mice were sacrificed at day 14 and tumors were removed and weighted. Tumors were divided in two parts. One part of the tumor was fixed in 4 % paraformaldehyde during 96 h and embedded in paraffin. Some tumor slides, chosen in three different levels (100 μm apart), were colored with hematotoxylin-phloxine-saffron (HPS) stain. The cavity area of colored slides was measured by ImageJ software at three levels in each tumor. For caspase-3 immunohistochemistry, we followed a method similar to that described in Bressenot et al. [22].

Statistical analyses

All results were analysed using ANOVA. Differences between two means were tested by the Fisher tests. Data are represented as means ± SEM. For each determination, two or three independent experiments were performed. The significance level was set at $P < 0.05$. For the proliferation experiments, we assessed the differences between treated cells and control cells at day 4 (D4). We also tested cell number reductions induced by NO-NSAID bi-therapies at D4 and D8 versus D0. For the immunoblotting analyses, we tested the differences between treated and control cells at D1 and D3. Moreover, for each NSAID/GTN combination (proliferation experiments at D4 and p73 expression at D3), we performed a two-factor variance analysis to assess the significance of NSAID or GTN effects individually and to test the presence of a NSAID/GTN interaction.

In the annexin V studies, a significant linear regression was obtained between apoptotic cell percentages and total number of cells, in controls: the apoptotic cell percentage increases when cell density grows. Thus, we compared the apoptotic cell percentage in each treated culture with a percentage (calculated with the regression) in a control containing the same total number of cells than the treated culture. For the *in vivo* experiment, we assessed the tumor volume growth and the mean differences between treatments by the two-factor analysis (time factor as repeated measures and treatment factor).

Results

Anti-proliferative effects of GTN, NSAID/GTN combinations and NO-indomethacin on TT cells

As previously reported, we observed that the NSAIDs celecoxib and indomethacin prevented the proliferation of TT cells: the cell number in treated samples was reduced by about 30 % at D2 and D4 versus controls (Fig. 1a and b). Moreover, we established that a NO-donor, GTN (100 μM), had a similar effect: the viable cell number was decreased by about 30 % versus controls (Fig. 1a and b). We revealed significant effects of each NSAID alone and GTN alone at D4. Interestingly, the combinations of one NSAID with GTN strongly increased the anti-tumoral action seen for each individual molecule at D4 (cell number diminution of 50 to 60 % versus controls). Significant reductions were observed between D0 and D4, $P < 0.05$, after celecoxib/GTN incubation and $P < 0.01$, after indomethacin-GTN treatment. The two-factor analysis of variance did not reveal an interaction between each NSAID and GTN; this result suggests the presence of additive effects. NO-indomethacin, NCX530, had the same anti-tumor action than the GTN and indomethacin incubation. The reduction of cell population treated with NCX 530 versus control was dose-dependent (Fig. 1c).

Continuous anti-tumor action of NSAID/GTN combinations and NO-indomethacin after long-time administration on TT cells

When cells were treated with NO-NSAID combinations until D8, the cell number reduction was prolonged from D4 to D8: $P < 0.05$ for indomethacin/GTN, $P < 0.01$ for celecoxib/GTN and NO-indomethacin alone (Fig. 2a). In another experiment, TT cells were incubated with NSAID/GTN combinations or NO-indomethacin during 7 days then, cultured in drug-free medium until D12. Under these conditions, no growth rebound was observed between D7 to D12 (Fig. 2b). Thus, the anti-tumoral action was amplified when treatments were prolonged and this beneficial effect was maintained after treatment cessation.

NSAIDs, GTN and NSAID/GTN bi-therapies reduce mitotic proliferation of TT cells. NSAID/GTN combined treatments only lead to cell death

PCNA is a nuclear antigen expressed during cell mitotic division. The effects of drug exposition on PCNA expression were investigated by western blot analysis. Figure 3a shows a significant decrease in PCNA levels in all 3-day-treated cells versus controls: celecoxib alone, $P < 0.0001$, indomethacin alone, $P < 0.0001$, GTN alone, $P < 0.0001$, NSAID/GTN combinations, $P < 0.0001$ (NCX 530, $P < 0.01$). Thus, all these treatments reduced the levels of TT cell mitotic divisions.

PARP is a substrate of caspase-3, cleaved early during cell apoptosis. Western blot analyses revealed that PARP was cleaved in TT cells incubated with drug combinations (or NO-indomethacin alone, data not shown) during 3 days: the levels of PARP full-length polypeptide were significantly decreased ($P < 0.05$ versus control cells) for all bi-therapies, (Fig. 3b). No effect appeared after one day of treatment (data not shown). Thus, the reduction of viable cell numbers receiving bi-therapies after D2 also resulted from apoptotic cell death induction.

Increased expression of the tumor suppressors p53 and p73

We investigated the expression of the tumor suppressors p53 and p73 in TT cells at basal levels and in response

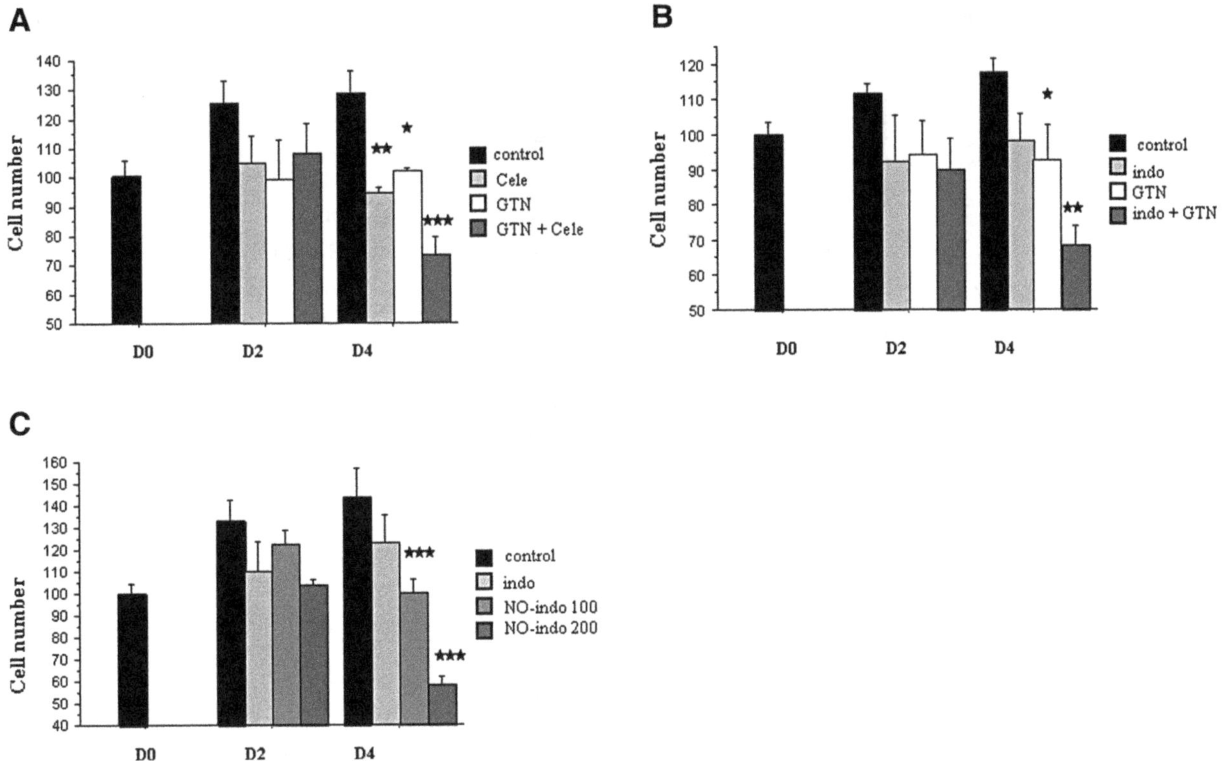

Fig. 1 **a** Evolution of the number of viable, control or treated TT cells: 25 μM celecoxib, (cele), 100 μM GTN or a combination of celecoxib plus GTN, during 4 days. **b** Evolution of viable TT cell number during 4-day treatments with 100 μM indomethacin (indo), 100 μM GTN or a bi-therapy of indomethacin plus GTN. **c** Effects of the conjugated molecule (NO-donor conjugated to indomethacin, NCX 530), 100 μM (NO-indo100) or 200 μM NO-indomethacin (NO-indo200), during the first 4 days of treatment. Representative graphs of three (**a**, **b**) or two (**c**) independent experiments performed in triplicates. Adherent cells were dissociated with trypsin-EDTA and count with an hemocytometer with blue trypan exclusion. * = $P < 0.05$, ** = $P < 0.01$, *** = $P < 0.001$ versus control (Fisher test)

to the different treatments by NSAIDs and NO. We found that this cell line expressed p53 and TAp73α at basal levels. ΔNp73 was not detected in control and treated TT cells. No change in p53 and p73 expressions was observed in 1-day treated cells (data not shown). Indomethacin, indomethacin plus GTN, and NO-indomethacin led to comparable increases in p53 levels at D3 while celecoxib and GTN had no effect (Fig. 3c).

In contrast, TAp73α expression increased by a factor two after 3-day NSAID/GTN combined treatments (Fig. 3d) or incubation with NO-indomethacin alone. These elevations were correlated with a reduction in PARP levels and TT cell number decrease between D2 and D4. The two-factor analysis of variance showed significant 50 %-increases of TAp73 level after 3-day treatments with NSAID alone or GTN alone: in the experiments with indomethacin plus GTN, $P = 0.05$ for indomethacin factor, $P = 0.01$ for GTN factor; in the experiment with celecoxib plus GTN, $P < 0.05$ for celecoxib and for GTN. No significant interaction between NSAIDs and GTN was revealed. Thus, additive effects lead to the strongest increases in TAp73 expression after 3-day combined treatments.

p73 siRNA transfection

Celecoxib/GTN combination induced a strong and significant increase of TAp73 expression in TT cells, after 2 days and 8 h of treatment ($P < 0.01$, Fig. 4a and b). Transfection of siRNA targeting TAp73 isoforms before this treatment, led to a significantly lower level of TAp73 (around minus 50 %, $P = 0.05$). We also observed a decrease of PARP heavy chain expression after the NSAID/GTN incubation ($P < 0.05$, Fig. 4a and c), while TAp73 siRNA suppressed this phenomenon. Thus, as suggested by the previously described correlation, the strong increase in p73 level must be responsible for PARP cleavage and cell apoptosis.

Confirmation of anti-proliferative effect of the indomethacin/GTN association on rMTC 6–23 cell cultures

Anti-proliferative actions of NO and indomethacin were also assessed by incubations with indomethacin alone (200 μM), GTN (100 μM) alone, or combinations of the two drugs in a second MTC cell line (Fig. 5). As observed in TT cells, indomethacine or GTN alone slowed the growth of rMTC 6–23 cell cultures; the combination amplified the anti-proliferative effect of each

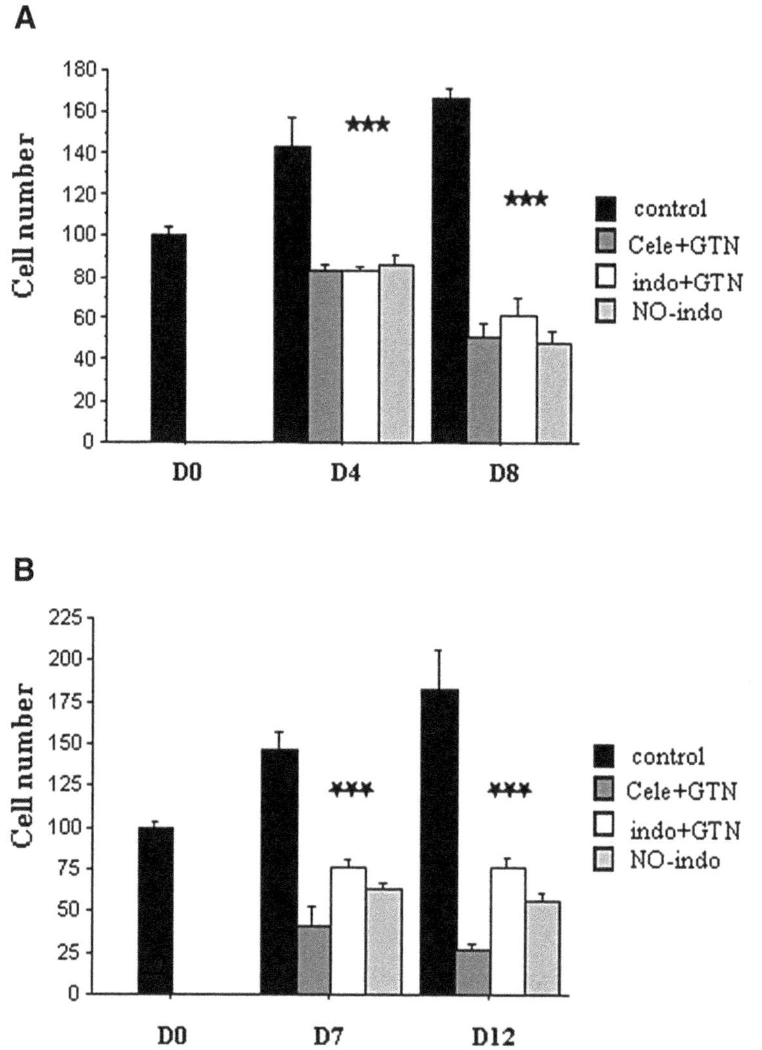

Fig. 2 a Evolution of viable TT cell number in control wells and in wells treated by NSAID/GTN combination: 25 μM celecoxib plus 100 μM GTN (cele + GTN), or 100 μM indomethacin plus 100 μM GTN (indo + GTN), or 150 μM NCX 530 (NO-indo), during 8 days. **b** Evolution of viable TT cell populations after cessation of treatments with NSAID/GTN bi-therapies or NCX 530 (25 μM celecoxib, 100 μM indomethacin, 100 μM GTN or 150 μM NCX 530). Representative graphs of two independent experiments performed in triplicates. Adherent cells were dissociated with trypsin-EDTA and count with a hemocytometer. *** = $P < 0.001$ versus control for each treatment (Fisher tests)

drug ($P < 0.01$ versus indomethacin alone, $P < 0.0001$ versus GTN alone, at D6) and even reduced the cell number at D6 versus D0 ($P < 0.05$). The apoptosis percentage was low, about 5 % in controls according to Annexin V staining and FACS analysis. Indomethacin did not produced significant change in apoptosis level versus control while GTN alone induced only a low elevation (145 %, $P < 0.05$) but the combination of both led to a stronger increase (308 %, $P < 0.001$), at D6. This ampification was significant ($P < 0.01$, combined treatment versus GTN incubation). Thus, also in this cell line, the strong anti-proliferative action of indomethacin/GTN association resulted from the promotion of apoptotic cell death.

Anti-tumoral action of combined administration of GTN plus indomethacin on established subcutaneous TT tumors in *nude* mice

Next, the *in vivo* activity of GTN alone or in combination with indomethacin was determined in *nude* mice. Figure 6 illustrated the effect of treatments on TT xenograft volumes. Subcutaneous injections of GTN did not significantly modified the growth of the subcutaneous tumors while the bi-therapy first slowed it down and then, stopped it from D7 to D12 (global analyses showed a significant effect of the bi-therapy versus control, $P < 0.0001$ and a significant effect of the combination versus GTN alone group, $P < 0.05$). Action on tumor weights at D14

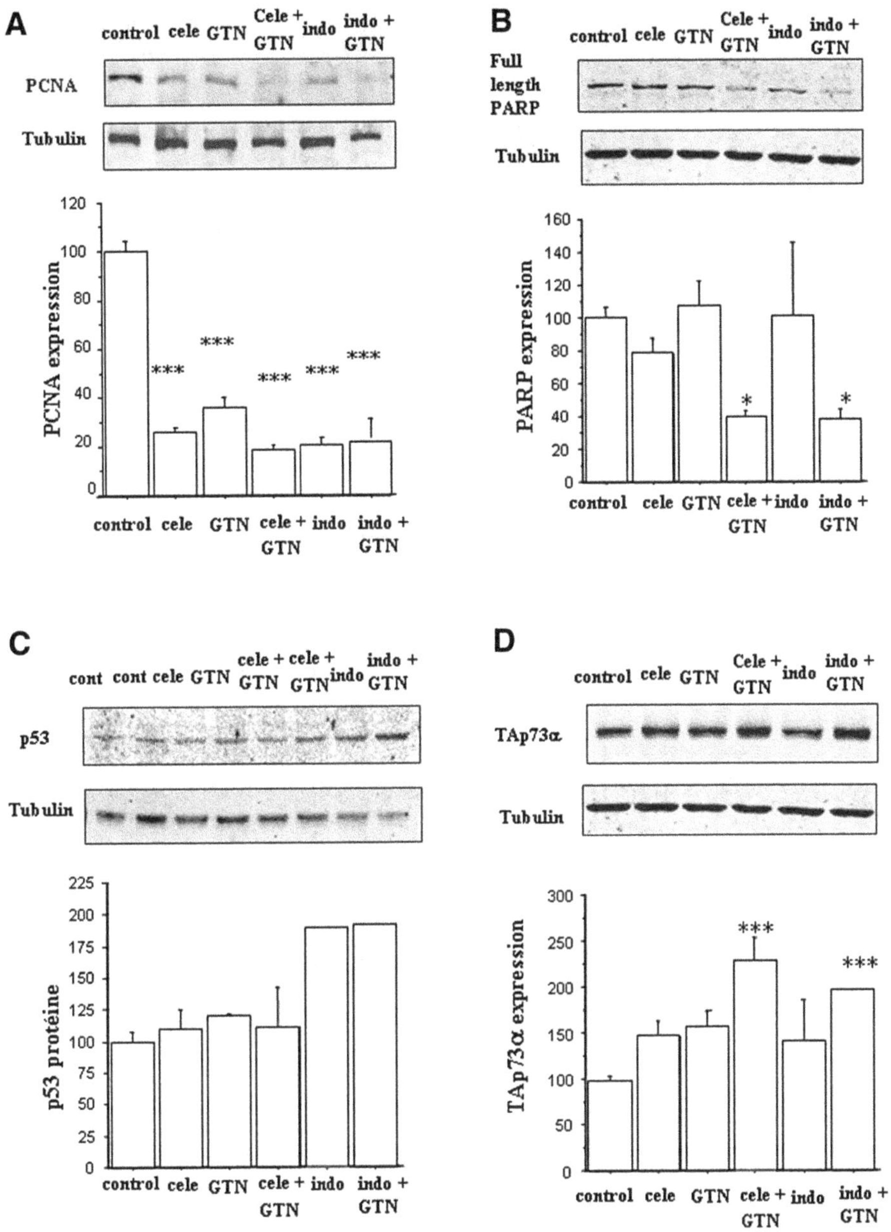

Figure 3 Expression of various proteins in TT cells after 3 days of exposition to 25 μM celecoxib (cele), 100 μM indomethacin (indo), 100 μM GTN or NSAID/GTN combinations. **a** PCNA protein. For each category, $n = 6$ to 3. **b** PARP heavy chain. For each category, $n = 4$ to 3. **c** Tumor suppressor p53. For each category, $n = 4$ to 2. **d** TAp73α. For each category, $n = 7$ to 4. Graphs obtained from associated results of two experiments on TT cells. Proteins from TT cell lysates were separated by SDS-PAGE using 10 % acrylamide gel and transferred onto nitro cellulose membranes. Immunoblots were probed with specific antibodies and a α-tubulin (internal control) antibody. * = $P < 0.05$, *** = $P < 0.001$ versus control (Fisher tests)

was strictly comparable to effect on tumor volumes at D12 (data not shown).

A HPS coloration of slides showed that control TT tumors were rather only composed of tumoral tissue. The GTN-treated tumors had the same appearance. On the contrary, numerous spaces empty of cancerous cells were visualized in tumors treated by the drug combination. The cavity area represented 19 ± 2.8 % of the total tumor surface. In agreement with these observations, we found numerous cleaved caspase-3 stained cells in these tumors indicating that the combination led to cell death, probably by apoptosis. Such immunostaining observations were rare in the GTN-treated and control groups. The tumor growth arrest with formation of cavities and presence of

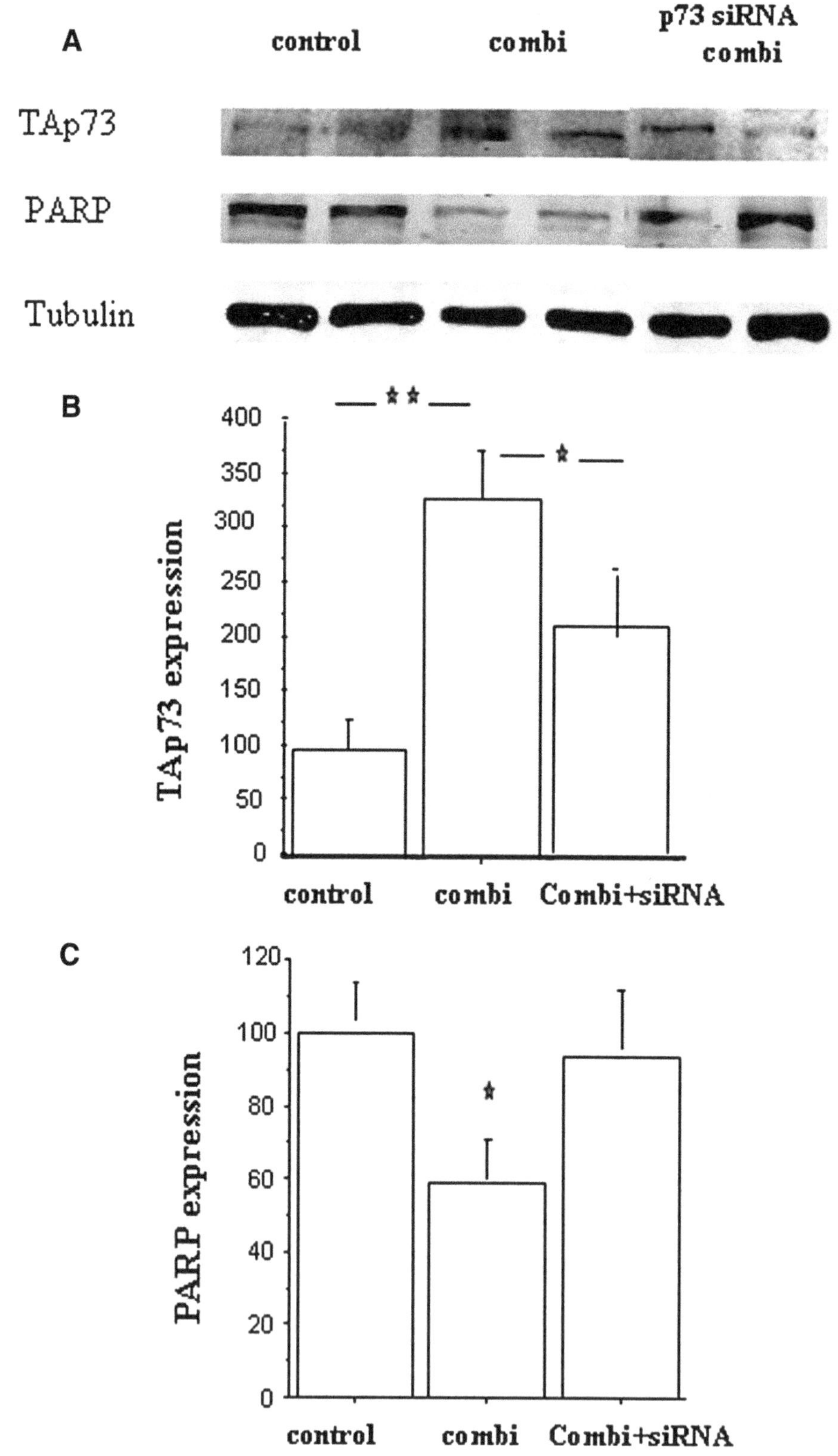

Fig. 4 **a** Effect of p73 siRNA pre-treatment on TAp73 and PARP expressions in TT cells receiving 25 μM celecoxib plus 100 μM GTN (combi) during 2 days and 8 h. **b** Effect of p73 siRNA pre-treatment on TAp73 expression in the same TT cells. **c** Effect of p73 siRNA pre-treatment on full length PARP expression in these cells. Graphs obtained from associated results of two experiments on TT cells. For each category, $n = 6$ to 4. Proteins from TT cell lysates were separated by SDS-PAGE using 10 % acrylamide gel and transferred onto nitro cellulose membranes. Immunoblots were probed with specific antibody and a α-tubulin (internal control) antibody. * = $P < 0.05$, ** = $P < 0.01$ (Fisher tests)

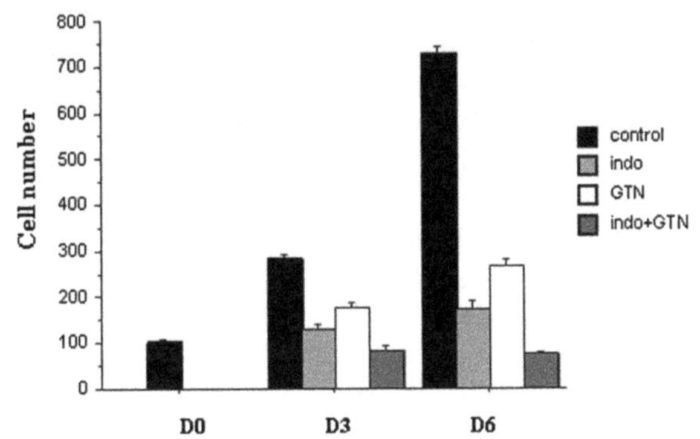

Fig. 5 Evolution of the number of viable, control or treated rMTC 6–23 cells: 200 μM indomethacin (indo), 100 μM GTN, or the combination of indomethacin plus GTN, during 6 days. Experiment performed in triplicates. Adherent cells were dissociated with trypsin-EDTA and their number was evaluated with a cell counter (blue trypan exclusion). Drug combination amplified the anti-proliferative effect of each drug ($P < 0.01$ versus indomethacin alone, $P < 0.0001$ versus GTN alone, at D6) and reduced the cell number at D6 versus D0 ($P < 0.05$, Fisher tests)

apoptotic cells suggested that the combined treatment reduced the cancer extension after D7 while GTN alone had no significant effect.

Discussion

In the present study we demonstrated the anti-proliferative value of NO donor plus NSAIDs on a human MTC cell line. The bi-therapies, celecoxib/GTN, indomethacin/GTN and NO-indomethacin amplified the anti-proliferative effects of each drug alone against TT cells. Indomethacin/GTN combination had the same action on the growth of rMTC 6–23 cells. Since the enhanced cytotoxicity of bi-therapies was correlated with increased expression of TAp73 in TT cells, we proposed that TAp73 might be implicated in the cytotoxic mechanism. In support of this hypothesis, knocking down TAp73 reduced PARP cleavage, a marker of apoptotic cell death. Interestingly, the indomethacin/GTN combination also produced a reduction of tumoral tissue extension and induced cell death, in the *in vivo* model. We have previously reported that the administration of indomethacin alone at the same dose only reduced TT xenograft growth [9].

It has been widely shown that NSAIDs and aspirin prevented the growth of numerous cancers and notably human cancers. The anti-tumor and pro-apoptotic potentials of NO have often been reported. During the last few years, authors have tested various conjugated molecules associating a NO-donor with a non-selective COX inhibitor, *i.e.* classical NSAID (NO-NSAID). They described that NO-NSAID have better anti-proliferative activity than the parent NSAID, *in vitro* and *in vivo*, and in particular, in colon, bladder and prostate cancer [23–26, 13]. Moreover, the administration of NO reduces the side effects of NSAID. Recently, the anti-proliferative action of nitro-oxy derivatives of the COX-2 selective inhibitor, celecoxib, has been assessed in various cell lines. These interesting derivatives of celecoxib which have less toxicity than the parent NSAID, showed an anti-tumor activity comparable to that of celecoxib [27, 28].

With respect to MTCs, our group has found that celecoxib at a low dose and the classical NSAID, indomethacin, reduced the development of tumors arising -from human TT cell injection in *nude* mice [10, 9]. Tomoda et al. [29] also reported that indomethacin have a strong anti-proliferative action on TT cells and two other MTC lines, due to mitotic division reduction without amplification of cell death level. Moreover, we have observed that three MTC cell lines were very sensitive to the anti-proliferative effect of a NO-donor [11]. The present publication reports that a pharmacological dose of GTN, a NO pro-drug used in cardiology, reduced significantly TT cell proliferation *in vitro* via mitotic division decrease.

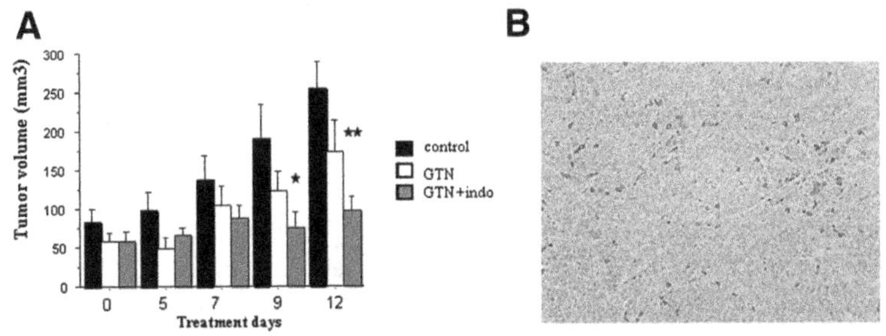

Fig. 6 *In vivo* effect of GTN plus indomethacin association on growth of TT xenografts in *nude* mice. Indomethacin was administrated in drinking water (2 mg/kg of body weight × day). Mice treated by GTN received Nitronal sc injections each two days (100 μl during the first week and 150 μl/20 g body weight the second week of treatment). **a** Effect on tumor volumes. The GTN-indomethacin/GTN association stopped the growth of TT tumors from D7 to D12. Significant differences were revealed between tumor volumes by ANOVAs ($P < 0.0001$ combination group versus control, $P < 0.05$ combination group versus GTN treated group; control group, $n = 5$, GTN treated group, $n = 5$ and indomethacin/GTN association, $n = 4$). * = $P < 0.05$, ** = $P < 0.01$ (Fisher tests versus control at D9 or D12). **b** A microphotography of immunostaining of caspase 3 protein revealed numerous apoptotic cells (dark dots) in indomethacin/GTN treated tumors. No staining was observed in the two other groups of tumor

As previously described for other cancer cells, incubation with NO and indomethacin strongly amplified the antitumoral effect of treatments alone in TT cell cultures. NO-indomethacin (NCX 530) had a stronger action than the individual NSAID. Interestingly, in our model, the association of GTN with celecoxib also increased the anti-proliferative activity of the drugs used as single agents. After analyses of the mitotic division and apoptosis markers, PCNA and PARP, we found that this phenomenon resulted from the induction of TT apoptotic cell death by combinations of a NO donor with each NSAID, while each molecule alone only acted on mitotic division.

In cancer biology, both positive and negative actions of NO have been reported. Low doses could promote cancer proliferation. Elevation of NO concentration can cause cell damage and apoptosis [15] and the tumor suppressor protein p53 have been implicated in the onset of cell death [16]. Recently, Tebbi et al. [20] described that NO induced the overexpression of the tumor suppressor isoform TAp73α in leukemia cells. In our model, the NO donor GTN, at low dose, did not increase p53 expression and only induced mitotic division reduction without apoptosis induction. This treatment moderately elevated TAp73α expression in TT cells but only after three days of exposition. The pathway leading to *in vitro* proliferation reduction remains unknown. Anyway, only a moderate, not significant growth reduction was obtained *in vivo*. This result could come from the difficulties to reveal a significant effect *in vivo* compared to *in vitro* experiment, from lower NO doses in tissues but also from the promotion of tumor angiogenesis which favors tumor cell proliferation.

The mechanisms of NSAID action are not completely elucidated. The anti-tumor effect of these drugs can result from the decrease of PG by inhibition of synthesis enzymes, COX 1 and/or 2. However, various mechanisms, independent of PG and COX have been also described [30, 31]. Increase of p53 expression was frequently observed after NSAID treatments of various models. In particular, Lau et al. [32] found that COX inhibitors induce apoptosis by increasing p53 stability and nuclear accumulation. Targeting p53 in MTCs may represent an attractive strategy since this protein is not mutated in these tumors [33]. In the present study, we found that only indomethacin increased p53 expression, in TT cells. Indomethacin alone acts on mitotic division [9]. However, p53 level elevation did not seem to intervene in the cell division reduction as this phenomenon appeared before p53 level increase.

Recently for the first time, Lau et al. [34] demonstrated the implication of p73 in the anti-tumor effect of a NSAID: the apoptotic response to celecoxib resulted from the increase of the TAp73β:ΔNp73 ratio in neuroblastoma cells. In our hand, both celecoxib and indomethacin increased the expression of the TAp73α isoform in TT cells. It is noteworthy that ΔNp73 and TAp73β were not detected in this cell line. The moderate elevation of TAp73α expression by a 1.5 factor did not promote the anti-mitotic action of the NSAIDs since this anti-tumor effect appeared during the first day of treatment while the variations in protein expression was only observed after more than two days. However we have not investigated post-translational modifications of TAp73α, such as phosphorylation that might be implicated in the anti-mitotic effects of these NSAIDs. Moreover, in our model, the increase of TAp73α after incubation with NSAIDs alone did not induce cell apoptosis. In fact, TAp73α would be a less potent apoptosis inducer than TAp73β [35].

Combinations of NO with one of the NSAIDs did not reinforce the cell division reduction as PCNA level in cells treated with only one simple drug was comparable to the protein expression in cells which have received combined treatment. But interestingly and for the first time, we observed the addition of NO and NSAID effects on TAp73α expression. Thus combinations led to a stronger elevation of this isoform level. Bi-therapies only promoted apoptosis resulting from the TAp73α expression increase as demonstrated by full length PARP western blot after TAp73α siRNA adjunction in TT cell cultures.

In the *in vitro* experiments, we used celecoxib and indomethacin doses that reproduced anti-tumor effects obtained for long term *in vivo* treatments; the NO-donor GTN was used at a pharmacological dose. Thus, the *in vitro* observations described here allow to study a phenomenon that can be also induced *in vivo* as demonstrated in our *in vivo* experiments. More *in vivo* validation has to be done but the bases are set to expect similar results. The expression of p73 must also be verified in human MTCs.

It could be of interest for many reasons to consider clinical studies with NSAID and/or NO-donor therapies. First, these drugs have a low cost and are currently used with many years of experience in healthy subjects. Second, these drugs could be used for a long period at all stage of the disease (advanced or not). Third, combined anti-proliferative actions of NO donor and NSAIDs demonstrated in this study seem independent of known actions of TKI and synergic actions with them could be of value [36]. Unfortunately, clinical experience with use of indomethacin in patients with recurrent or metastatic MTC has been limited to three cases. In only two out of three patients, indomethacin therapy for 3 or 4 months caused marked reduction in tumor mass as well as calcitonin levels [37]. The efficacy of these drugs remains to be determined by clinical trials.

Competing interests

The authors declare that they have no competing interests.

Authors' contribution

TR carried out rMTC 6.23 cell studies and FACS analyses, and participated to the redaction of the manuscript. CP and AP carried out the work on nude mice. RC gave medical advice. ML carried out his knowledge on p73, western blots, and siRNAs. SL conceived the global study, carried out works on TT cells and on histological and statistical analyses. SL wrote the manuscript with TR. All authors read and approved the final manuscript.

Acknowledgements

We thank Nicox SA for a gift of NCX 530 and Pfizer that gave us celecoxib. We also thank S. Dumont and F. Merabtene (plateforme d'histomorphologie, IFR 65, UPMC, Paris, France) and A. Rodenas (service d'anatomopathologie, Hôpital Tenon, Paris, France) for technical assistance in immunohistochemistry.

Author details

[1]UMR 8203, Gustave Roussy, Laboratoire de Vectorologie et de Thérapeutiques Anticancéreuses, Villejuif 94805, France. [2]UMR 8203, CNRS, Laboratoire de Vectorologie et Thérapeutiques Anticancéreuses, Villejuif 94805, France. [3]UMR 8203, Univ Paris-Sud, Laboratoire de Vectorologie et Thérapeutiques Anticancéreuses, Villejuif 94805, France. [4]Sorbonne Universités, UPMC University Paris 06, plateforme LIMP, Laboratoire d'Imagerie Médicale Positonique, Hôpital Tenon, Paris 75020, France. [5]Hopital Delafontaine, Endocrinology Unit, Saint Denis, France. [6]IBBMC, CNRS 8619, bat 430, Université Paris Sud XI, Orsay, Paris 91405, France.

References

1. Vitale G, Caraglia M, Ciccarelli A, Lupoli G, Abbruzzese A, Tagliaferri P, et al. Current approaches and perspectives in the therapy of medullary thyroid carcinoma. Cancer. 2001;91:1797–808.
2. Pacini F, Castagna MG, Cipri C, Schlumberger M. Medullary thyroid carcinoma. Clin Oncol. 2010;22(6):475–85.
3. Cohen R, Campos J, Salaün C, Heshmati H, Kraimps J, Proye C, et al. Preoperative calcitonin levels are predictive of tumor size and postoperative calcitonin normalization in medullary thyroid carcinoma. J Clin Endocrinol Metab. 2000;85:919–22.
4. Schlumberger M, Carlomagno F, Baudin E, Bidart J, Santoro M. New therapeutic approaches to treat medullary thyroid carcinoma. Nat Clin Pract Endocrinol Metab. 2008;4:22–32.
5. Wells Jr SA, Asa SL, Dralle H, Elisei R, Evans DB, Gagel RF, et al. Revised american thyroid association guidelines for the management of medullary thyroid carcinoma. Thyroid. 2015;25:567–610.
6. DuBois RN, Giardiello FM, Smalley WE. Nonsteroidal anti-inflammatory drugs, and colorectal cancer prevention. Gastroenterol Clin North Am. 1996;25:773–91.
7. Langman MJ, Cheng KK, Gilman EA, Lancashire RJ. Effect of anti-inflammatory drugs on overall risk of common cancer: case–control study in general practice research database. BMJ. 2000;320:1642–6.
8. Rothwell PM, Price JF, Fowkes FG, Zanchetti A, Tognoni G, Lee R, et al. Short-term effects of daily aspirin on cancer incidence, mortality, and non-cardiovascular death: analysis of the time course of risks and benefits in51 randomised controlled trials. Lancet. 2012;379:1602–12.
9. Quidville V, Segond N, Pidoux E, Cohen R, Jullienne A, Lausson S. Tumor growth inhibition by indomethacin in a mouse model of human medullary thyroid cancer: implication of cyclooxygenases and 15-hydroxyprostaglandin dehydrogenase. Endocrinology. 2004;145:2561–71.
10. Quidville V, Segond N, Tebbi A, Cohen R, Jullienne A, Lepoivre M, et al. Anti-tumoral effect of a celecoxib low dose on a model of human medullary thyroid cancer in nude mice. Thyroid. 2009;19:613–21.
11. Soler MN, Bobe P, Benihoud K, Lemaire G, Roos BA, Lausson S. Gene therapy of rat medullary thyroid cancer by naked nitric oxide synthase II DNA injection. J Gene Med. 2000;2:344–52.
12. Wallace JL, Del Soldato P. The therapeutical potential of NO-NSAIDs. Fundam Clin Pharmacol. 2003;17:11–20.
13. Rao CV, Reddy BS, Steele VE, Wang CX, Liu X, Ouyang N, et al. Nitric oxide-releasing aspirin and indomethacin are potent inhibitors against colon cancer in azoxymethane-treated rats: effects on molecular targets. Mol Cancer Ther. 2006;5:1530–8.
14. Ouyang N, Williams JL, Tsioulias GJ, Gao JJ, Iatropoulos MJ, Kopelovich L, et al. Nitric oxide-donating aspirin prevents pancreatic cancer in a hamster tumor model. Cancer Res. 2006;66:4503–11.
15. Akaike T, Fujii S, Kato A, Yoshitake J, Miyamoto Y, Sawa T, et al. Viral mutation accelerated by nitric oxide production during infection in vivo. Faseb J. 2000;14:1447–54.
16. Messmer UK, Ankarcrona M, Nicotera P, Brune B. p53 expression in nitric oxide-induced apoptosis. FEBS Lett. 1994;355:23–6.
17. Kaghad M, Bonnet H, Yang A, Creancier L, Biscan JC, Valent A, et al. Monoallelically expressed gene related to p53 at 1p36, a region frequently deleted in neuroblastoma and other human cancers. Cell. 1997;90:809–19.
18. Yang A, Kaghad M, Wang Y, Gillett E, Fleming MD, Dotsch V, et al. p63, a p53 homolog at 3q27-29, encodes multiple products with transactivating, death-inducing, and dominant-negative activities. Mol Cell. 1998;2:305–16.
19. Muller M, Schleithoff ES, Stremmel W, Melino G, Krammer PH, Schilling T. One, two, three–p53, p63, p73 and chemosensitivity. Drug Resist Updat. 2006;9:288–306.
20. Tebbi A, Guittet O, Cottet MH, Vésin F, Lepoivre M. TAp73 induction by nitric oxide. JBC. 2011;286:7873–84.
21. Guittet O, Tebbi A, Cottet MH, Vesin F, Lepoivre M. Upregulation of the p53R2 ribonucleotide reductase subunit by nitric oxide. Nitric Oxide. 2008;19:84–94.
22. Bressenot A, Marchal S, Bezdetnaya L, Garrier J, Guillemin F, Plénat F. Assessment of apoptosis by immunohistochemistry to active caspase-3, active caspase-7, or cleaved PARP in monolayer cells and spheroid and subcutaneous xenografts of human carcinoma. J Histochem Cytochem. 2009;57:289–300.
23. Kashfi K, Ryan Y, Qiao LL, Williams JL, Chen J, Del Soldato P, et al. Nitric oxide-donating non-steroidal anti-inflammatory drugs inhibit the growth of various cultured human cancer cells: evidence of a tissue type-independent effect. J Pharmacol Exp Ther. 2002;303:1273–82.
24. Huguenin S, Fleury-Feith J, Kheuang L, Jaurand MC, Bolla M, Riffaud JP, et al. Nitrosulindac (NCX 1102): a new nitric oxide- donating non steroidal anti-inflammatory drug (NO-NSAID), inhibits proliferation and induces apoptosis in human prostatic epithelial cell lines. Prostate. 2004;61:132–41.
25. Huguenin S, Vacherot F, Kheuang L, Fleury-Feith J, Jaurand MC, Bolla M, et al. Antiproliferative effect of nitrosulindac (NCX 1102), a new nitric oxide- donating non steroidal anti-inflammatory drug, on human bladder carcinoma cell lines. Mol Cancer Ther. 2004;3:291–8.
26. Fabbri F, Brigliadori G, Ulivi P, Tesei A, Vannini I, Rosetti M, et al. Pro-apototic effect of nitric oxide- donating NSAID, NCX 4040, on bladder carcinoma cells. Apoptosis. 2005;10:1095–103.
27. Bozzo F, Bassignana A, Lazzarato L, Boschi D, Gasco A, Bocca C, et al. Novel nitro-oxy derivatives of celecoxib for the regulation of colon cancer cell growth. Chem Biol Interact. 2009;182(2–3):183–90.
28. Bocca C, Bozzo F, Bassignana A, Miglietta A. Antiproliferative effects of COX-2 inhibitor celecoxib on human breast cancer cell lines. Mol Cell Biochem. 2011;350:59–70.
29. Tomoda C, Moatamed F, Naeim F, Hershman JM, Sugawara M. Indomethacin inhibits cell growth of medullary thyroid carcinoma by reducing cell cycle progression into S phase. Exp Biol Med. 2008;233:1433–40.
30. Kashfi K, Rigas B. Non-COX-2 targets and cancer: expanding the molecular target repertoire of chemoprevention. Biochem Pharmacol. 2005;70:969–86.
31. Grösch S, Maier T, Schiffmann S, Geisslinger G. Cyclooxygenase-2 (COX-2)-independent anticarcinogenic effects of selective COX-2 inhibitors. J Natl Cancer Inst. 2006;98:736–47.
32. Lau L, Hansford LM, Cheng LS, Hang M, Baruchel S, Kaplan DR. Cyclooxygenase inhibition modulate the p53/HDM2 pathway and enhance chemotherapy-induced apoptosis in neuroblastoma. Oncogene. 2007;26:1920–31.
33. Herfarth KKF, Wick MR, Marshall HN, Gartner E, Lum S, Moley JF. Absence of TP53 alterations in pheochromocytomas and medullary thyroid carcinomas. Genes Chromosom Cancer. 1997;20:24–9.
34. Lau LMS, Wolter JK, Lau JTML, Cheng LS, Smith KM, Hansford LM, et al. Cyclooxygenase inhibitors differentially modulate p73 isoforms in neuroblastoma. Oncogene. 2009;28:2024–33.
35. Gonzalez S, Perez-Perez MM, Hernando E, Serrano M, Cordon-Cardo C. P73beta-mediated apoptosis requires p57kip2 induction and IEX-1 inhibition. Cancer Res. 2005;65:2186–92.

33

Thyroid malignancy among patients with thyroid nodules in the United Arab Emirates

Eiman Alseddeeqi[1*], Raqwana Baharoon[2], Rawia Mohamed[3], Jenan Ghaith[4], Abeer Al-Helali[5] and Luai A. Ahmed[6]

Abstract

Objectives: Thyroid malignancy constitutes the sixth common cancer type in the United Arab Emirates (UAE). There are no epidemiological data outlining the prevalence of cancer in thyroid nodules, nor previous analysis of ultra-sonographic features correlating with thyroid malignancy in the UAE. This study aimed to estimate the prevalence of thyroid malignancy in patients with thyroid nodules and to describe the ultra-sonographic characteristics of thyroid nodules harbouring malignancy.

Methods: A retrospective electronic medical records review of all thyroid nodules in patients (aged 18 to 80 years) with normal thyroid-stimulating hormone (TSH) levels, who underwent ultrasound guided fine needle aspiration cytology (UG-FNA) at Sheikh Khalifa Medical City (SKMC) during 2011–2015.

Results: 436 patients with normal TSH underwent UG-FNA cytological examination of thyroid nodules ($n = 555$ nodules). The overall crude prevalence of thyroid cancer among patients was 10.1% (95% CI 7.5–13.3). The age-adjusted prevalence of thyroid cancer among UAE nationals, Arabs, Far East Asians, and Caucasians were 9.6% (3.6–15.6), 10.0% (6.2–13.8), 16.8% (4.5–29.0) and 16.3% (1.7–30.9), respectively. The crude prevalence was 14.5%(95% CI 6.2–22.8) in men, and 9.3%(95% CI 6.3–12.2) in women. The echogenicity features were significantly different between the cancerous and noncancerous nodules ($p = 0.025$). Cancerous nodules were relatively more hyper- and hypo-echoic, while noncancerous nodules were mostly complex.

Conclusion: We report a higher prevalence of thyroid malignancy among patients with thyroid nodules relative to that reported in other parts of the world. The rate of thyroid malignancy was higher in patients of Far-East Asian and Caucasian ethnic background.

Keywords: Thyroid, Thyroid nodules, Thyroid Cancer, Cancer, Prevalence, United Arab Emirates

Introduction

The overall worldwide incidence of thyroid malignancy has been increasing over the last four decades [1]. Ongoing research is aimed at exploring possible factors contributing to the formation of different thyroid cancer subtypes, to identify individuals at risk of thyroid malignancy [2].

Thyroid nodules are another common thyroid endocrinopathy with prevalence ranging from 1 to 5% in iodine-sufficient areas; this prevalence is significantly increased if nodules incidentally detected by ultrasound are included, reaching up to 68% [3]. Moreover, the overall number of thyroid nodules and malignancy cases reported in the last decade has increased due to widespread use of neck ultrasound [3].

The United Arab Emirates (UAE) is classified as an area with minimal iodine-deficiency with rate of households using iodized salt around 6% and a median urinary iodine excretion of 100 μg/l. Therefore, a high prevalence of

* Correspondence: ealseddeeqi@seha.ae
[1]Division of Endocrinology, Sheikh Khalifa Medical City, P.O. Box 51900, Abu Dhabi, UAE
Full list of author information is available at the end of the article

thyroid malignancy is not unexpected [4–7]. Thyroid malignancy is the most common endocrine malignancy in the UAE, and papillary thyroid cancer is the most common type of thyroid cancer [4]. It is reported as the sixth most common cancer type among UAE population and the second among UAE women [4].

There are no comprehensive epidemiological data outlining the prevalence of thyroid malignancy in thyroid nodules and its correlation with demographic data in UAE population (a heterogeneous population with multiple ethnic backgrounds). Moreover, there is no previous analysis of ultra-sonographic features correlating with thyroid malignant nodules in the UAE.

This study aimed to describe the prevalence of thyroid malignancy in euthyroid patients with thyroid nodules in the UAE population. The study also aims to analyse the distribution of thyroid malignancy by gender, age, ethnicity, cytological, and ultra-sonographic characteristics.

Methods

Study design and settings

This is a retrospective analysis of a cohort of patients (aged 18 years old and above with thyroid nodules and normal serum TSH) who underwent ultrasound guided fine needle aspiration (UG-FNA) cytology for the first time from January 2011 to December 2015, at Sheikh Khalifa Medical City (SKMC) in Abu Dhabi. SKMC is a tertiary centre and functioned as the referral centre for peripheral health care facilities during the study period. The normal reference range for TSH is 0.270–4.200 mIU/L and all TSH levels were measured at our institution. Neck ultrasound and reporting were performed by more than one radiologist while decision to perform aspiration cytology was made by endocrinologists based on ultrasound findings. The diagnosis of cancer was made following surgery by one experienced certified pathologist per each case. If features of malignancy are overlapping with benignity on histology specimens, a second opinion is sought through the monthly pathology meeting dedicated for such cases.

An institutional research board approval was obtained from SKMC.

All patients with known thyroid cancer history and abnormal TSH level were excluded.

Chart review data

Demographic characteristics of all patients who underwent cytological examinations were retrieved from their medical records. These included, age at the time of performing the fine needle aspiration, gender and ethnicity. Age was grouped as follows: 18–29, 30–39, 40–49, 50–59 and ≥ 60 years. Ethnicity was classified according to nationalities into six major groups: UAE nationals, Arabs (except UAE), Far-East Asians (Philippines, China), South-East Asians (India, Pakistan, Bangladesh, and Sri Lanka), Caucasians, and others.

UG-FNA was performed on all nodules sized ≥1 cm if they demonstrated worrisome ultra-sonographic features; and ultrasound features were reported according to the American Thyroid Association (ATA) clinical practice guidelines for assessment of thyroid nodule (2009) [8].

In case of a patient with more than one nodule, criteria for FNA selection were based on the size and presence of a worrisome feature on ultrasound as mentioned above. For each nodule, the size (in three dimensions with the greatest dimension used for data analysis) and echogenicity features (solid, cystic, or complex) were identified. For solid nodules, echogenicity was classified into either: is-echogenicity, hypo-echogenicity, or hyper-echogenicity. Other ultrasound features reported included the presence of nodal disease or calcifications.

Bethesda thyroid nodule cytological classification reporting system was used to report the cytopathology [9]. Nodules with Bethesda categories IV, V, and VI underwent lobectomy or total thyroidectomy with histological examination. For Bethesda III cytology result, a repeat fine needle aspiration cytology or lobectomy was recommended based on the presence of worrisome features on ultrasound. Thyroid malignancy was divided into subtypes as follows: classical papillary thyroid cancer (CPTC), follicular variant of papillary thyroid cancer (FvPTC), classical follicular thyroid cancer (FTC), Hurthle thyroid cancer and medullary thyroid cancer (MTC).

Statistical analysis

Data were analysed as per-patient and per-nodule basis. Demographic of the patients with nodules and the ultra-sonographic and cytological characteristics of the nodules were described. Categorical data were ex pressed as numbers and percentages. Continuous data were reported as means and standard deviations. Chi-squared or Fisher's tests were used to determine the statistical significance of the differences between the characteristics, when comparing cancerous and noncancerous nodules. The overall and gender-specific prevalence of cancerous nodules by demographic characteristics were estimated using logistic models and reported with 95% confidence intervals (CI). Stata 15 was used to perform the analysis. The significance level of the statistical tests was set at 5%.

Results

Demographics

Figure 1 shows the included numbers of patients and nodules in the analyses. 436 patients (367 women, 69 men) with normal TSH were included in the study. Table 1 shows the general characteristics of all patients. The overall mean age was 44.1 years (standard deviation

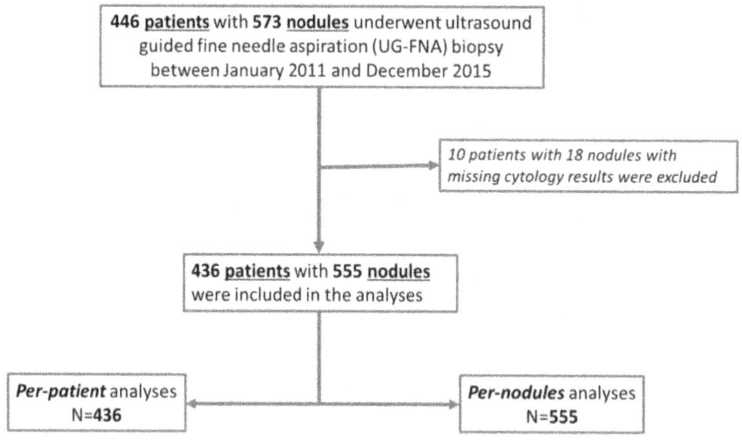

Fig. 1 Numbers of patients and thyroid nodules included in the analyses

(SD) 12.7 years). The mean (SD) age in women and men were 43.4 (12.7) and 47.8 (12.2), respectively ($p = 0.008$). Moreover, there were significant differences in the distribution of gender by age-groups ($p = 0.004$). 59.2% of women aged between 30 and 49 years whereas 58.3% of men aged between 40 and 59 years as illustrated in Fig. 2. Around 77% of the patients were of Arabic ethnicity (including UAE nationals).

Table 1 Characteristics of patients with thyroid nodules (N = 436) that underwent ultrasound guided fine needle aspiration (UG-FNA) cytology between January 2011 and December 2015 in a tertiary hospital in Abu Dhabi, United Arab Emirates

	Number *(%)*
N	
Gender	
Women	*367 (84.2)*
Men	*69 (15.8)*
Age *(years)* mean (SD)	*44.1 (12.7)*
Age groups	
18–29 years	*54 (12.4)*
30–39 years	*114 (26.2)*
40–49 years	*133 (30.5)*
50–59 years	*77 (17.7)*
≥ 60 years	*58 (13.3)*
Ethnicity[a]	
UAE	*95 (21.4)*
Arabs	*241 (55.4)*
Far-East Asians	*36 (8.3)*
South-East Asians	*29 (6.7)*
Caucasians	*26 (6.0)*
Others	*8 (1.8)*

[a]One patient with missing ethnicity

Prevalence

The overall crude prevalence of thyroid cancer in patients with thyroid nodules was 10.1% (95% CI 7.5–13.3). The crude prevalence was 9.3% (95% CI 6.3–12.2) in women, and 14.5% (95% CI 6.2–22.8) in men (Table 2). Similar to the crude prevalence, the overall age-adjusted prevalence was 10.0% (7.7–12.8), and 9.0% (6.0–11.9) in women; whereas slightly higher in men (15.1% (6.5–23.8)). Overall, there was no significant difference in age-adjusted thyroid cancer prevalence between women and men ($p = 0.117$).

The age-adjusted prevalence of thyroid cancer among UAE nationals, Arabs, Far East Asians, and Caucasians were 9.6% (3.6–15.6), 10.0% (6.2–13.8), 16.8% (4.5–29.0) and 16.3% (1.7–30.9), respectively; with relatively higher cancer prevalence in men. Only for Far-East Asians patients, the cancer prevalence was significantly higher in men compared to women ($p = 0.019$). No cancer was reported in thyroid nodules detected in South-East Asian or 'Other' ethnicities' patients.

Ultra-sonographic and cytological characteristics of the nodules

In total of 555 thyroid nodules underwent UG-FNA cytological examinations. As Table 3 shows, more than 60% of the nodules were sized 2 cm or more with no difference in the size distribution between the cancerous and noncancerous nodules ($p = 0.176$). Around 54% of the nodules were of complex echogenicity. The echogenicity features were significantly different between the cancerous and noncancerous nodules ($p = 0.025$). Cancerous nodules were relatively more hyper- and hypo-echoic, while noncancerous nodules were mostly complex. Although 70% of the nodules had no calcifications, coarse calcification occurred more frequently with cancerous nodules compared to noncancerous nodules ($p < 0.001$). Around 79% of all

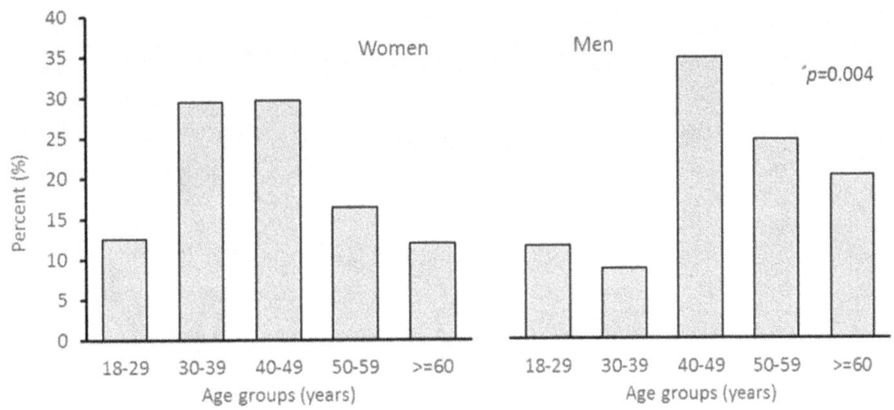

Fig. 2 Age and gender distribution of patients with thyroid nodules ($N = 555^*$) who underwent ultrasound guided fine needle aspiration (UG-FNA) cytology between January 2011 and December 2015 in a tertiary hospital in Abu Dhabi, United Arab Emirates (*471 nodules in women and 84 nodules in men)

the nodules were classified as Bethesda II while cancerous nodules were more frequently classified as Bethesda IV, V, or VI compared to noncancerous nodules ($p < 0.001$).

Among the cancerous thyroid nodules, 47% were PTC while 35% were FvPTC (Fig. 3). No significant histological differences were found between women and men in cancerous nodules ($p = 0.443$).

Discussion

This study is the first to estimate the prevalence of thyroid cancer among thyroid nodules in the UAE and

Table 2 Crude and age-adjusted overall and gender-specific thyroid cancer prevalence (95% CI) among patients with thyroid nodules who underwent ultrasound guided fine needle aspiration (UG-FNA) biopsy between January 2011 and December 2015 in a tertiary hospital in Abu Dhabi, United Arab Emirates

	Crude Cancer Prevalence % *(95% CI)*			
	Overall	Women	Men	*p*-value*
N (cancer/No cancer)	44/392	34/333	10/59	
All thyroid nodules	10.1 (7.5–13.3)	9.3 (6.3–12.2)	14.5 (6.2–22.8)	*0.186*
Age (years)				
18–29 years	16.7 (6.7–26.6)	15.2 (4.8–25.6)	25.0 (0.0–55.0)	*0.493*
30–39 years	8.8 (3.6–14.0)	8.3 (3.1–13.5)	16.7 (0.0–46.5)	*0.482*
40–49 years	12.0 (6.5–17.6)	11.0 (5.1–16.9)	16.7 (1.8–31.6)	*0.441*
50–59 years	5.2 (0.2–10.2)	5.0 (0.0–10.5)	5.9 (0.0–17.1)	*0.885*
≥ 60 years	8.6 (1.4–15.8)	6.8 (0.0–14.3)	14.3 (0.0–32.6)	*0.386*
Ethnicity**				
UAE	9.5 (3.6–15.4)	7.7 (1.8–13.6)	17.6 (0.0–35.8)	*0.204*
Arabs	10.4 (6.5–14.2)	*10.1 (5.9–14.3)*	*11.6 (2.0–21.2)*	*0.766*
Far-East Asians	16.7 (4.5–28.8)	*12.1 (1.0–23.3)*	*66.7 (13.3–99.9)*	*0.015*
Caucasians	15.4 (1.5–29.3)	*16.0 (1.6–30.4)*	*0*	
	Age-adjusted Cancer Prevalence % *(95% CI)*			
All thyroid nodules	10.0 (7.7–12.8)	9.0 (6.0–11.9)	15.1 (6.5–23.8)	*0.117*
Ethnicity[a]				
UAE	9.6 (3.6–15.6)	7.7 (1.8–13.7)	18.7 (0.0–37.9)	*0.166*
Arabs	10.0 (6.2–13.8)	*9.7 (5.5–13.8)*	*10.9 (1.5–20.4)*	*0.799*
Far-East Asians	16.8 (4.5–29.0)	*12.3 (1.0–23.6)*	*65.1 (10.4–99.9)*	*0.019*
Caucasians	16.3 (1.7–30.9)	*17.0 (1.8–32.1)*	*0*	

*p-value comparing women vs men

[a]No cancerous nodules in patients of South-East Asians/Other ethnicities

Table 3 Characteristics of thyroid nodules ($N = 555$) that underwent ultrasound guided fine needle aspiration (UG-FNA) biopsy between January 2011 and December 2015 in a tertiary hospital in Abu Dhabi, United Arab Emirates

	Total N (%*)	Cancer status		p-value**
		Cancer N (%[a])	No cancer N (%[a])	
N	555 (100)	49 (100)	506 (100)	
Nodule size	535 (100)	48 (100.0)	487 (100.0)	0.176
< 1 cm	*27 (5.1)*	*5 (10.4)*	*22 (4.5)*	
1 – < 2 cm	*174 (32.5)*	*17 (35.4)*	*157 (32.2)*	
2–4 cm	*222 (41.5)*	*20 (41.7)*	*202 (41.5)*	
> 4 cm	*112 (20.9)*	*6 (12.5)*	*106 (21.8)*	
Echogenicity	531 (100)	47 (100.0)	484 (100.0)	0.025
Cystic	*15 (2.8)*	*1 (2.1)*	*14 (2.9)*	
Complex	*287 (54.1)*	*17 (36.2)*	*270 (55.8)*	
Hyper-echoic	*18 (3.4)*	*4 (8.5)*	*14 (2.9)*	
Hypo-echoic	*124 (23.4)*	*17 (36.2)*	*107 (22.1)*	
Isoechoic	*87 (16.4)*	*8 (17.0)*	*79 (16.3)*	
Calcification	547 (100)	48 (100.0)	499 (100.0)	< 0.001
Coarse	*25 (4.6)*	*14 (29.2)*	*11 (2.2)*	
Yes	*125 (22.9)*	*10 (20.8)*	*115 (23.0)*	
No	*397 (72.6)*	*24 (50.0)*	*373 (74.8)*	
Lymphadenopathy	554 (100)	49 (100)	505 (100)	0.999
No	*530 (95.7)*	*47 (95.9)*	*483 (95.6)*	
Yes	*24 (4.3)*	*2 (4.1)*	*22 (4.4)*	
FNA Cytology	551 (100)	49 (100)	502 (100)	< 0.001
Bethesda, I	*29 (5.3)*	*1 (2.0)*	*28 (5.6)*	
Bethesda II	*435 (79.0)*	*4 (8.2)*	*431 (85.9)*	
Bethesda III	*32 (5.8)*	*6 (12.2)*	*26 (5.2)*	
Bethesda IV	*25 (4.5)*	*17 (34.7)*	*8 (1.6)*	
Bethesda V	*16 (2.9)*	*12 (24.5)*	*4 (0.8)*	
Bethesda VI	*14 (2.5)*	*9 (18.4)*	*5 (1.0)*	

[a]Column percent. **p-value comparing cancerous vs noncancerous groups
(20, 24, 8, 1, & 4 nodules were missing size, echogenicity, calcification, lymphadenopathy, & FNA cytology information, respectively)

covered the period from 2011 to 2015. Relatively high prevalence ranging between 9 to 15% were found in women and men. High malignancy rates were found in nodules with sizes between 2 and 4 cm.

The overall cancer crude prevalence of 10.1% which was found among thyroid nodules in our study is relatively high compared to the prevalence reported in some Western countries. The prevalence of thyroid malignancy in a single nodule in a study performed in the United States was 5% [6]. Finding of a similar study conducted in Italy supported the same lower prevalence (3.3%) of thyroid malignancy among thyroid nodules [6]. A study by Santos J. et al. found an association between increased risk of thyroid nodules and thyroid malignancy in iodine-deficient areas [5]. Another regional study reported the same association of increased malignant thyroid nodules among iodine-deficient subjects [10]. This could explain the relatively higher malignancy formation in thyroid nodules found in our study as most of the study population descend from iodine deficient parts of the world. However, the rate found in our study was more or less similar to other reported prevalence in Saudi Arabia, Cyprus, and Taiwan, where thyroid cancer rates among thyroid nodules ranged from 7 to 15% [11–13].

We found an 10.0% overall age-adjusted prevalence of thyroid cancer; with 9.0% in women and 15.1% in men. This gender differences with higher rate in men is consistent with findings from an Asian population study [8]. In this study, although the highest proportions of thyroid and cancerous nodules occurred among subjects aged 40–49 years, thyroid malignancy prevalence was highest among thyroid nodules in women aged 18–29 years and men aged 30–39 years. An increased unmet demand of iodine during pregnancy in the reproductive age group

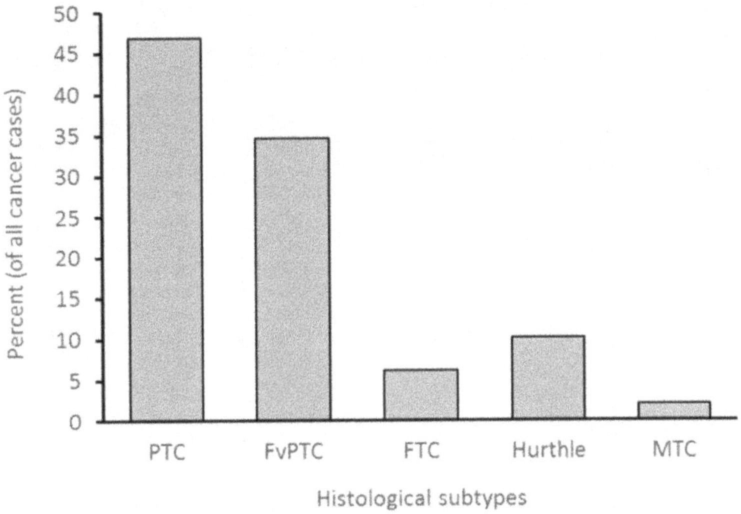

Fig. 3 Distribution of histological subtypes of cancerous thyroid nodules ($N = 49$) underwent ultrasound guided fine needle aspiration (UG-FNA) cytology between January 2011 and December 2015 in a tertiary hospital in Abu Dhabi, United Arab Emirates. *(PTC: Papillary Thyroid cancer, FvPTC: Follicular Variant of Papillary Thyroid Cancer, FTC: Follicular Thyroid Cancer, MTC: Medullary Thyroid Cancer)*

may explain the increased frequency of thyroid nodules with a younger age presentation in women; and hence, the associated occurrence of malignancy in women compared to men [5, 14, 15]. Another possible factor for the earlier presentation in women during the childbearing years is the associated level of oestrogen which is known to induce thyroid cancer in mice [16].

Interestingly, the prevalence of thyroid malignancy in this study varies between patients of different ethnic backgrounds. It was found to be highest among Far-East Asians and among Caucasian populations presenting with thyroid nodules. Higher rates of thyroid malignancy were reported previously among Far-East Asians in North America [17]. A similar study was performed in North America where it was found that thyroid cancers were proportionally higher in both foreign- and United States-born Arabs compared with other metropolitan ethnicities [18]. Further research to identify risk factors influencing malignancy occurrence in certain ethnic groups is warranted. Ultrasound examination is readily available in the UAE in secondary care centres; therefore, the increased detection rate of thyroid nodules by ultrasound might have contributed to the increased prevalence of thyroid malignancy in this study. Therefore, we speculate that ethnicity, iodine-deficiency (which leads to the formation of multinodular goiters), and the wide spread use of ultrasound, led to the detection of relatively higher prevalence of thyroid cancer in our study.

Most nodules in this study were classified as Bethesda II cytology type (76.6%), in which thyroid malignancy is not common. Conventional PTC was found in 46.9% of all cancer types while FvPTC constituted 34.7% of all thyroid malignancies in our study. This result is consistent with reports from different parts of the world that PTC constitutes 80–90% of all thyroid malignancy types [1, 19]. In terms of ultrasound characteristics, around 41.3% of nodules with a size of between 2 and 4 cm was associated with the occurrence of thyroid malignancy in our study. This result is consistence with other studies demonstrating similar association with size [20, 21]. Even the most recent ATA guidelines (2015) showed that the potential of malignancy in nodules < 2 cm is low in the absence of other worrisome features [22]. Therefore, FNA of thyroid nodules is indicated for all thyroid nodules above 2 cm. An exception to that is a nodule that is purely cystic or that has a spongiform pattern on ultrasound [22]. The presence of such ultra-sonographic worrisome features could indicate the need to decrease the threshold required for performing thyroid nodule FNA, especially in certain ethnic groups or in all ethnicities when certain size criteria is met.

Limitations and strengths

This retrospective data analysis occurred in a single centre. The analysis was performed on nodules managed according to the ATA 2009 standard of practice guidelines for managing thyroid nodules. Referrals to our tertiary centre could have created a referral bias, however, FNA indication was based on certain clinical criteria. Since histological confirmation was not performed on all thyroid nodules, the rates of thyroid malignancy could have been underestimated. Among the strength of this study is the large sample size of patients and nodules included. Moreover, all patients included in the study had normal TSH to ensure validity of the results because patients from iodine-deficient areas exhibit more autoimmune thyroid conditions as well as increased risk of thyroid malignancy when presenting with high TSH [14].

Conclusion

The prevalence of thyroid malignancy in this study is higher relative to that reported in other parts of the world. Far-East Asian and Caucasian ethnic groups were found to have higher rates of thyroid malignancy.

Abbreviations

ATA: American Thyroid Association; CPTC: Conventional papillary thyroid cancer; FTC: Classical follicular thyroid cancer; FvPTC: Follicular variant of papillary thyroid cancer; MTC: Medullary thyroid cancer; SKMC: Sheikh Khalifa Medical City; TSH: Thyroid-stimulating hormone; UAE: United Arab Emirates; UG-FNA: Ultrasound guided fine needle aspiration

Acknowledgments

Not Applicable

Funding

This research received no specific grant from any funding agency in the public, commercial or not-for-profit sectors.

Authors' contributions

EA, RB, AA, RM, JG, and LAA conceptualized and designed the study. EA, RB, AA, RM, and JG obtained the data. LAA analysed the data. EA and LAA drafted the manuscript. EA, RB, AA, RM, JG, and LAA critically revised the manuscript. EA, RB, AA, RM, JG, and LAA approved the final submission of the manuscript.

Consent for publication

No individual person's data were included in the manuscript.

Competing interests

The authors declare that they have no competing interests.

Author details

[1]Division of Endocrinology, Sheikh Khalifa Medical City, P.O. Box 51900, Abu Dhabi, UAE. [2]Division of Nuclear Medicine, Sheikh Khalifa Medical City, Abu Dhabi, UAE. [3]Division of Pathology, Sheikh Khalifa Medical City, Abu Dhabi, UAE. [4]Division of Internal Medicine, Sheikh Khalifa Medical City, Abu Dhabi, UAE. [5]Division of Radiology, Sheikh Khalifa Medical City, Abu Dhabi, UAE. [6]Institute of Public Health, College of Medicine and Health Sciences, United Arab Emirates University, Al Ain, UAE.

References

1. Siegel RL, Miller KD, Jemal A. Cancer statistics, 2016. CA Cancer J Clin. 2016;66:7–30.
2. Alzahrani AS, Alomar H, Alzahrani N. Thyroid cancer in Saudi Arabia: a histopathological and outcome study. Int J Endocrinol. 2017;2017:8423147. https://doi.org/10.1155/2017/8423147. Epub 2017 Feb 27.
3. Guth S, Theune U, Aberle J, et al. Very high prevalence of thyroid nodules detected by high frequency (13 MHz) ultrasound examination. Eur J Clin Invest. 2009;39:699–706.
4. Al-Zaher N, Al-Salam S, El Teraifi H. Thyroid carcinoma in the United Arab Emirates: perspectives and experience of a tertiary care hospital. Hematol Oncol Stem Cell Ther. 2008;1:14–21.
5. Santos JE, Kalk WJ, Freitas M, et al. Iodine deficiency and thyroid nodular pathology--epidemiological and cancer characteristics in different populations: Portugal and South Africa. BMC Res Notes. 2015;8:284.
6. Brito JP, Yarur AJ, Prokop LJ, et al. Prevalence of thyroid cancer in multinodular goiter versus single nodule: a systematic review and meta-analysis. Thyroid. 2013;23:449–55.
7. Mohammadi M, et al. Iodine deficiency status in the WHO eastern Mediterranean region: a systematic review. Environ Geochem Health. 2018; 40(1):87-97. https://doi.org/10.1007/s10653-017-9911-z. Epub 2017 Feb 21.
8. Cooper D, et al. Revised American Thyroid Association management guidelines for adult patients with thyroid nodules and differentiated thyroid cancer: the American Thyroid Association guidelines task force on thyroid nodules and differentiated thyroid cancer. Thyroid. 2009;19(11):1167–214.
9. Cibas E, Ali S. The Bethesda system for reporting thyroid cytopathology. Thyroid. 2009;19(11):1159-65. https://doi.org/10.1089/thy.2009.0274.
10. Al-Salamah SM, Khalid K, Bismar HA. Incidence of differentiated cancer in nodular goiter. Saudi Med J. 2002;23:947–52.
11. Lin JD, Chao TC, Huang BY, et al. Thyroid cancer in the thyroid nodules evaluated by ultrasonography and fine-needle aspiration cytology. Thyroid. 2005;15:708.
12. Werk EE Jr, Vernon BM, Gonzalez JJ, et al. Cancer in thyroid nodules. A community hospital survey. Arch Intern Med. 1984;144:474–6.
13. Hadjisavva I, et al. Prevalence of Cancer in patients with thyroid nodules in the island of Cyprus: predictive value of ultrasound features and thyroid autoimmune status. Eur Thyroid J. 2015;4:123–8.
14. Belfiore A, Giuffrida D, La Rosa GL, et al. High frequency of cancer in cold thyroid nodules occurring at young age. Acta Endocrinol. 1989;121:97–202.
15. Harding KB, Peña-Rosas JP, Webster AC, et al. Iodine supplementation for women during the preconception, pregnancy and postpartum period. Cochrane Database Syst Rev. 2017;3:CD011761. https://doi.org/10.1002/14651858.CD011761.pub2.
16. Hussain F, Iqbal S, Mehmood A, et al. Incidence of thyroid cancer in the Kingdom of Saudi Arabia, 2000-2010. Hematol Oncol Stem Cell Ther. 2013;6:58–64.
17. Laudico AV, Mirasol-Lumague MR, Mapua CA, et al. Cancer incidence and survival in metro Manila and Rizal province, Philippines. Jpn J Clin Oncol. 2010;40:603–12.
18. Khan F, Ruterbusch JJ, Gomez SL, et al. Differences in the cancer burden among foreign-born and US-born Arab Americans living in metropolitan Detroit. Cancer Causes Control. 2013;24:1955–61.
19. Vaccarella S, Franceschi S, Bray F, et al. Worldwide thyroid-cancer epidemic? The increasing impact of overdiagnosis. N Engl J Med. 2016;375:614–7.
20. Smith-Bindman R, Lebda P, Feldstein VA, et al. Risk of thyroid cancer based on thyroid ultrasound imaging characteristics: results of a population-based study. JAMA Intern Med. 2013;173:1788–96.
21. Cappelli C, Castellano M, Pirola I, et al. The predictive value of ultrasound findings in the management of thyroid nodules. Q J Med. 2007;100:29–35.
22. Haugen BR, Alexander EK, Bible KC, et al. 2015 American Thyroid Association management guidelines for adult patients with thyroid nodules and differentiated thyroid cancer: the American Thyroid Association guidelines task force on thyroid nodules and differentiated thyroid cancer. Thyroid. 2016;26:1–33.

Permissions

All chapters in this book were first published in TR, by BioMed Central; hereby published with permission under the Creative Commons Attribution License or equivalent. Every chapter published in this book has been scrutinized by our experts. Their significance has been extensively debated. The topics covered herein carry significant findings which will fuel the growth of the discipline. They may even be implemented as practical applications or may be referred to as a beginning point for another development.

The contributors of this book come from diverse backgrounds, making this book a truly international effort. This book will bring forth new frontiers with its revolutionizing research information and detailed analysis of the nascent developments around the world.

We would like to thank all the contributing authors for lending their expertise to make the book truly unique. They have played a crucial role in the development of this book. Without their invaluable contributions this book wouldn't have been possible. They have made vital efforts to compile up to date information on the varied aspects of this subject to make this book a valuable addition to the collection of many professionals and students.

This book was conceptualized with the vision of imparting up-to-date information and advanced data in this field. To ensure the same, a matchless editorial board was set up. Every individual on the board went through rigorous rounds of assessment to prove their worth. After which they invested a large part of their time researching and compiling the most relevant data for our readers.

The editorial board has been involved in producing this book since its inception. They have spent rigorous hours researching and exploring the diverse topics which have resulted in the successful publishing of this book. They have passed on their knowledge of decades through this book. To expedite this challenging task, the publisher supported the team at every step. A small team of assistant editors was also appointed to further simplify the editing procedure and attain best results for the readers.

Apart from the editorial board, the designing team has also invested a significant amount of their time in understanding the subject and creating the most relevant covers. They scrutinized every image to scout for the most suitable representation of the subject and create an appropriate cover for the book.

The publishing team has been an ardent support to the editorial, designing and production team. Their endless efforts to recruit the best for this project, has resulted in the accomplishment of this book. They are a veteran in the field of academics and their pool of knowledge is as vast as their experience in printing. Their expertise and guidance has proved useful at every step. Their uncompromising quality standards have made this book an exceptional effort. Their encouragement from time to time has been an inspiration for everyone.

The publisher and the editorial board hope that this book will prove to be a valuable piece of knowledge for researchers, students, practitioners and scholars across the globe.

List of Contributors

Katarzyna Wojciechowska-Durczyńska and Andrzej Lewiński
Department of Endocrinology and Metabolic Diseases, Polish Mother's Memorial Hospital Research Institute, Medical University of Lodz, Rzgowska St. No. 281/289, 93-338 Lodz, Poland

Adam Durczyński and Janusz Strzelczyk
Department of General and Transplant Surgery, Medical University of Lodz, Barlicki University Hospital, Lodz, Poland

Stanisław Sporny
Department of Dental Pathology, Medical University of Lodz, The Clinical- Didactic Centre, Lodz, Poland

Mario Vaisman
Hospital Clementino Fraga Filho, Universidade Federal do Rio de Janeiro, Rua Prof. Rodolpho Paulo Rocco 255, Cidade Universitária, CEP 21941-913, Rio de Janeiro-RJ, Brazil

Rosita Fontes
Diagnósticos da América SA, Rio de Janeiro, Brazil

Claudia Regina Coeli and Fernanda Aguiar
Núcleo de Estudos de Saúde Coletiva, Universidade Federal do Rio de Janeiro, Rio de Janeiro, Brazil

Janina Krupińska, Grzegorz Kulig, Elżbieta Sowińska-Przepiera, Elżbieta Andrysiak-Mamos and Anhelli Syrenicz
Department of Endocrinology, Metabolic Diseases and Internal Diseases, Pomeranian Medical University, Szczecin, Poland

Waldemar Urbanowicz
Department of Infectious Diseases and Hepatology, Pomeranian Medical University, Szczecin, Poland

Mariusz Kaczmarczyk
Institute of Clinical Biochemistry and Molecular Diagnostics, Pomeranian Medical University, Szczecin, Poland

Yosuke Wakita, Toshiki Nagasaki, Yuki Nagata, Yasuo Imanishi, Shinsuke Yamada, Koichiro Yoda, Masanori Emoto, Eiji Ishimura and Masaaki Inaba
Department of Metabolism, Endocrinology and Molecular Medicine, Osaka City University Graduate School of Medicine, 1-4-3, Asahi-machi, Abeno-ku, Osaka-city 545-8585, Japan

Adam Gesing
Department of Oncological Endocrinology, Medical University of Lodz, 7/9 Zeligowski St., 90 752, Lodz, Poland

Andrzej Lewiński
Department of Endocrinology and Metabolic Diseases, Medical University of Lodz, Lodz, Poland
Department of Endocrinology and Metabolic Diseases, Polish Mother's Memorial Hospital, Research Institute, Lodz, Poland

Małgorzata Karbownik-Lewińska
Department of Oncological Endocrinology, Medical University of Lodz, 7/9 Zeligowski St., 90 752, Lodz, Poland
Department of Endocrinology and Metabolic Diseases, Polish Mother's Memorial Hospital, Research Institute, Lodz, Poland

Paweł Szychta
Department of Oncological Endocrinology, Medical University of Lodz, 7/9 Zeligowski St., 90 752, Lodz, Poland
Department of Oncological Surgery and Breast Diseases, Polish Mother's Memorial Hospital, Research Institute, Lodz, Poland

Wojciech Szychta
Department of Oncological Endocrinology, Medical University of Lodz, 7/9 Zeligowski St., 90 752, Lodz, Poland
1st Department of Cardiology, Medical University of Warsaw, Warsaw, Poland

Melissa Ardley, Thomas McCorquodale, Hooshang Lahooti and Bernard Champion
The Department of Medicine, The University of Sydney, Nepean Hospital, Penrith, NSW 2751, Australia

Jack R Wall
The Department of Medicine, The University of Sydney, Nepean Hospital, Penrith, NSW 2751, Australia
University of Sydney, Western Clinical School, Nepean Hospital, Penrith, NSW 2751, Australia

Ovie Edafe
Department of Oncology, University of Sheffield, Beech Hill Road, Sheffield S10 2RX, UK

Sabapathy P Balasubramanian
Department of Oncology, University of Sheffield, Beech Hill Road, Sheffield S10 2RX, UK
Endocrine Surgical Unit, Sheffield Teaching Hospitals NHS Foundation Trust, Sheffield, UK

Jonathan Wadsley
Department of Oncology, Weston Park Hospital, Sheffield, UK

Barney J Harrison
Endocrine Surgical Unit, Sheffield Teaching Hospitals NHS Foundation Trust, Sheffield, UK

Zbigniew Adamczewski
Department of Endocrinology and Metabolic Diseases, Medical University of Lodz, Polish Mother's Memorial Hospital - Research Institute, Rzgowska 281/ 289, 93-338, Lodz, Poland

Jan Stepniak
Department of Oncological Endocrinology, Medical University of Lodz, 7/9 Zeligowski St, Lodz 90-752, Poland

Andrzej Lewinski
Department of Endocrinology and Metabolic Diseases, Medical University of Lodz, 281/289 Rzgowska St, Lodz 93-338, Poland
Polish Mother's Memorial Hospital - Research Institute, 281/289, Rzgowska St, Lodz 93-338, Poland

Malgorzata Karbownik-Lewinska and Agnieszka Kokoszko-Bilska
Department of Oncological Endocrinology, Medical University of Lodz, 7/9 Zeligowski St, Lodz 90-752, Poland
Polish Mother's Memorial Hospital - Research Institute, 281/289, Rzgowska St, Lodz 93-338, Poland

Kimberly N Walter, Jan Ulbrecht, Jeanette M Bennett, Courtney A Whetzel and Laura Cousino Klein
Department of Biobehavioral Health, 219 Biobehavioral Health Bldg, The Pennsylvania State University, University Park, PA 16802, USA

Elizabeth J Corwin
Nell Hodgson Woodruff School of Nursing, Emory University, Atlanta, GA 30322, USA

Laurence M Demers
Department of Biobehavioral Health, 219 Biobehavioral Health Bldg, The Pennsylvania State University, University Park, PA 16802, USA
Department of Pathology, H158 Pathology, The M.S. Hershey Medical Center, Hershey, PA 17033, USA

Abdelaziz Belkadi
INSERM U694, Institut Biologie Santé (IBS), rue des Capucins, F-49100 Angers, France
University of Angers, rue de Rennes, F-49045 Angers, France
Laboratory of human genetics of infectious diseases Necker Branch, INSERM, U980 Paris, France

Caroline Jacques, Frédérique Savagner and Yves Malthièry
University of Angers, rue de Rennes, F-49045 Angers, France
Laboratory of human genetics of infectious diseases Necker Branch, INSERM, U980 Paris, France

Yannis M Paulus, Mona M Sabra, Robert Michael Tuttle and Marcia F Kalin
Memorial Sloan-Kettering Cancer Center, Department of Medicine, 1275 York Avenue, New York, NY 10065, USA

Elyn R Riedel
Memorial Sloan-Kettering Cancer Center, Department of Epidemiology and Biostatistics, 1275 York Avenue, New York, NY 10065, USA

Hidetaka Hamasaki and Hidekatsu Yanai
Department of Internal Medicine, National Center for Global Health and Medicine Kohnodai Hospital, Chiba, Japan

Taro Yoshimi
Department of Psychiatry, National Center for Global Health and Medicine Kohnodai Hospital, Chiba, Japan

Jonathan D Boyd
Department of Pathology & Laboratory Medicine, Vidant Medical Center and Brody School of Medicine, East Carolina University, Greenville, NC, USA

Ridas Juskevicius
Department of Pathology & Laboratory Medicine, Vidant Medical Center and Brody School of Medicine, East Carolina University, Greenville, NC, USA
Department of Pathology & Laboratory Medicine, Brody School of Medicine, East Carolina University, 600 Moye Blvd, Brody Medical Sciences Building 7S18, Greenville, NC 27858-4353, USA

Kae Hamamoto, Masaaki Inaba, Shinsuke Yamada, Maki Yoda, Koichiro Yoda and Hitoshi Goto
Department of Nephrology, Department of Metabolism, Endocrinology and Molecular Medicine, Osaka City University Graduate School of Medicine, 1-4-3, Asahi-machi, Abeno-ku, Osaka 545-8585, Japan

Masafumi Kurajoh and Hidenori Koyama
Department of Internal Medicine, Division of Diabetes, Endocrinology and Metabolism, Hyogo College of Medicine, Mukogawa-cho 1-1, Nishinomiya, Hyogo 663-8501, Japan

Zahid Ali Memon
Senior Registrar, Surgical Unit 1, Civil Hospital, Karachi, Pakistan

Gulrayz Ahmed, Sarah Rafi Khan and Mahvesh Khalid
Dow Medical College, DUHS, D - 31, Block 8, Gulshan-e-Iqbal, Karachi, Pakistan

Naheed Sultan
Dean Surgery and Allied, Incharge Surgical Unit 1, Dow University of Health Sciences, Civil Hospital, Karachi, Pakistan

Claudia Campomenosi, Stefano Gay and Eleonora Monti
Endocrine Unit, IRCCS Azienda Ospedaliera Universitaria San Martino - IST Istituto Nazionale per la Ricerca sul Cancro, Genoa, Italy

Barbara Massa
Cytopathology and Pathology Unit, IRCCS Azienda Ospedaliera Universitaria San Martino - IST Istituto Nazionale per la Ricerca sul Cancro, Genoa, Italy

Enzo Silvestri and Giovanni Turtulici
Radiology Unit, Ospedale Evangelico, Genoa, Italy

Massimo Giusti
Endocrine Unit, IRCCS Azienda Ospedaliera Universitaria San Martino - IST Istituto Nazionale per la Ricerca sul Cancro, Genoa, Italy
UO Clinica Endocrinologica, Viale Benedetto XV, 6, I-16100 Genoa, Italy

Jing Yang, Carmen Sarita-Reyes, David Kindelberger and Qing Zhao
Department of Pathology and Laboratory Medicine, Boston University Medical Center, 670 Albany St. Biosquare III, Boston, MA 02118, USA

Saroj Khatiwada
Department of Biochemistry, Modern Technical College, Lalitpur, Nepal

Basanta Gelal, Nirmal Baral and Madhab Lamsal
Department of Biochemistry, B P Koirala Institute of Health Sciences, Ghopa, Dharan, Nepal

J. Colin Boyd
Dalhousie Medical School, Dalhousie University, 5849 University Avenue, Halifax, NS B3H 4H7, Canada

Blair A. Williams, Matthew H. Rigby, Jonathan R. B. Trites, S. Mark Taylor and Robert D. Hart
Division of Otolaryngology - Head and Neck Surgery, Department of Surgery, Dalhousie University, Halifax, NS, Canada

Katharina Kieser
Department of Obstetrics and Gynecology, Dalhousie University, Halifax, NS, Canada

Saul Offman and Hemlata Shirsat
Department of Pathology, Dalhousie University, Halifax, NS, Canada

Christina Tugendsam, Karin Rudolph and Georg Zettinig
Schilddruesenpraxis Josefstadt, Laudongasse 12/8, Vienna AT-1080, Austria

Veronika Petz
Division of Nuclear Medicine, Department of Biomedical Imaging and Image-guided Therapy, Medical University of Vienna, Vienna, Austria

Wolfgang Buchinger
Schilddrueseninstitut Gleisdorf, Gleisdorf, Austria

Brigitta Schmoll-Hauer
Schilddruesenpraxis Josefstadt, Laudongasse 12/8, Vienna AT-1080, Austria
Department of Nuclear Medicine, Krankenanstalt Rudolfstiftung, Vienna, Austria

Iris Pia Schenk
Schilddruesenpraxis Josefstadt, Laudongasse 12/8, Vienna AT-1080, Austria
Department of Nuclear Medicine, Sozialmedizinisches Zentrum Hietzing, Vienna, Austria

Michael Krebs
Schilddruesenpraxis Josefstadt, Laudongasse 12/8, Vienna AT-1080, Austria
Clinical Division of Endocrinology, Department of Medicine III, Medical University of Vienna, Vienna, Austria

Kaoru Kobayashi, Mitsuyoshi Hirokawa, Tomonori Yabuta, Mitsuhiro Fukushima, Hiroo Masuoka, Takuya Higashiyama, Minoru Kihara, Yasuhiro Ito, Akihiro Miya, Nobuyuki Amino and Akira Miyauchi
Kuma Hospital, 8-2-35 Shimoyamate-dori, Chuo-ku, Kobe-City 650-0011, Japan

Honglai Zhang
Department of Thyroid Surgery, the affiliated Hospital of Qingdao University, Qingdao, Shandong, China

Dong Chen
Department of General Surgery, the affiliated Hospital of Qingdao University, Qingdao, Shandong, China

Georgia Geller, Janessa Laskin and Cheryl Ho
Medical Oncology, British Columbia Cancer Agency, 600 W 10th Avenue, Vancouver, BC V5Z 4E6, Canada

Winson Y. Cheung
Medical Oncology, Tom Baker Cancer Centre, Calgary, AB, Canada

Naoki Edo, Koji Morita, Miki Sakamoto, Erina Okamura, Masumi Ogawa, Kazuhisa Tsukamoto, Hiroko Okinaga and Toshio Ishikawa
Department of Internal Medicine, Teikyo University School of Medicine, 2-11-1, Kaga, Itabashi, Tokyo 173-0003, Japan

Tatsuro Kaminaga
Department of Radiology, Teikyo University School of Medicine, 2-11-1, Kaga, Itabashi, Tokyo 173-0003, Japan

Hiromi Edo
Department of Radiology, Toho University Ohashi Medical Center, 2-22-36, Ohashi, Meguro, Tokyo, Japan

Simon H. S. Pearce
Institute of Genetic Medicine and Queen Elizabeth Hospital, International Centre for Life, Newcastle University, Central Parkway, Newcastle upon Tyne NE1 3BZ, UK

Salman Razvi
Institute of Genetic Medicine and Queen Elizabeth Hospital, International Centre for Life, Newcastle University, Central Parkway, Newcastle upon Tyne NE1 3BZ, UK
Department of Endocrinology, Queen Elizabeth Hospital, Gateshead NE9 6SX, UK

Lorna Ingoe
Department of Endocrinology, Queen Elizabeth Hospital, Gateshead NE9 6SX, UK

Vicky Ryan
Institute of Health & Society, Newcastle University, Baddiley Clark Building, Richardson Road, Newcastle upon Tyne NE2 4AX, UK

Scott Wilkes
Department of Pharmacy, Health and Wellbeing, Faculty of Applied Sciences, University of Sunderland, Sunderland SR1 3SD, UK

Manish M George, Jay Goswamy and Susannah E Penney
Department of Otolaryngology-Head and Neck Surgery, Manchester Royal
Infirmary, Oxford Road, Manchester M13 9WL, United Kingdom

Rumi Hino
Department of Sports and Health Science, Daito Bunka University, 560 Iwadono, Higashimathuyama-shi, Saitama 355-8501, Japan
Department of Pathology, Toranomon Hospital, Tokyo 105-0001, Japan

Naoko Inoshita, Toyoki Yoshimoto and Makiko Ogawa
Department of Pathology, Toranomon Hospital, Tokyo 105-0001, Japan

Daishu Miura
Akasaka Miura Clinic, Tokyo 107-0052, Japan

Ryoko Watanabe and Kenta Watanabe
Department of Otolaryngology, Toranomon Hospital, Tokyo 105-0001, Japan

Mako Kamiya
Graduate School of Medicine, The University of Tokyo, Tokyo 113-0033, Japan
PRESTO, Japan Science and Technology Agency (JST), Saitama 332-0012, Japan

Yasteru Urano
Graduate School of Medicine, The University of Tokyo, Tokyo 113-0033, Japan
Graduate School of Pharmaceutical Sciences, The University of Tokyo, Tokyo 113-0033, Japan
AMED CREST, Japan Agency for Medical Research and Development, Tokyo 100-0004, Japan

Hernando Vargas-Uricoechea
Department of Internal Medicine, Division of Endocrinology and Metabolism, Universidad del Cauca, Popayán, Colombia

Ivonne Meza-Cabrera
Laboratory of Pathology, Hospital Universitario San José, Popayán, Cauca, Colombia

Jorge Herrera-Chaparro
Department of surgery, Universidad del Cauca, Carrera 6 No 41 N-135 apto 202B terrazas del campestre, Popayán, Cauca, Colombia

Yuji Oto, Koji Muroya, Junko Hanakawa, Yumi Asakura and Masanori Adachi
Department of Endocrinology and Metabolism, Kanagawa Children's Medical Center, Mutsukawa 2-138-4 Minami-ku, Yokohama 232-8555, Japan

Tomoe Nakao, Mitsushige Nishikawa, Mako Hisakado, Toshihiko Kasahara, Takumi Kudo, Eijun Nishihara, Mitsuru Ito, Shuji Fukata and Hirotoshi Nakamura
Department of Internal Medicine, Kuma Hospital, Centre for Excellence in Thyroid Cares, 8-2-35 Shimoyamate-dori, Chuo-ku, Kobe 650-0011, Japan

Mitsuyoshi Hirokawa
Department of Diagnostic Pathology and Cytology, Kuma Hospital, Centre for Excellence in Thyroid Cares, 8-2-35 Shimoyamate-dori, Chuo-ku, Kobe 650-0011, Japan

Akira Miyauchi
Department of Surgery, Kuma Hospital, Centre for Excellence in Thyroid Care, 8-2-35 Shimoyamate-dori, Chuo-ku, Kobe 650-0011, Japan

Thierry Ragot
UMR 8203, Gustave Roussy, Laboratoire de Vectorologie et de Thérapeutiques Anticancéreuses, Villejuif 94805, France
UMR 8203, Univ Paris-Sud, Laboratoire de Vectorologie et Thérapeutiques Anticancéreuses, Villejuif 94805, France

Claire Provost, Aurélie Prignon and Sylvie Lausson
Sorbonne Universités, UPMC University Paris 06, plateforme LIMP, Laboratoire d'Imagerie Médicale Positonique, Hôpital Tenon, Paris 75020, France

Régis Cohen
Hopital Delafontaine, Endocrinology Unit, Saint Denis, France

Michel Lepoivre
IBBMC, CNRS 8619, bat 430, Université Paris Sud XI, Orsay, Paris 91405, France

Eiman Alseddeeqi
Division of Endocrinology, Sheikh Khalifa Medical City, Abu Dhabi, UAE

Raqwana Baharoon
Division of Nuclear Medicine, Sheikh Khalifa Medical City, Abu Dhabi, UAE

Rawia Mohamed
Division of Pathology, Sheikh Khalifa Medical City, Abu Dhabi, UAE

Jenan Ghaith
Division of Internal Medicine, Sheikh Khalifa Medical City, Abu Dhabi, UAE

Abeer Al-Helali
Division of Radiology, Sheikh Khalifa Medical City, Abu Dhabi, UAE

Luai A. Ahmed
Institute of Public Health, College of Medicine and Health Sciences, United Arab Emirates University, Al Ain, UAE

Index

R

S

T

U

V

www.ingramcontent.com/pod-product-compliance
Lightning Source LLC
LaVergne TN
LVHW080905210926
848485LV00004B/600